Headache

NEUROLOGY IN PRACTICE:

SERIES EDITORS:

ROBERT A. GROSS, DEPARTMENT OF NEUROLOGY, UNIVERSITY OF ROCHESTER MEDICAL CENTER, ROCHESTER, NY, USA

JONATHAN W. MINK, DEPARTMENT OF NEUROLOGY, UNIVERSITY OF ROCHESTER MEDICAL CENTER, ROCHESTER, NY, USA

Headache

EDITED BY

Matthew S. Robbins, MD
Brian M. Grosberg, MD
Richard B. Lipton, MD

Montefiore Headache Center
Saul R. Korey Department of Neurology
Albert Einstein College of Medicine
Bronx, NY, USA

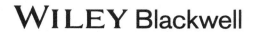

Contents

Contributor List

Jessica Ailani, MD
Assistant Professor, Department of Neurology
Director, Georgetown University Headache
Center
Georgetown University Hospital
Washington, DC, USA

Frank Andrasik, PhD
Distinguished Professor and Chair
Department of Psychology
University of Memphis
Memphis, TN, USA

Sait Ashina
Headache Program, Director
Assistant Professor of Neurology and
Anesthesiology
Department of Pain Medicine and Palliative
Care
Department of Neurology
Beth Israel Medical Center
Albert Einstein College of Medicine
New York, NY, USA

Karen Ballaban-Gil, MD
Professor of Clinical Neurology and Clinical
Pediatrics
Albert Einstein College of Medicine
Montefiore Medical Center
Bronx, NY, USA

Lars Bendtsen, MD, PhD
Associate Professor
Danish Headache Center and Department of
Neurology,
University of Copenhagen, Glostrup Hospital,
Glostrup, Copenhagen, Denmark

Marcelo E. Bigal, MD, PhD
Head of the Merck Investigator Studies Program,
Scientific Engagements and Education (MISP/
SEE)
North Wales, PA, USA, and
Clinical Associate Professor, The Saul R. Korey
Department of Neurology, Albert Einstein
College of Medicine
Bronx, NY, USA

Dawn C. Buse, PhD
Associate Professor, Department of Neurology
Albert Einstein College of Medicine of Yeshiva
University,
Assistant Professor, Clinical Health Psychology
Doctoral Program
Ferkauf Graduate School of Psychology of
Yeshiva University
Bronx, NY, and
Director of Behavioral Medicine
Montefiore Headache Center
Bronx, NY, USA

Luzma Cardona, MD
Instructor in Neurology
Harvard Medical School
Boston, MA, and
Staff Physician
Graham Headache Centre
Faulkner Hospital
Boston, MA, USA

Sara C. Crystal, MD
Clinical Assistant Professor
Department of Neurology
NYU School of Medicine
New York Headache Center
New York, NY, USA

Hans-Christoph Diener, MD, PhD
Department of Neurology and Headache Center
University Duisburg-Essen
Essen, Germany

Benjamin W. Friedman, MD
Attending Physician, Department of Emergency
Medicine
Montefiore Medical Center, Bronx, NY, and
Associate Professor of Emergency Medicine
Albert Einstein College of Medicine
Bronx, NY, USA

Deborah I. Friedman, MD, MPH
Professor, Department of Neurology &
Neurotherapeutics and Ophthalmology
University of Texas Southwestern
Dallas, TX, USA

Peter J. Goadsby, MD, PhD
Headache Group, Department of Neurology
University of California, San Francisco
UCSF Headache Center
San Francisco, CA, USA

Brian M. Grosberg, MD
Associate Professor of Neurology
Albert Einstein College of Medicine, and
Co-Director, Montefiore Headache Center
Director, Headache and Facial Pain Fellowship
Montefiore Headache Center
Bronx, NY, USA

Katherine A. Henry, MD
Associate Professor
Department of Neurology
New York University School of Medicine
New York, NY, USA

Dagny Holle, MD
Department of Neurology and Headache Center
University Duisburg-Essen
Essen, Germany

Richard B. Lipton, MD
Edwin S. Lowe Professor and Vice Chair of
Neurology
Professor of Epidemiology and Population
Health,
Professor of Psychiatry and Behavioral Science
Albert Einstein College of Medicine, and
Co-Director, Montefiore Headache Center
Bronx, NY, USA

Elizabeth W. Loder, MD, MPH
Associate Professor of Neurology
Harvard Medical School
Boston, MA, USA, and
Chief, Division of Headache and Pain
Department of Neurology
Brigham and Women's/Faulkner Hospitals
Boston, MA, USA

Dawn A. Marcus, MD
Professor, Department of Anesthesiology
University of Pittsburgh
Pittsburgh, PA, and
Headache Clinic
University of Pittsburgh
Pittsburgh, PA, USA

Vince Martin, MD
Professor, Department of Internal Medicine,
University of Cincinnati
and
Headache Clinic,
University of Cincinnati
Cincinnati, OH, USA

Arne May, MD
Professor of Neurology
Department of Systems Neuroscience
Universitäts-Krankenhaus Eppendorf (UKE)
Hamburg, Germany

Uri Napchan, MD
Middletown Medical
Middletown, NY, USA

Robert A. Nicholson, PhD
Associate Professor of Research
Department of Neurology & Psychiatry and
School of Public Health
Saint Louis University School of Medicine, and
Senior Research Methodology Advisor
Mercy Health Research & Ryan Headache
Center
St. Louis, MO, USA

Lucille A. Rathier, PhD
Clinical Assistant Professor
Psychiatry and Human Behavior
Warren Alpert Medical School, Brown
University, and
Staff Psychologist
Behavioral Medicine Clinical Services
The Miriam Hospital
Providence, RI, USA

Matthew S. Robbins, MD
Assistant Professor of Neurology
Albert Einstein College of Medicine
Chief of Service—Neurology
Einstein Division of Montefiore Medical Center,
and
Director of Inpatient Services
Montefiore Headache Center
Bronx, NY, USA

Oranee Sanmaneechai, MD
Fellow in Child Neurology
Albert Einstein College of Medicine, and
Assistant Professor of Pediatrics
Division of Neurology, Department of Pediatrics
Siriraj Hospital, Mahidol University
Bangkok, Thailand

C. Mark Sollars, MS
Research Coordinator
Montefiore Headache Center
Bronx, NY, USA

Seymour Solomon, MD
Director Emeritus, Montefiore Headache Center
Montefiore Medical Center, Bronx, NY, and
Professor of Neurology
Albert Einstein College of Medicine
Bronx, NY, USA

Sarah Vollbracht, MD
Assistant Professor of Neurology
Albert Einstein College of Medicine
Montefiore Headache Center
Bronx, NY, USA

William B. Young, MD, FAHS, FAAN
Professor of Neurology
Thomas Jefferson University
Philadelphia, PA, USA

Series Foreword

The genesis for this book series started with the proposition that, increasingly, physicians want direct, useful information to help them in clinical care. Textbooks, while comprehensive, are useful primarily as detailed reference works but pose challenges for uses at the point of care. By contrast, more outline-type references often leave out the "hows and whys"—pathophysiology, pharmacology—that form the basis of management decisions. Our goal for this series is to present books, covering most areas of neurology, that provide enough background information to allow the reader to feel comfortable, but not so much as to be overwhelming; and to associate that with practical advice from experts about care, combining the growing evidence base with best practices.

Our series will encompass various aspects of neurology, with topics and the specific content chosen to be accessible and useful.

Chapters cover critical information that will inform the reader of the disease processes and mechanisms as a prelude to treatment planning. Algorithms and guidelines are presented, when appropriate. "Tips and Tricks" boxes provide expert suggestions, while other boxes present cautions and warnings to avoid pitfalls. Finally, we provide "Science Revisited" sections that review the most important and relevant science background material, and "Bibliography" sections that guide the reader to additional material.

We welcome feedback. As additional volumes are added to the series, we hope to refine the content and format so that our readers will be best served.

Our thanks, appreciation, and respect go out to our editors and their contributors, who conceived and refined the content for each volume, assuring a high-quality, practical approach to neurological conditions and their treatment.

Our thanks also go to our mentors and students (past, present, and future), who have challenged and delighted us; to our book editors and their contributors, who were willing to take on additional work for an educational goal; and to our publisher, Martin Sugden, for his ideas and support, for wonderful discussions and commiseration over baseball and soccer teams that might not quite have lived up to expectations. We would like to dedicate the series to Marsha, Jake, and Dan; and to Janet, Laura, and David. And also to Steven R. Schwid, MD, our friend and colleague, whose ideas helped to shape this project and whose humor brightened our lives, although he could not complete this goal with us.

Robert A. Gross
Jonathan W. Mink
Rochester, NY, USA

Preface

The practice of clinical neurology has changed remarkably over the last 25 years, transforming from a diagnosis-oriented specialty into a discipline with many dynamic therapeutic opportunities. The subspecialty of headache medicine exemplifies this transformation as insights from genetics, imaging, and animal models have supported the development of specific treatments for migraine and other headache disorders. As a consequence, clinicians have an unparalleled opportunity to relieve pain, restore function, and improve quality of life for our patients.

Headache is such an extraordinarily common complaint encountered in medical settings, having the unusual duality of often being both intimidating and disregarded. In some patients, headaches may be an infrequent nuisance, which responds well to over-the-counter medications. In others, headaches may occur on a daily basis and completely disrupt educational, occupational, and social function, despite treatment. Diagnosis is complicated by the hundreds of different etiologies, both benign and life-threatening, that give rise to headache.

In this volume, we present a practical overview of headache disorders, designed to address the needs of both neurologists and general practitioners alike. Our authors include both research experts from the laboratory and practitioners who are "in the trenches." In the first section, we review the principles of headache medicine by focusing on the classification and diagnostic approach of both primary and secondary headache disorders.

The second section features a comprehensive, multifaceted appraisal of migraine, the most common headache disorder that presents to medical attention. Tension-type headache is the focus of the third section, a disorder that is usually quite benign although enigmatic, but in some patients can require significant multidisciplinary treatment. We then present the trigeminal autonomic cephalalgias, which while uncommon are the most distinctive group of headache disorders and require some expertise in diagnosis and treatment.

In the fifth section, we review uncommon and unusual primary headache disorders, including new daily persistent headache and hemicrania continua. We conclude by detailing the approach to managing headache disorders in specific populations, including women, children, and the elderly.

Numerous volumes addressing headache have been published previously. The goal of this work is to present a crisp, practical approach to headache disorders that has been written by a diverse group of experienced clinicians and scientists. We hope our approach resonates with both trainees, newly credentialed practitioners, and experienced clinicians in the many medical fields where headache is encountered.

Matthew S. Robbins, MD
Brian M. Grosberg, MD
Richard B. Lipton, MD

Acknowledgments

The successes and accomplishments of the authors would not have been possible without the support and sacrifices of many other people. All three authors would like to thank their colleagues at the Montefiore Headache Center: Seymour Solomon, Dawn Buse, Sarah Vollbracht, Jelena Pavlovic and Mark Sollars for their friendship and brilliance.

Matthew Robbins thanks his lovely wife Hilary for her supreme devotion, partnership, support, wisdom, and guidance in all aspects of life, and for sharing in the joy of raising their magnificent children Zoe and Dylan. His parents Mitchell and Debra, brother David, and grandmother Rose have remarkably provided an unparalleled lifetime of love and cheerleading. His co-editors of this volume have been two of his major professional mentors and he expresses eternal gratitude towards them.

Brian Grosberg would like to thank his mentors Seymour Solomon, Richard Lipton, and Deborah Friedman for teaching him with untiring enthusiasm and for encouraging him to be the best he can be. He is amazingly grateful to his family: his parents Carole and Lee Grosberg and his brother Michael for their unending love and support, his children Noah and Talia for the joy they bring him every moment of every day and who have been waiting patiently for Daddy to finish this book and be able to see their names in print, and most of all he acknowledges the love, support, companionship, sacrifice and encouragement of his wife Jennifer who is the love of his life and makes everything he does possible.

Richard Lipton thanks Amy, his wife and partner for 36 years, for being his compass, for giving him deep roots, wonderful children and so much love. He thanks his children, Lianna and Justin, for the joyful chapters lived together and for all the promise contained in their every smile. He thanks his research mentor, Philip Holzman, for teaching him what it means to be a scientist and his clinical mentor, Seymour Solomon, for teaching him the ways and pleasures of relieving pain. He also thanks his many collaborators in headache medicine, particularly Walter Stewart, Marcelo Bigal, Dawn Buse and Daniel Serrano for teaching him the joys of shared discovery. Finally, he thanks his co-editors of this volume for being inspirational clinicians and teachers and for their infinite patience and hard work in bringing this book to fruition.

Part I

Principles of Headache: Primary and Secondary Headache Disorders

The Basics of Headache Classification and Diagnosis

Seymour Solomon[1,2] and Richard B. Lipton[1,2]

[1]Montefiore Headache Center, Bronx, NY, USA
[2]Albert Einstein College of Medicine, Bronx, NY, USA

Introduction

The causes of headache range from the short-lived and trivial (e.g., a hangover headache) to the intermittent and quality-of-life threatening (migraine), to the unremitting and life-threatening (subarachnoid hemorrhage headache). This broad range of etiologies is matched by the very high prevalence of headache in the general population. In combination, the diversity of causes and high prevalence mandate a systematic approach to classification and diagnosis. Classification refers to a set of categories with diagnostic rules that provide the framework for a clinical approach. Diagnosis is the process of applying the rules to individual patients, defining their place in the classification.

In this chapter, we present an approach to both headache classification and diagnosis. We begin by describing the classification for headache disorders (see Tables 1.1, 1.2, 1.3, and 1.4 in the relevant sections). We recommend a three-step diagnostic process. First, we emphasize the identification or exclusion of secondary headache disorders by history, physical examination, and judicious use of diagnostic tests (see Table 1.5 and Figure 1.1). Second, we consider four groups of primary headache disorders that are defined

based on headache frequency and duration (see Table 1.6) and refer to these as primary headache syndromes. Finally, we emphasize the identification of specific disorders within syndromic groups.

Approach to classification

The classification system for headache disorders has evolved over the past 50 years. Good classification systems should be valid, reliable, generalizable, and complete. A valid system provides categories that correspond, as much as possible, to biologic reality. As a practical matter, a valid system should usefully predict prognosis, response to treatment, and pathobiology. In a reliable system, two clinicians seeing the same patient should assign the same diagnoses. A generalizable system should work in a variety of settings including population studies, primary care, specialty care, and clinical trials. Finally, a complete system has an appropriate category for every headache type.

The first modern attempt at headache classification, sponsored by the National Institute of Health in 1962, was undertaken by the Ad Hoc Committee on Headache Classification of Headache [1]. While the Ad Hoc Committee's

Headache, First Edition. Edited by Matthew S. Robbins, Brian M. Grosberg, and Richard B. Lipton.
© 2013 John Wiley & Sons, Ltd. Published 2013 by John Wiley & Sons, Ltd.

descriptions of headache types, for the most part, stand to this day, disorders were described in terms of their typical features without explicit operational rules regarding the characteristics required to diagnose or exclude particular disorders. In the absence of such rules, diagnostic reliability is not possible.

For the past 25 years, headache classification efforts have been led by the International Headache Society, which has published two editions of its International Classification of Headache Disorders (known as ICHD-1 and -2) [2, 3]. A third edition (ICHD-3) is in development. Learning the lessons taught by the Diagnostic and Statistical Manual of Mental Disorders system in psychiatry, the ICHD system provides clear boundaries among the primary headache disorders (Table 1.1). Although it is based on both evidence and expert opinion, the effort to be explicit inevitably leads to rules that are somewhat arbitrary. For example, to diagnose migraine without aura, at least five headache attacks are required. A patient

Table 1.1. The classification system (modified) (numbers refer to the ICHD-2 code)

A. Primary headache disorders
1. Migraine
    1.1.   Migraine without aura
    1.2.   Migraine with aura
    1.3.   Childhood periodic syndromes that are commonly precursors with migraine
    1.4.   Retinal migraine
    1.5.   Complications of migraine
    1.6.   Probable migraine
2. Tension-type headache
    2.1.   Infrequent episodic tension-type headache
    2.2.   Frequent tension-type headache
    2.3.   Chronic tension-type headache
    2.4.   Probable tension-type headache
3. Cluster headache and other trigeminal autonomic cephalalgias (TAC)
    3.1.   Cluster headache
           3.1.1. Episodic cluster headache
           3.1.2. Chronic cluster headache
    3.2.   Paroxysmal hemicrania
           3.2.1. Episodic paroxysmal hemicrania
           3.2.2. Chronic paroxysmal hemicrania
    3.3.   Short-lasting unilateral neuralgiform headache attacks with conjunctival injection and tearing (SUNCT)
    3.4.   Probable TAC
4. Other primary headaches
    4.1.   Primary stabbing headache
    4.2.   Primary cough headache
    4.3.   Primary exertional headache
    4.4.   Primary headache associated with sexual activity
    4.5.   Hypnic Headache
    4.6.   Primary thunderclap headache
    4.7.   Hemicrania continua
    4.8.   New daily persistent headache (NDPH)

B. Secondary headache disorders
5. Headache attributed to head and/or trauma
    5.1.   Acute post-traumatic headache
    5.2.   Chronic post-traumatic headache

Table 1.1. (*Continued*)

6. Headache attributed to cranial or cervical vascular disorder
   6.1.   Headache attributed to ischemic stroke or transient ischemic attack
   6.2.   Headache attributed to non-traumatic intracranial hemorrhage
   6.3.   Headache attributed to unruptured vascular malformation
   6.4.   Headache attributed to arteritis
   6.5.   Carotid or vertebral artery pain
   6.6.   Headache attributed to cerebral venous thrombosis
   6.7.   Headache attributed to other intracranial vascular disorder
7. Headache attributed to non-vascular intracranial disorder
   7.1.   Headache attributed to high cerebrospinal fluid pressure
   7.2.   Headache attributed to low cerebrospinal fluid pressure
   7.3.   Headache attributed to non-infectious inflammatory disease
   7.4.   Headache attributed to intracranial neoplasm
   7.5.   Headache attributed to intrathecal injection
   7.6.   Headache attributed to epileptic seizure
   7.7.   Headache attributed to Chiari malformation type I
   7.8.   Syndrome of transient headache and neurologic deficits with cerebrospinal fluid lymphocytosis
   7.9.   Headache attributed to other non-vascular intracranial disorder
8. Headache attributed to a substance or its withdrawal
   8.1.   Headache induced by acute substance use or exposure
   8.2.   Medication-overuse headache (MOH)
   8.3.   Headache as an adverse event attributed to chronic medication
   8.4.   Headache attributed to substance withdrawal
9. Headache attributed to infection
   9.1.   Headache attributed to intracranial infection
   9.2.   Headache attributed to systemic infection
   9.3.   Headache attributed to HIV/AIDS
   9.4.   Chronic post-infection headache
10. Headache attributed to disorder of homeostasis
   10.1.   Headache attributed to hypoxia and/or hypercapnia
   10.2.   Dialysis Headache
   10.3.   Headache attributed to hypertension
   10.4.   Headache attributed to hypothyroidism
   10.5.   Headache attributed to fasting
   10.6.   Cardiac cephalalgia
   10.7.   Headache attributed to other disorder of homeostasis

C. Headache or facial pain attributed to disorder of cranial structures, psychiatric disorders, cranial neuralgias

11. Headache or facial pain attributed to disorder of cranium, neck, eyes, ears, nose, sinuses, teeth, mouth or other facial or cranial structures
   11.1.   Headache attributed to disorder of cranial bone
   11.2.   Headache attributed to disorder of neck
   11.3.   Headache attributed to disorder of eyes
   11.4.   Headache attributed to disorder of ears
   11.5.   Headache attributed to rhinosinusitis
   11.6.   Headache attributed to disorder of teeth, jaws or related structures
   11.7.   Headache or facial pain attributed to temporomandibular joint disorder
   11.8.   Headache attributed to other disorder of cranium, neck, eyes, ears, nose sinuses, teeth, mouth or other facial or cervical structures

(Continued)

Table 1.1. (*Continued*)

   12. Headache attributed to psychiatric disorder
        12.1. Headache attributed to somatisation disorder
        12.2. Headache attributed to psychotic disorder
   13. Cranial neuralgias and central causes of facial pain
        13.1. Trigeminal neuralgia
        13.2. Glossopharyngeal neuralgia
        13.3. Nervus intermedius neuralgia
        13.4. Superior laryngeal neuralgia
        13.5. Nasociliary neuralgia
        13.6. Supraorbital neuralgia
        13.7. Other terminal branch neuralgias
        13.8. Occipital neuralgia
        13.9. Neck-tongue syndrome
        13.10. External compression headache
        13.11. Cold-stimulus headache
        13.12. Constant pain caused by compression, irritation or distortion of cranial nerves or upper cervical roots by structural lesions
        13.13. Optic neuritis
        13.14. Ocular diabetic neuropathy
        13.15. Head or facial pain attributed to herpes zoster
        13.16. Tolosa-Hunt syndrome
        13.17. Ophthalmoplegic "migraine"
        13.18. Central causes of facial pain
        13.19. Other cranial neuralgia or other centrally mediated facial pain
   14. Other headache, cranial neuralgia, central or primary facial pain
        14.1. Headache not elsewhere classified
        14.2. Headache unspecified

with four typical attacks of migraine and a family history of migraine almost certainly has migraine, although they may not meet full criteria for the disorder.

Since ICHD-1, the criteria have evolved, based on formal field testing and clinical experience [3]. Major improvements have been made in the area of completeness as important disorders not included in ICHD-1, such as chronic migraine, new daily persistent headache, and hypnic headache were added to ICHD-2, published in 2004 [3]. In the years that followed, as field testing revealed limitations to ICHD-2, proposed revisions have been published, which will culminate in ICHD-3. This chapter is based on ICHD-2 and the published proposals for revision that will inform the shape of ICHD-3.

The ICHD approach to classification defines three overarching categories: primary headache disorders, secondary headache disorders, and cranial neuralgias and facial pains. For the primary disorders, the headache disorder is the problem; there is no underlying disease. For secondary headaches, the headache is attributed to an underlying cause. In this chapter, the discussion of secondary headaches will deal mainly with the features that differentiate them from the primary headaches, i.e., the "red flags" that indicate the need for further diagnostic evaluation. The primary headaches are divided into four broad groups: migraine, tension-type headache (TTH), trigeminal autonomic cephalalgias (TACs; including cluster headache), and other uncommon primary headaches.

Approach to diagnosis

Headache history

Because most patients seeing their doctor for headache have normal medical and neurologic examinations, the history is essential for accurate diagnosis. We recommend beginning with an open-ended statement such as, "Tell me about your headaches and how they affect your life." Although many clinicians fear that such an open-ended statement will generate a very long and unhelpful narrative, most patients speak for less than 90 seconds and usually provide useful information about both the headache's features and the impact on their life. Studies show that the use of open-ended questions makes headache visits shorter and increases both clinician and patient satisfaction with the visit.

After the patient's narrative, directed questions are used to fill in the details. The age of onset of the headache and the accompanying circumstances are important. Ask about the features of the head pain, including the location (unilateral, bilateral, or focal), quality (throbbing, stabbing, or steady ache), and intensity of the pain (on a scale of 1 to 10). The duration and frequency of headaches are important. The timing of attacks may assist both diagnosis and therapy. What time in the 24-hour day do they occur; are they associated with menstruation; do they cluster in time?

★ TIPS AND TRICKS

Patients often first describe their worst or most recent headache. They may rate the intensity as 10 on a scale of 1 to 10, and the duration as constant since last Tuesday. Ask about the range of intensity and the typical duration. Similarly, they may state that the headache lasts for 3 days and occurs three times per week. It then is useful to determine the number of headache-free days per week or per month.

Ask about possible warning or premonitory symptoms that typically precede the onset of the headache by hours or days. Typical premonitory features include changes in mood such as irritability, food cravings, and neck stiffness among others. Auras are focal neurologic symptoms that usually begin 15–60 minutes before the headache. Premonitory features and auras are most typical of migraine although not entirely specific. Symptoms accompanying the headache may include nausea, vomiting, photophobia, and phonophobia as well as tearing of the eye, conjunctival injection, and nasal discharge among others.

It is also helpful to understand factors associated with an increased chance of headache onset (triggers). Avoidance or management of triggers becomes a therapeutic strategy. Aggravating factors increase the severity of a pre-existing headache but are not associated with an increased rate of headache initiation. Ameliorating factors provide diagnostic clues. For example, hibernation in a dark, quiet room suggests a diagnosis of migraine. Understanding the effects of treatment and the course of the headache over time is also helpful.

★ TIPS AND TRICKS

Patients often list their prescription medication, but fail to mention the over-the-counter (OTC) medications they use. OTC medications and dietary caffeine are important causes of medication overuse headache. After the history of the present illness has been obtained, other historical factors should be elicited. Is there a past history of illness, surgery, trauma, depression, or anxiety? Family history should include questions on other members with headache. Social history factors relating to marital status, education, occupation, interests, habits (alcohol, nicotine, and illicit drugs), sleep patterns, childhood abuse, and past and present stressors may all be relevant.

Diagnosing headache is as easy as 1, 2, 3

The first step in evaluating a patient with headache is to differentiate primary from secondary headaches. Secondary headaches are attributable to an underlying neurologic, medical, or psychiatric illness (Figure 1.1). Secondary headache is suspected if red flags on the history or examination suggest it. Primary headache disorders are likely if red flags are absent or if diagnostic testing excludes secondary headache. In addition, if a

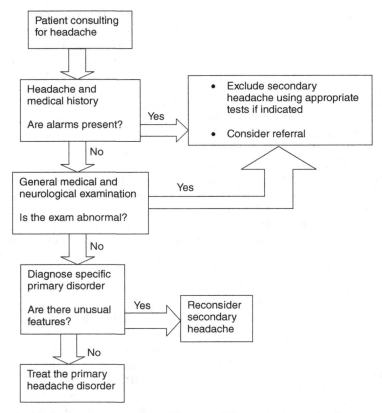

Figure 1.1. Headache diagnosis. (Reproduced from *Wolff's Headache and Other Pain*, 8th edition by Lipton et al. (2008) [15]. By permission of Oxford University Press, USA.)

secondary cause of headache is present but temporally remote from a pre-existing headache disorder, both primary and secondary headaches are likely. Consider a woman with typical attacks of migraine with aura from age 10 who develops a new form of daily headache at age 70. The MRI reveals a meningioma. Most likely, the patient has migraine with aura and a secondary headache attributed to her meningioma.

> ★ **TIPS AND TRICKS**
>
> When a headache changes in intensity or frequency, or in another feature, it may be a worsening of the primary headache, but one must always consider the superimposition of a new secondary headache. Searching for a new potential cause is warranted.

In making the diagnosis of a primary headache, the history and physical and neurologic examinations do not suggest secondary headache, or the latter can be ruled out either by investigations or by a distant temporal relationship (see Table 1.5). Symptoms that point to a specific primary headache but may not include all of the diagnostic criteria listed in ICHD-2 are preceded by the title "probable," for example "probable migraine." If the patient has two or more types of headache contemporaneously, all should be classified. The presence of a primary headache does not, of course, exclude the development of a secondary headache. Inattention to that obvious fact is a common and sometimes fatal error.

After excluding a secondary headache disorder, the next step is to identify a primary headache syndrome. Common headache syndromes and the specific disorders to consider within each syndromic group are summarized in Table 1.6.

These syndromes are defined based on the number of headache days per month and on the average duration of attacks. Based on headache days, two examples with long and short frequencies are chronic TTH, with 15 or more days per month, and episodic TTH with fewer than 15 headache days per month. Based on duration, we consider short-duration attacks as lasting less than 4 hours and long-duration attacks as lasting for 4 hours or more, for example cluster headache and chronic migraine, respectively. Some ICHD-2 defined disorders are included in more than one syndromic group. Most people with migraine have episodic headache of a long duration, but a clinically important subgroup have chronic migraine, the most important cause of chronic daily headache with a long attack duration.

Having identified the syndrome, the next task is to diagnose the specific disorder within the syndromic group. In the sections that follow, we discuss a number of specific primary headache disorders.

Migraine (ICHD-2 1.0)

Migraine is divided into two categories based on the characteristics of the attack: migraine without aura and migraine with aura. Attacks typically occur from less than once to several times a month. Migraine is also categorized based on headache days per month. When migraine occurs on 15 or more days per month for at least 3 months, the term "chronic migraine" is applied. The term "chronic" has several possible meanings in ordinary English and in medicine. As applied to migraine and TTH, it has the very specific meaning of headaches occurring on more days than not over at least 3 months. There are rare variants of migraine: retinal migraine, familial or sporadic hemiplegic migraine, and basilar-type migraine. Migraine is a very common phenomenon, affecting 12% of the population—18% of women and 6% of men in any given year. In contrast to past concepts, epidemiologic studies have shown that the prevalence of migraine varies inversely with socioeconomic status [4].

Migraine without aura

Migraine without aura (ICHD-2 1.1) represents about 75%–80% of all migraineurs. The criteria for migraine without aura are listed in Table 1.2. The typical features of an attack are a headache that is one-sided, pulsating, moderate or severe in pain intensity, lasting for hours, and associated with nausea and/or vomiting, photophobia, and phonophobia. In children, the duration is often shorter, 1 or 2 hours, and the associated features of nausea or vomiting or both are sometimes more prominent than the headache. Migraine attacks may not be typical but still fulfill the diagnostic criteria. For example, the location is often bilateral, and the quality may be a steady ache rather than pulsating. In the absence of these two features, the diagnosis is still appropriate if the two other features of the headache are present (pain of moderate or severe intensity and aggravation by physical activity) and other criteria are fulfilled. Similarly, only one of the two associated features—nausea and sensitively to light and sound—need be present. The frequency of attacks may vary from one per week to one per year. When the frequency increases to more than 15 days per month, the additional classification of chronic migraine is applied.

Migraine with aura

Migraine with aura (ICHD-2 1.2) (Table 1.2) occurs in about 20% of people with migraine. The most common aura of migraine is a positive homonymous visual phenomenon, a scintillating arc of zigzag lines that occurs for minutes before the onset of the headache and then completely disappears. Any neurologic symptom or sign may be an aura of migraine, but unusual conditions are more specifically subclassified as hemiplegic migraine, basilar-type (brainstem dysfunction) migraine, or retinal migraine (see "Subtypes of migraine"). The symptoms are usually positive, such as flickering lights or tingling sensations, in contrast to negative symptoms such as loss of vision or impaired sensation. The visual symptoms are typically homonymous, and the sensory symptoms usually affect the hand and face. These focal symptoms are most often on the side opposite the headache. Dysphasic speech is the least common aura manifestation. The aura usually evolves gradually and lasts from 5 to 60 minutes. Headache with features of migraine without aura usually begins as soon as the aura stops but sometimes begins at the same time as the aura and may begin as long as 1 hour after the aura. The aura may occur without headache, especially during middle or late age. Typical auras

Table 1.2. Diagnostic criteria for migraine without and with aura

ICHD-2 diagnostic criteria for 1.1 migraine without aura

A. At least 5 attacks fulfilling criteria B–D
B. Headache attacks last 4–72 hours (untreated or unsuccessfully treated)
C. Headache has at least 2 of the following characteristics:
   1. Unilateral location
   2. Pulsating quality
   3. Moderate or severe pain intensity
   4. Aggravation by, or causing avoidance of, routine physical activity (e.g., walking or climbing stairs)
D. During the headache attack, at least 1 of the following:
   1. Nausea and/or vomiting
   2. Photophobia and phonophobia
E. Symptoms not attributed to another disorder

ICHD-2 diagnostic criteria for 1.2 migraine with aura (modified)

A. At least 2 attacks fulfilling criteria B–D
B. Aura consists of at least 1 of the following:
   1. Fully reversible visual symptoms
   2. Fully reversible sensory symptoms
   3. Fully reversible dysphasic speech disturbance
      (not motor weakness)
C. At least 2 of the following:
   1. Homonymous visual symptoms and/or unilateral sensory symptoms
   2. At least one aura symptom develops gradually over more than 5 minutes and/or different aura symptoms occur in succession over 25 minutes
D. Headache fulfills criteria B–D for 1.1 migraine without aura
E. Symptoms not attributed to another disorder

sometimes occur with nonmigraine headaches and have been reported with cluster headache, chronic paroxysmal hemicranias, and hemicrania continua.

Cerebrovascular disease, especially transient ischemic attacks, may closely resemble the aura of migraine. Features that differentiate the two entities are the aura's slow evolution and the positive nature of the visual and sensory symptoms (e.g., scintillating scotomas rather than blindness). Investigations to rule out cerebrovascular disease are warranted if the symptoms are of rapid onset (less than 5 minutes), the visual or sensory symptoms are negative (blindness or sensory loss), the aura is prolonged (more than 1 hour), or the patient has risk factors for vascular disease including onset after the age of 50 [5].

Subtypes of migraine

There are several unusual forms of migraine named for the area of the affected nervous system. In all cases, the manifestation of these unusual auras is reversible.

Familial hemiplegic migraine (FHM) (ICHD-2 1.2.4), as the name implies, is manifested by hemiparesis sometimes with hemisensory impairment. Ataxia or other features of basilar-type migraine may occur. Unlike a typical aura, the hemiparesis may last for hours. This is the first headache syndrome linked to genetic polymorphisms. The loci for the condition are on chromosomes 1, 2, or 19 [6]. One or more first-degree relatives have similar attacks. People without a family history but otherwise meeting the criteria are classified as having sporadic hemiplegic migraine. The genetics of FHM are discussed in detail in Chapter 6.

In patients with *basilar-type migraine* (ICHD-2 1.2.6), the symptoms associated with the headache implicate the posterior fossa. The ICHD-2 classification requires at least two of the following aura symptoms: vertigo, tinnitus, decreased hearing, double vision, visual defects in both the temporal and nasal fields of both eyes, ataxia, dysarthria, bilateral paresthesias, or decreased consciousness.

Retinal migraine (ICHD-2 1.4) is manifested by scintillation, other positive visual symptoms, or more likely scotomas or partial or complete blindness limited to one eye (in contrast to common homonymous symptoms). Many of these patients experience a permanent partial defect representing retinal infarction [7]. Other causes of monocular visual loss (transient ischemic attacks, optic neuropathy, and retinal detachment) must be considered.

Childhood periodic syndromes are often precursors of migraine. *Cyclic vomiting* (ICHD-2 1.3.1) is manifested by intractable recurrent vomiting lasting for hours or days. Pallor and lethargy are usually associated. There is no evidence of gastrointestinal disease. Patients with *abdominal migraine* (ICHD-2 1.3.2) have attacks of abdominal pain associated with anorexia or nausea, with or without vomiting, and pallor. The ICHD-2 criteria require at least two of the three associated symptoms. Again, examination and studies rule out gastrointestinal disease. In patients with *benign paroxysmal vertigo of childhood* (ICHD-2 1.3.3), there are recurrent attacks (at least five) of severe vertigo that may last for minutes to hours; the attacks resolve spontaneously. Neurologic and vestibular functions are normal between attacks, as are imaging studies and electroencephalography. When this condition occurs after childhood, the patients often have bouts of migraine during or independent of vertigo. "Migrainous vertigo" or "vertiginous migraine" are not accepted entities in the ICHD-2 classification. Benign recurrent vertigo may occur at any age and often coexists with migraine. It is considered a comorbid condition.

Complications of migraine

Chronic migraine (ICHD-2 1.5.1) is defined as migraine headaches (usually without aura) or TTHs recurring on more than 15 days per month for more than 3 months [8]. At least 50% of the headaches should be migraine based on the presence of migraine features or response to migraine treatment. Chronic migraine evolves from episodic migraine. Many risk factors contribute to the evolution of chronic migraine from episodic migraine (see Chapter 5). Risk factors include frequent episodic headaches, high levels of disability, allodynia, depression, traumatic head injury, and overuse of drugs, most importantly opioid- and barbiturate-containing analgesics. The diag-

nosis of chronic migraine in the setting of medication overuse is complex (see Chapter 10). In practice, we treat medication overuse as a modifier, I.e., chronic migraine with medication overuse.

Status migrainosus (ICHD-2 1.5.2) is a term used for a severe and disabling migraine that lasts for more than 3 days. *Prolonged aura* is an extension of the patient's typical aura for more than 1 hour but less than 1 week. *Persistent aura without infarction* (ICHD-2 1.5.3) refers to persistence of an aura for more than 1 week. The aura is otherwise typical of past attacks. Evaluations do not reveal cerebral infarction. *Migrainous infarction* (ICHD-2 1.54) rarely occurs. The typical aura symptom or symptoms persist beyond 1 hour, and neurologic examination or neuroimaging or both confirms cerebral infarction. Other causes of stroke must be excluded.

Many patients exhibit all but one of the criteria for migraine. The term "probable migraine" (ICHD-2 1.6) is then appropriate.

TTH (ICHD-2 2.0)

This term replaces the former names of "tension headache" (implying emotional stress) and "muscle contraction headache" (implying a muscular origin of the headache). Although TTH is the most common primary headache, its mechanism is the least well understood. Many believe that TTHs are fragments of migraine. The diagnostic criteria are listed in Table 1.3. The headache characteristics are purposely nonmigrainous. The location is bilateral, the quality is nonpulsating, the intensity is mild to moderate, and the headache is not aggravated by physical activity. Similarly, there is a paucity of associated symptoms: no nausea or vomiting, although either photophobia or phonophobia may be present, but not both. There may or may not be associated pericranial tenderness.

TTHs are classified into episodic (fewer than 15 attacks per month) and chronic (more than 15 attacks per month). Episodic TTH is further subdivided into *infrequent episodic TTH* (ICHD-2 2.1) (less than 1 day per month) and *frequent episodic TTH* (ICHD-2 2.2) (1–14 days per month). *Chronic TTH* (ICHD-2 2.3) usually evolves from the episodic form and in its purest form should not be diagnosed in patients overusing acute medication. In practice, patients with medication overuse headache (a secondary headache)

Table 1.3. ICHD-2 Diagnostic criteria for 2.0 tension-type headache (TTH) (modified)

A. Episodes occuring in frequencies below (see 2.1, 2.2 and 2.3A)
B. Headache lasting from 30 minutes to 7 days
C. Headache has at least 2 of the following characteristics:
   1. Bilateral location
   2. Pressing/tightening (non-pulsating) quality
   3. Mild or moderate intensity
   4. Not aggravated by routine physical activity, such as walking or climbing upstairs
D. Both of the following:
   1. No nausea or vomiting (anorexia may occur)
   2. No more than one of the following: photophobia or phonophobia
E. Symptoms not attributed to another disorder

2.1 Infrequent episodic TTH
At least 10 episodes occurring on <1 day per month on average (<12 days per year) and fulfilling criteria B–D

2.2 Frequent episodic TTH
At least 10 episodes occurring on ≥1 but <15 days per month for at least 3 months (≥12 and <180 days per year) and fulfilling criteria B–D

2.3 Chronic TTH
A. Headache occurring on >15 days per month on average for >3 months (>180 days per year) and fulfilling criteria C–E (above)
B. Headache lasts hours or may be continuous

usually manifest the features of chronic TTH. As with the classification of migraine, the diagnosis of *probable TTH* (ICHD-2 2.4) is warranted if all but one of the ICHD-2 criteria are met. Another headache that phenotypically may resemble chronic TTH is new daily persistent headache (see "Other primary headaches").

TACs (ICHD-2 2.3.0)

The group of primary headaches known as TACs are characterized by trigeminal activation with unilateral pain typically affecting one orbit and ipsilateral autonomic activation (predominantly parasympathetic) [9]. The pain may spread to adjacent areas of one side and is usually locked to the same side on repeated attacks.

   Cluster headache (ICHD-2 3.1) is the best known of the TACs, and the criteria for diagnosing it are noted in Table 1.4. The pain, usually in or around one orbit, is excruciating and is typically boring, sharp, or stabbing. It begins quickly and lasts from 15 minutes to 3 hours. During the attack, one or more of the following associated features are present: ipsilateral redness and tearing of the eye, clogging or drainage from the nostril, and ptosis and miosis. The attacks may occur between one and eight times per day, often

Table 1.4. ICHD-2 diagnostic criteria for cluster headache

3.0 Cluster headache (modified)
A. At least 5 attacks fulfilling criteria B–D
B. Severe or very severe unilateral orbital, supraorbital and/or temporal pain lasting 15–180 minutes if untreated
C. Headache is accompanied by at least 1 of the following:
   1. Ipsilateral conjunctival injection and/or lacrimation
   2. Ipsilateral nasal congestion and/or rhinorrhea
   3. Ipsilateral eyelid edema
   4. Ipsilateral forehead and facial sweating
   5. Ipsilateral miosis and/or ptosis
   6. A sense of restlessness or agitation
D. Attacks have a frequency from one every other day to 8 per day
E. Not attributed to another disorder

3.1 Episodic cluster headache occurs in periods lasting 7 days to 1 year

3.2 Chronic cluster headache occurs for more than 1 year without remission

awakening the patient from sleep. During the headache, in contrast to the behavior during migraine, the patient cannot lie still but is impelled to move about or sit and rock. Cluster headaches affect men more than women. These people are often heavy smokers.

The most common subtype is *episodic cluster headache* (ICHD-2 3.1.1), recurring every day for weeks or months (in clusters), and then remitting for one or more months annually, often recurring during the same season or seasons every year. During these cluster periods, alcoholic beverages and other vasodilating agents may trigger an attack. The unfortunate individuals who do not experience a remission within a year or have only a brief remission of less than 1 month are classified as having *chronic cluster headache* (ICHD-2 3.1.2).

Paroxysmal hemicranias, as the name implies, are unilateral headaches that are of short duration (2–30 minutes) and occur more than five times per day [9]. Associated with these are some or all of the autonomic features of cluster headache. The headaches invariably respond to prophylactic doses of indomethacin. The headaches usually occur without remission: *chronic paroxysmal hemicrania* (ICHD-2 3.2.2). Less frequent are remissions of 1 month or more: *episodic paroxysmal hemicrania* (ICHD-2 3.2.1).

Short-lived unilateral neuralgiform headache attacks with conjunctival injection and tearing (SUNCT) syndrome (ICHD-2 3.3)—the name of this syndrome tells it all [10]. The headache and autonomic features are again similar to those of cluster headaches and paroxysmal hemicranias, but the duration is shorter (5 seconds to 4 minutes) and the frequency is higher (3–200 attacks per day).

Other primary headaches

Hemicrania continua (ICHD-2 4.7) is a daily and continuous unilateral headache that always responds to therapeutic doses of indomethacin [11]. The daily pain is of moderate intensity, but superimposed exacerbations often occur and may mimic migraine or cluster headache. Patients sometimes complain only of the migraine or cluster headache symptoms. A sensation of conjunctival irritation is often noted. Without inquiring about lesser daily headaches, the diagnosis of hemicrania continua may be missed.

> ⭐ **TIPS AND TRICKS**
>
> Patients often describe the headache that is most intense or disabling, such as migraine. Ask whether or not some headache or discomfort is present between the severe attacks. This may lead to the diagnosis of hemicrania continua with exacerbations that resemble a migraine-like headache.

Primary stabbing headaches (ICHD-2 4.1) are manifested by episodes of localized stabs of pain [12]. Formerly called "jabs and jolts," the pains last only one or a few seconds and occur at random without a consistent location. The frequency may range from a few per day to a few per month. Associated symptoms are lacking. These headaches are not uncommon in people with migraine.

Other primary headaches may be triggered by *cough, exertion,* or *sexual activity* (ICHD-2 4.2, ICHD-2 4.3, ICHD-2 4.4) and are labeled as such. Organic disease may cause headache evoked by these activities. Neuroimaging with special attention to the posterior fossa is mandatory to rule out cerebral aneurysm, subarachnoid hemorrhage, arterial dissection, and Arnold–Chiari malformation. Headache associated with sexual activity may be preorgasmic, causing a dull ache in the head and neck, or orgasmic, which often has an explosive quality.

Primary thunderclap headache (ICHD-2 4.6) is a severe headache of sudden onset [13]. The attack mimics the pain of subarachnoid hemorrhage, which must be excluded. The headache lasts from 1 to 10 days and may recur at random over weeks or months.

Hypnic headaches (ICHD-2 4.7) awaken patients from sleep, often at the same time each night. The pain is not specific and is without associated symptoms. Usually mild to moderate in intensity, the headache lasts about 30 minutes. It occurs mainly in late middle age or beyond.

New daily persistent headache (ICHD-2 4.8) was initially thought to mainly resemble chronic TTH. Recent evaluation, however, has revealed that most people with this condition have many features of migraine, and a modified classification has been proposed [14]. Patients can often identify the exact day or days of onset. The headaches begin within 3 days of the noted day and are constant for more than 3 months. Acute medication overuse must be first considered, and chronic migraine should also be ruled out before the diagnosis is made.

Headache diagnosis

In beginning to formulate a diagnosis, the few steps in the algorithm of Figure 1.1 should be helpful. As noted before, headaches secondary to organic disease or dysfunction must be ruled out before a diagnosis of primary headache disorder is established. Neurologic workup is not necessary with every new patient, but if the headache is atypical or has recently changed or there is a history of red flags, a search for underlying disease is warranted (Table 1.5).

In formulating the differential diagnoses of the primary headaches, it is useful to follow a sequence of steps (Table 1.6). First, classify the headaches into low or high frequency (less or more than 15 headache days per month). Second, divide the headaches into those of short or long

Table 1.5. Alarms warranting further consideration

Red flag	Consider	Possible investigation(s)
Sudden-onset headache	Subarachnoid hemorrhage, bleed into mass or AVM, mass lesion (especially posterior fossa), pituitary apoplexy	Neuroimaging Lumbar puncture (after neuroimaging evaluation)
Worsening-pattern of headache (change in frequency or character)	Subdural hematoma, other mass lesion, medication overuse	Neuroimaging
Headache with systemic illness (fever, neck stiffness, rash)	Meningitis, encephalitis, Lyme disease, systemic infection, collagen vascular disease, arteritis	Neuroimaging Lumbar puncture Biopsy Blood tests
Focal neurologic signs, or symptoms other than typical visual or sensory aura	Mass lesion, AVM, collagen vascular disease	Neuroimaging Lumbar puncture (after neuroimaging evaluation) Blood tests
Papilledema	Mass lesion, idiopathic intracranial hypertension, encephalitis, meningitis	Neuroimaging Lumbar puncture (after neuroimaging evaluation)
Triggered by cough, exertion or sexual activity	Subarachnoid hemorrhage, mass lesion	Neuroimaging Consider lumbar puncture
Headache during pregnancy or post-partum	Cortical vein/cranial sinus thrombosis, carotid dissection, pituitary apoplexy	Neuroimaging
New headache type in a patient with cancer	Metastasis	Neuroimaging Lumbar puncture
Lyme disease	Meningoencephalitis	Neuroimaging Lumbar puncture
HIV	Opportunistic infection, tumor	Neuroimaging Lumbar puncture
Age of onset over 50	Organic disease: e.g., giant cell arteritis, mass lesion	Neuroimaging Erythrocyte sedimentation rate

AVM, arteriovenous malformation.

Table 1.6. Primary headache diagnosis by syndromic group

Frequency	Short duration (<4 hours)	Long duration (4 hours or more)
Low to moderate (<15 days per month)	Primary stabbing headache Thunderclap headache SUNCT syndrome Hypnic headache	Migraine Episodic TTH
Chronic (15 or more days per month)	Cluster headache and other TACs Paroxysmal hemicrania Primary stabbing headache Thunderclap headache SUNCT syndrome Hypnic headache	Chronic migraine Chronic TTH Hemicrania continua New daily persistent headache

duration (less than or more than 4 hours). Finally, consider headaches of short duration of low or high frequency and the presence or not of triggering factors. This approach should lead to the correct diagnosis for almost all patients.

References

1. Ad Hoc Committee on Classification of Headaches. Classification of headache. *JAMA* 1962;**179**:717–8.
2. Headache Classification Committee of the International Headache Society. Classification and diagnostic criteria for headache disorders, cranial neuralgias and facial pain. *Cephalalgia* 1988;**8**(Suppl. 7):1–96.
3. Headache Classification Committee of the International Headache Society. The International Classification of Headache Disorders. *Cephalalgia* 2004;**24**:1–160.
4. Lipton RB, Stewart WF, Diamond S, et al. Prevalence and burden of migraine in the United States: data from the American Migraine Study II. *Headache* 2001;**41**:646–57.
5. Fisher CM. Late life migraine accompaniments as a cause of unexplained transient ischemic attacks. *Can J Neurol Sci* 1980;**7**:9–17.
6. Ducros A, Denier C, Joutel A, et al. The clinical spectrum of familial hemiplegic migraine associated with mutations in a neuronal calcium channel. *N Engl J Med* 2001;**345**:17–24.
7. Grosberg BM, Solomon S, Friedman DI, et al. Retinal migraine reappraised. *Cephalalgia* 2006;**26**:1275–86.
8. Silberstein SD, Lipton RB, Sliwinski M. Classification of daily and near daily headaches: field trial of revised IHS criteria. *Neurology* 1996;**47**:871–5.
9. Goadsby PJ, Lipton RB. A review of paroxysmal hemicranias, SUNCT syndrome and other short-lasting headaches with autonomic features, including new cases. *Brain* 1997;**120**:193–209.
10. Sjaastad O, Saunte C, Salvesen R, et al. Short-lasting unilateral neuralgiform headache attacks with conjunctival injection, tearing, sweating, and rhinorrhea. *Cephalalgia* 1989; **9**:147–56.
11. Sjaastad O, Spierings EL. Hemicrania continua: another headache absolutely responsive to indomethacin. *Cephalalgia* 1984;**4**:65–70.
12. Pareja JA, Rujiz J, Deisla C, et al. Idiopathic stabbing headache (jabs and jolt syndrome). *Cephalalgia* 1996;**16**:93–6.
13. Day JW, Raskin NH. Thunderclap headache: symptom of unruptured cerebral aneurysm. *Lancet* 1986;**2**:1247–8.
14. Robbins MS, Grosberg BM, Napchan U, et al. Clinical and prognostic subforms of new daily persistent headache. *Neurology* 2010;**74**:1358–64.
15. Lipton RB, Silberstein SD, Dodick D. Overview of diagnosis and classification. In Silberstein SD, Lipton RB, & Dodick DW (eds.), *Wolff's Headache and Other Head Pain* (8th edn). New York: Oxford University Press; 2008: p. 38.

Approach to the Patient with Headache

Brian M. Grosberg, Benjamin W. Friedman, and Seymour Solomon

Albert Einstein College of Medicine, Bronx, NY, USA

Introduction

Headache is one of the most common complaints presenting to primary care physicians and neurologists. Although the vast majority of headache syndromes are benign, clinicians are faced with the crucial task of differentiating benign headache disorders from potentially life-threatening conditions. Given the broad range of disorders that present with headache, a focused and systematic approach is necessary to facilitate the prompt diagnosis and treatment of various kinds of head pain.

In managing a patient with chronic, recurrent primary headaches, there must be a positive interrelationship between patient and doctor. Some patients sit back and say "I'm here. It's your job to cure me." Some doctors quickly prescribe an analgesic and give the patient short shrift. During the initial evaluation, the patient and the doctor should get to know one another. Patients want their doctor to take an interest in them as a person. They want to know why they have a headache and what is causing it. The doctor wants not only to make a diagnosis, but also to judge the patient's personality and needs. Effective communication and interpersonal skills are integral to the care of headache patients [1].

There are several steps in patient management. First, of course, is the history and examination. One must differentiate primary from secondary headaches. If worrisome features or "red flags" are present either in the history or on examination, diagnostic testing may be necessary to exclude secondary headache disorders. A summary of these red flags is listed in Table 2.1 [2]. Having determined that the condition is a primary headache, the specific headache type must be diagnosed. Once a diagnosis has been established, the general therapeutic options should be outlined in a treatment plan tailored to the patient. By taking into account the patient's headache diagnosis or diagnoses, frequency of headache attacks, headache-related functional impairment, comorbid medical conditions, frequency of acute medication use, health-related quality of life, and treatment preferences, clinicians can then develop an optimal treatment plan for each patient. One should emphasize the need for the patient to be active in his or her own care. Realistic expectations should be established, and rarely will the initial plan be perfect. Follow-up visits are scheduled to modify the therapy and, if necessary, to reassess the diagnosis.

Headache, First Edition. Edited by Matthew S. Robbins, Brian M. Grosberg, and Richard B. Lipton.
© 2013 John Wiley & Sons, Ltd. Published 2013 by John Wiley & Sons, Ltd.

Table 2.1. Worrisome red flags for headache ("SNOOP")

- Systemic symptoms (fever, stiff neck, weight loss, rash, chills, night sweats)
- Secondary headache risk factors (e.g., HIV, cancer)
- Seizures
- Neurologic symptoms or abnormal signs (e.g., confusion, impaired alertness, loss of consciousness, or focal signs)
- Onset: sudden, abrupt, or first headache, triggered by a Valsalva maneuver or position change
- Older: new-onset and progressive headache, especially in middle age >50 years (e.g., giant cell arteritis)
- Progression of headache (e.g., change in attack frequency, severity, or clinical features)
- Positional change (e.g., headache worsens with assuming an erect position or with recumbency)
- Papilledema
- Precipitated by cough, exertion, sexual activity, Valsalva maneuver, or sleep

Adapted from [2].

Headache history

Given the usual paucity of findings on physical and neurologic examination, the most important tool for making a correct headache diagnosis is a detailed history [3]. Without an adequate history, unnecessary diagnostic and treatment interventions may be performed or, alternatively, crucial testing may not be obtained. Taking the headache history provides an opportunity to establish a rapport with the patient that will serve as the basis for an ongoing therapeutic relationship. The goal of the headache history is to provide a comprehensive view of the patient's headache(s) and any associated comorbidities or problems that might influence diagnosis or treatment.

Headache descriptors should first be sought with open-ended statements such as "Tell me about your headaches and how they impact your life." Out of a concern for a lengthy visit, physicians are often hesitant to use open-ended questions. However, this technique usually takes no more than 2 minutes. Physicians can then follow up the patient's account with a series of directed close-ended questions to target missing information. History-taking is often complicated by the presence of more than one type of headache or by a change in the headache pattern over time. It is often helpful to begin with the current headache of greatest concern to the patient and subsequently explore other headache patterns and the evolution of those patterns.

In addition to the history of present illness, the doctor must know about the patient's past medical history as well as their social and psychological background. The doctor will have a general idea about the degree of disability after speaking to the patient. More specifically, we want to know how the headaches are impacting on family life, schoolwork or occupation, and social life. To save the physician's time, detailed intake forms may be completed by patients before the initial appointment.

Age at onset and at presentation

Most of the primary headache disorders begin in childhood or early adult life. Like migraine, tension-type headache and cluster headache may start in early childhood or later in life, but commonly occur between the ages of 20 and 30 years.

✋ CAUTION!

Headaches that begin after the age of 50 years are more likely to be due to serious conditions, such as giant cell arteritis, mass lesions, or cerebrovascular disease [4]. With advancing age, headache or facial pain may result from medications, systemic disorders, postherpetic neuralgia, trigeminal neuralgia, or disorders of the head, neck, eyes, ears, or nose. For these reasons, testing is indicated when older patients present with headaches of recent onset, headaches that have changed from a pre-existing pattern, or headaches that are associated with an abnormal examination. In these circumstances, an MRI of the brain and erythrocyte sedimentation rate should be obtained as an initial workup to help identify or exclude structural disease and giant cell arteritis.

Location and character of the headache

The location and sidedness of the pain can be helpful in distinguishing between different headache disorders. The pain of migraine often affects the right or left frontal and temporal regions of the head but may involve any region of the head and neck; occipitonuchal and frontotemporal pain is not uncommon. The location of headache in a patient with migraine may fluctuate over the course of an attack and between attacks.

> ★ **TIPS AND TRICKS**
>
> Headache "locked to one side" on repeated attacks may be a symptom of underlying organic disease but is not rare in patients with migraine and is typical of cluster headache and other trigeminal autonomic cephalalgias (TACs).

Cluster headache and TACs predominantly affect the orbit and adjacent areas. Holocephalic or band-like pressure is characteristic of tension-type headache. Infratentorial, occipitonuchal, and cervical spine pathology can refer pain to the forehead or eye because of the convergence of cervical nociceptive afferents at the second and third cervical levels with trigeminal afferents in the caudal trigeminal nucleus of the brainstem. As blood or pus tracks down the subarachnoid space, the acute headache of a subarachnoid hemorrhage or meningitis may be followed by pain that travels down the spinal column to the interscapular region or lower back.

Pulsatile or throbbing headaches are typical of migraine. Tension-type headache is pressure-like or aching. Cluster headache is described as a boring, drilling, or lancinating pain. Attacks of trigeminal neuralgia are momentary paroxysms of electric-like pain.

Burning or pulsating ocular or periorbital pain may reflect incipient ischemia in the vertebrobasilar territory, an expanding skull base aneurysm, extracranial or intracranial vascular dissection, dural sinus occlusion, or inflammation in the cavernous sinus. Nonvascular causes include cluster headache, short-lasting unilateral neuralgiform headache with conjunctival injection and tearing (SUNCT), ophthalmic disorders, and inflammatory meningeal syndromes.

Duration, frequency, and timing of attacks

The duration of primary headaches is short: seconds to minutes for TACs, and hours for migraine and tension-type headaches. However, the latter two headache types may last for days or may evolve into a chronic form (i.e., on more than 15 days per month) or become continuous. Frequency of headache within an individual episode can be many times per day, as with some of the TACs, many times over the course of weeks, as with cluster headache, or several per week or month, as with attacks of migraine or tension-type headache. The timing of headaches within a diurnal, monthly, or annual cycle is particularly important in the diagnosis of cluster headache.

Changes in the frequency of headache may be the cause of the visit to the physician, as when relatively well-controlled attacks of migraine increase in frequency or transform into a daily or near-daily headache. Frequent episodic and chronic headaches are managed differently from a rarely occurring headache.

Time to peak severity is also useful information. Vascular etiologies of headache, such as aneurysmal subarachnoid hemorrhage, pituitary apoplexy, and reversible cerebral vasoconstriction syndrome, usually present with a thunderclap headache [5]. The frequency and timing of headache attacks within a longer period of time, such as months or a year or more, allow an understanding of the burden of headache for the individual.

Pain intensity

Pain severity can be used to differentiate primary headache types. Ask the patient to grade the intensity on a scale of 1 to 10, with 1 as pain that can barely be appreciated and 10 as the worst pain possible. The intensity of a tension-type headache is rarely more than moderate, migraine is usually moderate to severe, and cluster headaches are unbearably severe.

Premonitory and aura symptoms

Patients with migraine can often predict the arrival of a headache because of premonitory symptoms that may occur hours or days preceding the headache. These include changes in mood, appetite, concentration, and sleep patterns [6].

Premonitory symptoms are distinct from the aura. The latter precede the headache by minutes or as much as an hour, whereas sometimes the aura begins with the headache.

Any condition that affects the brain may be an aura; most common are visual and sensory phenomena, whereas motor and speech disturbances are rare. These symptoms may be disturbing by themselves or because of what they herald. Visual and sensory auras consist of positive or negative symptoms. Positive visual symptoms may be bright or complex patterns, such as zigzag scintillating scotomas, or photopsia such as floaters and flashes. Negative symptoms include visual field defects, blank scotomas, or blurring. Similarly, sensory auras may consist of hypersensitivity or paresthesias.

Transient visual symptoms support a diagnosis of migraine. However, progressive impairment of visual acuity with transient visual obscurations (with or without visual field cuts or papilledema) may be seen in patients with headaches caused by raised intracranial pressure. Amaurosis occurs in patients with anterior ischemic optic neuropathy secondary to vasculitis (e.g., giant cell arteritis) or retinal emboli from an atherosclerotic or dissecting carotid artery. Diplopia with head pain may be a manifestation of basilar-type migraine but often signifies a parasellar mass or a posterior communicating artery aneurysm. Cheiro-oral paresthesias, which "march" from a hand to the face, are common with migraine but may be a manifestation of a partial sensory seizure or a transient ischemic attack.

Temporal profile

The onset of the headache and its course over time has diagnostic and therapeutic implications. The rapid onset of pain associated with cluster headaches, SUNCT syndrome, and trigeminal neuralgia rarely poses a diagnostic quandary as the characteristics of each of these are distinctive. Primary stabbing headaches ("jabs and jolts") are fleeting, often multifocal cranial pains, which, despite their intensity, are benign. Abrupt-onset headaches suggest a vascular mechanism such as subarachnoid hemorrhage. Some infections and ophthalmologic headache syndromes may also begin suddenly. Usually, features on examination will distinguish between these serious conditions. Other headaches, despite their cataclysmic onset, have a benign prognosis. Examples of this include headaches associated with sexual activity, cough, and exertion.

A chronic recurrent or long-standing daily headache usually represents a primary disorder such as migraine, cluster headache, or tension-type headache. Migraine and other primary headache disorders may only be diagnosed in retrospect after their episodic course becomes manifest and there is no evidence of an underlying lesion. The intensity and quality of the pain may evolve during the course of an attack (i.e., from a bland sensation to a more typical presentation). Migraine and tension-type headaches tend to dissipate over many years. Some physicians inform their female patients with migraine that their headaches will completely cease once they have reached menopause. In truth, the natural history of migraine varies from one person to another; occasionally, migraine may even start at menopause.

> **⚜ CAUTION!**
>
> Progressively worsening headaches (over weeks to months) suggest increasing intracranial pressure, medication overuse headache, or systemic disease. Patients with idiopathic intracranial hypertension, bilateral subdural hematomas, midline obstructive lesions, and chronic meningitic syndromes may exhibit a subacute progressive headache.

Associated features

Noting the associated features of headache, or their absence, and their temporal relationship to the headache provides essential features of the history. Nausea and vomiting are common with migraine and help confirm the diagnosis. They are not pathognomonic for migraine as elevated intracranial pressure, disturbances to the area postrema of the medulla, and systemic infection can cause vomiting. Similarly, phonophobia, photophobia, and osmophobia often accompany migraine, although these symptoms may also occur with meningitis. Cluster headache is associated with one or more ipsilateral autonomic symptoms such as lacrimation, conjunctival injection, nasal congestion, rhinorrhea, ptosis, miosis, eyelid edema, and facial or forehead perspiration. Visual disturbances are often associated with migraine but should also raise concerns of ischemic brain pathology. Pituitary adenoma or idiopathic intracranial hypertension may cause visual field cuts. Symptoms of an upper respiratory infection or toothache may be indicative of acute sinusitis as the cause of the headache, but nasopharyngeal symptoms are often misdiagnosed as "sinus headache" rather than migraine. On the other hand, sphenoid sinusitis may present with headache without nasal symptoms. The physician should differentiate between symptoms that are due to the underlying headache disorder and those due to treatment. For example, ergot agents and nonsteroidal anti-inflammatory drugs may cause nausea.

Aggravating or precipitating factors

Patients often have an understanding of headache triggers even before the visit to the healthcare provider. If the patient is not aware of specific triggers, headache diaries are helpful at elucidating them. When the headaches are associated with menses, ovulation, stress, hormonal supplements, fatigue, depression, food deprivation, or food sensitivity, migraine is likely. Similarly, environmental factors such as fumes, glare or flickering lights, perfume or chemical smells, or exercise may influence the headache pattern. Daily patterns may be triggered by caffeine withdrawal or sleep deprivation. Alcohol is a notorious trigger of cluster headache, and red wine is a classic instigator of migraine. A change in sleep habits may be associated with headache exacerbation; sleep apnea may cause early-morning headaches. Headaches aggravated by an upright posture suggest intracranial hypotension, which can occur spontaneously or iatrogenically. The supine position, or a change in position, may worsen the headaches of intracranial hypertension. Headaches due to elevated intracranial pressure, third ventricular colloid cyst, and Arnold–Chiari malformation are characteristically exacerbated by coughing or Valsalva maneuvers, although migraine and primary cough headache may be similarly triggered. Headaches associated with sexual activity should raise a red flag for intracranial aneurysm, although more often than not it is a recurrent benign headache.

Relieving factors

Typically, migraine is relieved by sleep or rest in a dark and quiet room. Cluster headache, on the other hand, induces patients to be active, typically pacing to and fro. Patients may use a variety of techniques to relieve their headaches, ranging from home remedies, such as cold or warm compresses and relaxation techniques, to herbs, prescription medications, and over-the-counter medications.

Social history

Understanding the patient's social environment is key to understanding the milieu of the primary headache disorders. One should learn of the patient's home life and their responsibilities at home, in the community, and at work. The patient's marital status, education, occupation, and interests are also helpful information.

> ### ✋ CAUTION!
> A history of childhood abuse is more common in patients with chronic migraine or tension-type headache than in the general population.

Stressors at home, at school, and at work should be understood, although the practitioners should not attribute a primary headache disorder solely to stress. Alcohol, tobacco, and street drugs may contribute to headache pathogenesis. Practitioners should only cautiously prescribe triptans or ergotamines to patients who smoke cigarettes or use cocaine.

Family history

Many migraineurs report extended family members with migraine. Migraine has a genetic component although, except for rare familial hemiplegic migraine, convergence within families is inconsistent. Secondary causes of headache, such as cerebral aneurysms, may cluster within families.

> ### ✋ CAUTION!
> A family history of intracranial saccular aneurysms, polycystic kidney disease, or brain tumors should prompt investigations.

Past history of headache

Integral to any headache history is an understanding of what diagnostic testing and what treatment the patient has previously undergone or is currently utilizing. A list of present and past medications is essential. Medications may have been effective but are no longer prescribed because of a change in healthcare provider or a change of insurance. Previously ineffective treatments may have been due to an inadequate dose or duration of trial and may be worth restarting. The headache may have increased or decreased in frequency at various points in the patient's life, and understanding why may help identify triggers or give other useful information. Finally, determine whether biofeedback, psychotherapy, relaxation techniques, or alternative or complementary therapies have been tried.

Impact of and disability from headache

The patient should be given the opportunity to explain how the headache has impacted his or her life. Is the headache intermittent and easily treated with medication, or is it pervasive, destroying relationships, interfering with employment, and always to the forefront in the patient's life? The impact of the headache in the patient's life can be measured using published scales such as the Migraine Disability Assessment questionnaires (MIDAS score) or the Headache Impact Test, both of which are available online. These scales provide a numerical accounting of the patient's suffering and can be used throughout treatment as a reference point.

General medical history and review of systems

A general medical history and a careful review of systems are essential in history-taking. An underlying history of carcinoma should prompt the clinician to consider a metastatic lesion. The most common culprits are cancers of the breast, lung, and kidney, and melanoma. Head trauma may predispose the patient to post-traumatic headaches, a subdural hematoma, or extracranial arterial dissection. A wide variety of disorders associated with dental, sinus, ear, or nose abnormalities may present as headache. A history of headaches in an individual with repeated spontaneous abortions or thromboembolic events suggests an associated antiphospholipid syndrome. Nitrates and antihistamines can cause headache, as can oral contraceptives and hormone replacement therapy.

Understanding a patient's use of medication, including over-the-counter medication, is important. Some people do not consider headache pills bought at the supermarket to be medication.

> ⭐ **TIPS AND TRICKS**
>
> Frequent use of analgesic medication can trigger medication overuse headache and cause episodic headache to evolve to a chronic form.

Chronic daily headache may be the initial component of depression. Depression and epilepsy often occur comorbidly with migraine. Comorbidities are important factors when choosing acute or preventive therapy.

> ✋ **CAUTION!**
>
> Cardiovascular risk factors or other atherosclerotic vascular diseases preclude the use of triptans or ergotamines.

Asthma may require the avoidance of beta-blockers while comorbid hypertension may warrant a beta-blocker as a preventive agent. Comorbid depression may make amitriptyline a good choice as a preventive.

Physical and neurologic examinations

The physical and neurological examinations are essential components of the headache encounter. Although the majority of headache patients will have normal examinations, those with an abnormality on examination usually warrant imaging or other studies. It is the patient with a normal examination who requires an astute diagnostician.

Note the weight of the patient; obesity is a risk factor for migraine. Elevated blood pressure and headache have long been linked in the public mind, although usually there is no relationship. However, when blood pressure rises to high levels very quickly, as in hypertensive encephalopathy, headache will occur. Severe pain itself can elevate a blood pressure. Fever usually accompanies acute infectious etiologies of headache, but an elevated temperature should not be used to explain the etiology of a recurrent headache disorder. Skin changes may be associated with a variety of etiologies for headache. Café-au-lait spots suggest neurofibromatosis associated with intracranial meningiomas and schwannomas. Dry skin, alopecia, and swelling are seen with hypothyroidism. Malignant melanotic lesions may be associated with metastatic disease to the brain.

Auscultation of bruits over the carotid and vertebral arteries and the orbit can alert the clinician to potential arterial stenosis or dissection, or an arteriovenous malformation. Trigger points, areas of tenderness, masses or other skull defects, hematomas, and bruises are detected by inspection and palpation of the head and neck. Temporomandibular joint problems may be associated with headache and should be considered if there is tenderness or limitation of movement of the joints. Palpation of the scalp and face, and tapping of the teeth, may trigger the pain of trigeminal neuralgia, or suggest local pathology in these structures. Acute sinusitis usually presents with tenderness over the involved sinus. Especially in patients 50 years and older, palpation of the superficial temporal arteries may reveal thickened, enlarged vessels with a diminished pulse and tenderness or redness of the scalp, indicative of temporal (giant cell) arteritis. Tenderness over the cervical spine may be associated with muscle spasm and a diminished range of motion, suggesting a cervicogenic cause for the headache. Nuchal rigidity due to meningeal irritation, found with subarachnoid hemorrhage and meningitis, needs prompt measures [7].

The mental status of the patient may be assessed by his or her ability to concentrate and recall details of past history; there may be accompanying difficulties in comprehension or with speech. If impairment is suspected while taking the history, a mental status examination should be pursued, beginning with the Mini Mental Status Examination. Similarly, the physician will be able to make a rough assessment of the patient's psychological status after discussing the history. The intake history form can be useful in making an initial assessment; the Patient Health Questionnaire (PHQ-9) and Generalized Anxiety Disorder (GAD-7) scales may be incorporated into the form [8, 9].

Cranial nerve examination may yield clues regarding the etiology of the headache. While disruption of smell is most often due to incidental nasal pathology or to remote head trauma, it may reflect symptoms of olfactory groove or frontotemporal tumors. On fundoscopic examination, evidence of hemorrhage or papilledema warrants prompt imaging to rule out a space-occupying lesion. A visual field examination may reveal bitemporal visual field defects in patients with a pituitary tumor. During cluster headache attacks, patients may present with ipsilateral lacrimation, rhinorrhea, ptosis, miosis, and facial sweating. A painful Horner syndrome may signify a carotid artery dissection and should trigger an emergency diagnostic evaluation. Ocular movement abnormalities may be due to raised intracranial pressure with secondary involvement of the oculomotor nerves. Other cranial nerves can be affected by a wide variety of causes. If the involvement is patchy, asymmetric, and progressive, infiltrative causes such as neoplasm, tuberculous meningitis, and sarcoidosis should be considered.

The motor examination can be divided into categories of bulk, power, tone, involuntary movements, and coordination. Lesions of the brain and spinal cord manifest increased tone, weakness, and hyper-reflexia, while weakness, atrophy, fasciculations, and diminished tendon reflexes suggest a lesion of the nerve root, nerve plexus, or peripheral nerve. Evidence of truncal instability suggests a midline cerebellar lesion, whereas limb incoordination is indicative of ipsilateral cerebellar hemispheric lesions. Impairment of sensory discrimination is typical of parietal sensory dysfunction. Midline sensory defects usually reflect a central etiology. Glove and stocking sensory defects are noted in patients with peripheral neuropathies but may also be psychogenic.

The presence of reflex asymmetry may be clinically significant, but it must be assessed in the context of other findings. Focal deficits on examination prompt further workup.

Categorizing the primary headache disorder

The first step toward arriving at a diagnosis is the division of headaches into primary and secondary disorders. If primary, decide whether the headache is of long duration (>4 hours) or short duration (<4 hours) and whether it is episodic or chronic. The term "chronic" is used in several forms. Chronic may refer to the time since onset, as in chronic post-traumatic headache, more than 3 months. Alternatively, chronic may refer to frequency, as in chronic migraine (i.e., more than 15 days of headache per month), or to an unremitting course, as in chronic cluster headache. If the headache does not fit into any clear diagnostic category of a primary headache, a secondary cause of headache should be strongly considered. If the patient is seen within the throes of a first acute attack or with a history of a single recent attack, an initial diagnosis may not be feasible. There is a tendency to diagnose common secondary causes of headache such as sinusitis or hypertension when the patient usually has a primary headache disorder.

Diagnosing the specific primary headache disorder

Once it has been determined that the patient has a recurrent primary headache disorder, a specific headache diagnosis may be made. The diagnostic criteria are discussed in Chapter 1 using the International Classification of Headache Disorders. In brief, a cluster headache is characterized by severe unilateral pain, lasting from 15 to 180 minutes, and is associated with ptosis, miosis, ipsilateral lacrimation, and nasal congestion. Attacks of cluster can occur from one to eight times a day over a period of weeks or months. Migraine presents as a recurrent, pulsating, unilateral, functionally disabling pain lasting from 4 to 72 hours, associated with nausea and photophobia. A tension-type headache is characterized by a bilateral ache or pressure-like pain of mild to moderate intensity. Migraine is not as prevalent as tension-type headache but it is the most common cause of a functionally disabling headache. Various diagnostic aides are available for use in the primary setting. The POUNDing mnemonic and ID Migraine (Table 2.2) have good positive predictive value [10, 11]. The rare and more esoteric headaches can usually be diagnosed by a careful description of the patient's symptoms.

Therapy

A wide variety of medications and other treatments are available for managing primary headache disorders. An evidence-based treatment plan incorporates an analysis of the patient's needs. One must understand how the headaches

Table 2.2. The POUNDing mnemonic and ID Migraine

POUNDing mnemonic
- **P**ulsating
- Duration of 4–72 h**O**urs
- **U**nilateral
- **N**ausea
- **D**isabling

If 4 of the 5 criteria are met, the positive likelihood ratio for diagnosing migraine is 24.

ID Migraine

Do you have headaches that limit your ability to work, study, or enjoy life?

Do you want to talk to your health care professional about your headaches?

Please answer these questions and give your answers to your health care professional.

During the last 3 months, did you have the following with your headaches:

1. You felt nauseated or sick to your stomach
   ( ) Yes   ( ) No
2. Light bothered you (a lot more than when you don't have headaches)
   ( ) Yes   ( ) No
3. Your headaches limited your ability to work, study, or do what you needed to do for at least one day
   ( ) Yes   ( ) No

The ID Migraine can diagnose migraine with a sensitivity of 81% and a specificity of 75%.

affect the patient's life; does the patient require acute treatment once every few months, or is the headache a constant daily and unremitting presence in the patient's life? Is it the nausea or the photophobia rather than the headache itself that most annoys the patient?

★ TIPS AND TRICKS

For acute medication, it is best to start with the higher dose of the most potent medication. For prophylaxis, it is best to start low and go slow, gradually increasing the dose every 1, 2, or 3 months until maximum efficacy is attained.

Using a patient's diary and the MIDAS score, a summation of the patient's headaches and related disability over the previous 3 months can be seen. Medications can be delivered in a variety of formats including pills, injections, nasal sprays, and suppositories. The patient's preference and the absence or presence of nausea can be used to determine the optimal route of therapy. For some patients, complementary and alternative medicines may have appeal. For most others, biofeedback and cognitive therapy are more appropriate. Injections and cognitive therapy may be more effective than pills.

Different patients may respond differently to the same medication. Fortunately, there are multiple classes of acute and chronic medication, any of which may turn out to be the appropriate therapy for the individual patient. Patients need to be encouraged to "hang in there for the long haul." The most common failing of prophylactic medication is not attaining a high enough dosage over a sufficient period of time. For some patients, eliminating triggers, defeating a reliance on daily analgesics, and identifying good habits may have near-magical results. Patients will respond best by being active participants in their treatment plan—completing headache diaries, practicing biofeedback, and choosing the therapeutic mode that most appeals to them. Those patients who want the healthcare provider to make all the decisions (i.e., "Just give me a prescription") will not do well.

Educating the patient

Talking to the patient about their specific diagnosis and discussing general treatment options is what most patients look forward to. Headache sufferers often fear that their headaches are a result of a brain tumor or aneurysm. For some patients, reassurance is most important; it should alleviate unfounded concern once secondary disorders have been excluded. The healthcare practitioner may ask an open-ended question to solicit the patient's opinion: "So, what do you think about your headaches?" The patient's answer may serve as a starting point for a discussion of headache diagnosis and treatment. The question will also help frame the patient's expectations and understanding of the healthcare provider's role. Does the patient expect the doctor to solve the patient's headaches, or does the patient understand that she or he is a partner with the doctor in headache management?

Many patients are more interested in having a discussion on the cause of pain than in pain relief per se. Briefly discuss the mechanics of migraine or cluster headache, or admit medical science's ignorance of the etiology of other primary headaches. Patients appreciate learning the rationale for the therapy. Discuss the therapeutic plan, involving pharmacologic agents, injections, and cognitive-behavioral therapies. It is useful to discuss any information or misinformation that the patient has acquired during his or her own research. It is wise to correct misconceptions found on the Internet or acquired from friends.

Note that many of the "alternative treatments" and expensive "cures" seen on the Internet are ineffective or evoke a favorable response by their placebo effect. Emphasize the patient's obligation to make changes, if necessary, in their lifestyle. Compliance with pharmacologic therapy is a major responsibility. Medication may be required for more than pain control. For example, the nausea and vomiting of migraine may be more disabling than the pain.

> ★ TIPS AND TRICKS
>
> In developing a treatment plan, one must take into consideration other medical problems and their therapies, comorbid conditions, and past use (likes and dislikes) of medications.

Discuss potential side effects of the medication. Often the adverse effects are slight and of short duration and do not warrant discontinuation of medication. In any case, the medication should not be discontinued without a discussion with the doctor.

> ★ TIPS AND TRICKS
>
> Because primary headaches cannot be cured, realistic expectations should be discussed, and reasonable goals should be set. The value of acute medication should be evaluated after at least three trials before changing to another agent. With regard to prophylactic medications, we hope to reduce headache frequency by 50% or more. It often takes months to reach that goal by gradually increasing the dose of the preventive medication.

A cure for headache is not realistic, but the ability to abort or ameliorate the acute attack, decrease headache frequency, and improve quality of life are usual attainable goals.

Follow-up

Follow-up care is essential for chronic illnesses. Re-evaluations are necessary at appropriate times depending upon the patient's headache frequency. At the time of revisits, one must determine whether the current therapy has to be adjusted, a different therapy needs to be initiated, or the diagnosis requires reassessment.

Headache diaries or calendars require patients' positive participation and allow doctors a bird's-eye view of headache frequency and intensity, potential headache triggers, and assessment of therapeutic benefits (or not). Patients can be informed that medications are usually not a life-long burden. Once the frequency of headache has decreased to a reasonable level, prophylactic medication may be tapered off without exacerbation of the headache.

✋ CAUTION!

If treatment is suboptimal, physicians should consider other possible causes of failure (i.e., the diagnosis is incomplete or incorrect, important exacerbating factors have been missed, pharmacotherapy has been inadequate, nonpharmacologic treatment has been inadequate, or the patient has unrealistic expectations).

Reconsider the diagnosis if treatment has failed. The headache phenotype may evolve, or a more precise description may become available. Comorbid conditions such as medication overuse or intercurrent infection may become apparent. Healthcare providers need to determine whether the patient is taking the medication as prescribed. There may be barriers to healthcare access. For example, medications may be too expensive for the patient to afford. Cost may also make the patient reluctant to use acute medication at its most effective early stage before the headaches become unbearable. Conversely, has the patient been taking over-the-counter pills, often considered not to be "real medicine?" Patients may overly rely on pills and not focus on identifying and eliminating the potential triggers; patients and physicians should search for occult exacerbating factors. Pharmacotherapy may have been too little (dosage) or for too short a trial. Non-pharmacologic therapy or injection therapies may not have been adequately implemented. Even if a long course of therapy has not reached favorable goals, persistent trials of therapy and interaction are warranted. Even if the patient's headaches appear to be intractable, it is important for the physician to project a positive attitude as this assures the patient that someone is interested in them and will continue to try to improve their life.

Conclusion

Headaches are a common condition, always annoying, sometimes functionally disabling, and occasionally life-threatening. There are many causes of headache. By utilizing a thorough history, a focused examination, and a knowledge of diagnostic criteria, the precise headache type can usually be identified. With the patient as a partner, the healthcare provider can develop an appropriate treatment plan that addresses both the pain of the headache and how the headache affects the patient's daily life.

References

1. Buse DC, Lipton RB. Facilitating communication with patients for improved migraine outcomes. *Curr Pain Headache Rep* 2008;**12**: 230–6.
2. Dodick D. Pearls: Headache. *Semin Neurol* 2010;**30**:74–81.
3. Silberstein SD, Lipton RB, Dalessio DJ. Overview, diagnosis, and classification. In Silberstein SD, Lipton RB, Dalessio DJ (eds), *Wolff's Headache and Other Head Pain* (7th edn). Oxford: Oxford University Press; 2001: p. 6–26.
4. Edmeads J. Headaches in older people. How are they different in this age-group? *Postgrad Med* 1997;**101**(5):91–100.
5. Schwedt TJ, Matharu MS, Dodick DW. Thunderclap headache. *Lancet Neurol* 2006;**5**(7): 621–31.
6. Giffin NJ, Ruggiero L, Lipton RB. Premonitory symptoms in migraine: an electronic diary study. *Neurology* 2003;**60**(6):935–40.

7. Edmeads J. Emergency management of headache. *Headache* 1988;**28**:675–9.

8. Kroenke K, Spitzer RL, Williams JB. The PHQ-9: validity of a brief depression severity measure. *J Gen Intern Med* 2001;**16**(9): 606–13.

9. Spitzer RL, Kroenke K, Williams JB, Lowe B. A brief measure for assessing generalized anxiety disorder: the GAD-7. *Arch Intern Med* 2006;**166**(10):1092–7.

10. Detsky ME, McDonald DR, Baerlocher MO, Tomlinson GA, McCrory DC, Booth CM. Does this patient with headache have a migraine or need neuroimaging? *JAMA* 2006;**296**(10): 1274–83.

11. Lipton RB, Dodick D, Sadovsky R, et al. A self-administered screener for migraine in primary care: the ID Migraine validation study. *Neurology* 2003;**61**(3):375–82.

Secondary Headache Disorders Encountered in Clinical Practice

Deborah I. Friedman

University of Texas Southwestern, Dallas, TX, USA

Brain tumor

Diagnosis

Approximately 43,800 new cases of benign and malignant brain tumors are diagnosed in the USA each year, including 3410 cases in children and adolescents; the incidence of brain tumors is 14.8 per 100,000 person–years, with half being histologically benign [1]. Headache is the most common presenting symptom, occurring in 35% of patients. It is very unusual for headache to be the sole manifestation of a brain tumor [2, 3]. Other symptoms and signs, such as nausea, vomiting, ataxia, blurred vision, visual field defect, papilledema, personality changes, seizures, endocrinologic abnormalities, and focal neurologic dysfunction coexist with headache in 90% of cases [4]. Early-morning vomiting and gait ataxia are more frequent symptoms in children with high-grade or infratentorial tumors [4].

There is no defining characteristic of brain tumor-associated headache. The headache may be located in the frontal, parietal, or occipital areas, may be unilateral or bilateral, and is most frequently described as dull, resembling tension-type headache [3]. It is usually not a daily headache and is only infrequently continuous. The location of the headache often bears no relationship to the location of the tumor, although infratentorial tumors tend to produce more posterior pain, and supratentorial tumors often produce vertex and frontal pain [2, 3]. The headache tends to occur ipsilateral to the tumor, particularly in the absence of increased intracranial pressure. The "classic" brain tumor headache, with early-morning awakening, nausea, and vomiting, occurred in only 17% of patients in one large series [5].

★ **TIPS AND TRICKS**

The following features of headache raise the possibility of a brain tumor:

- A change in a pre-existing headache pattern
- The development of persistent headaches in a patient with no personal or family history of migraine
- A rapid onset of headache after strenuous exercise
- Headaches not resembling primary headache disorders
- A progressive escalation in the intensity or duration of the headache without medication overuse

Headache, First Edition. Edited by Matthew S. Robbins, Brian M. Grosberg, and Richard B. Lipton.
© 2013 John Wiley & Sons, Ltd. Published 2013 by John Wiley & Sons, Ltd.

The likelihood of diagnosing a brain tumor in a patient with a typical history of migraine and a normal neurologic examination is so small that neuroimaging is not recommended in such patients [6]. The trigeminal autonomic cephalalgias (cluster headache, paroxysmal hemicrania, and short-lasting neuralgiform headache attacks with conjunctival injection and tearing) differ from migraine in this respect [7]. These headache types may be associated with vascular abnormalities, such as carotid and vertebral artery dissection, intracranial aneurysm, intracranial and arterial thrombosis, demyelinating disease, trigeminal nerve tumors, and pituitary gland tumors [8]. The cranial autonomic symptoms tend to be ipsilateral to the tumor in patients with a pituitary adenoma, whose headaches often resemble those of chronic migraine [7].

Pathophysiology

The pain of a brain tumor is in most cases ascribed to its mass effect. Traction of intra- and extracranial pain-sensitive structures may be produced by a tumor mass, edema, or hemorrhage. The brain parenchyma is insensitive to pain because it lacks free nerve endings. Pain-sensitive structures include the venous sinuses, arteries, dura, skin, subcutaneous and muscle tissue, and cranial periosteum [2]. Acute headaches may arise in the setting of increased intracranial pressure during abnormal pressure ("plateau") waves characterized by an increase in blood volume and vasodilatation, decreased cerebral perfusion pressure, and a sharp rise in intracranial pressure. The classic "early-morning" brain tumor headache results from increased brain edema in the morning after lying supine, coupled with increased vasodilation from a high pCO_2 occurring during sleep. Rapidly expanding tumors tend to produce pain more frequently than slow-growing tumors because the brain cannot rapidly adapt to the increased pressure.

Pituitary region tumors may produce pain by stretching of the dura or invasion of pain-producing structures around the cavernous sinus. However, cases of pituitary gland microadenomas associated with headaches are not rare. Elevated prolactin levels are associated with headaches even in the absence of a mass effect, and somatostatin analogs may be effective in aborting the headache in patients with acrome-galy [7, 9]. Similarly, patients with microadenomas and migraine who developed severe headaches and increased prolactin levels following a thyrotropin-releasing hormone test frequently showed improvement with dopamine agonist treatment [10].

Headaches may also complicate the treatment of brain tumors. Surgical resection, chemotherapy, and radiation therapy are often employed. Radiotherapy may produce white matter edema and headaches, and headaches are a side effect of many chemotherapeutic agents. Post-craniotomy pain is reported in up to 60% of patients and is more common with a suboccipital or subtemporal surgical approach. The pain resolves in most patients within a few months of surgery.

Management

Headaches associated with edematous brain tumors often improve rapidly after the initiation of corticosteroid treatment. Surgical resection and procedures that normalize intracranial pressure often cure the headache. Patients with residual pain may be treated with headache preventives and analgesics. The long-term prognosis varies with the type of tumor.

Idiopathic intracranial hypertension

Diagnosis

The typical patient with idiopathic intracranial hypertension (IIH) is an overweight female of childbearing age [11]. When the syndrome arises from a secondary cause, it is termed "pseudotumor cerebri"; children, males, and normal-weight individuals may be affected in this scenario.

The most common symptom is headache, although the character of the headache is variable. It is often described as a "pressure" or "explosive" headache located frontally, retro-orbitally, or globally, but some patients experience more neck, back, and shoulder pain than headache. The headache may be constant or intermittent, and it is sometimes hemicranial, simulating migraine. There may be associated photophobia, phonophobia, nausea, and vomiting. IIH is in the differential diagnosis of new daily persistent headache, and should be suspected in patients with unexplained worsening of a pre-existing headache disorder. Episodes of transient obscurations of vision are common, leading to partial or

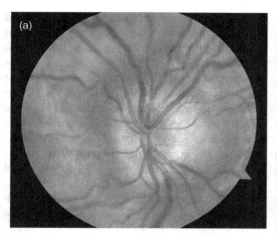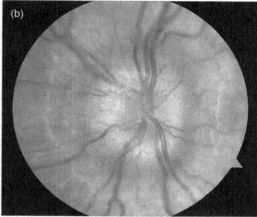

Figure 3.1. Papilledema in a patient with IIH in the right (a) and left (b) eye.

complete visual loss lasting less than a minute that are often provoked by a postural change. Many patients experience pulsatile tinnitus in one or both ears. Ataxia, torticollis, and facial paresis occur more frequently in children. There may be a bulging fontanel in young children prior to closure of the cranial sutures. Other symptoms include blurred vision, diplopia, radicular pain, and peripheral edema.

Papilledema is the hallmark of IIH (Figure 3.1). The severity of optic disc edema varies, and it may be asymmetric or unilateral. Visual field defects commonly occur, such as enlargement of the physiologic blind spot (reflecting optic disc swelling), inferonasal loss, generalized constriction, and central scotomas. Diplopia is produced by a unilateral or bilateral abducens palsy.

★ TIPS AND TRICKS

Direct ophthalmoscopy is one of the most difficult aspects of the physical examination and requires practice to achieve a comfort level with the technique. Helpful strategies for using the direct ophthalmoscope include the following:

- Darken the room lights and instruct the patient to focus straight ahead in the distance.
- Perform ophthalmoscopy while standing in order to change the viewing angle easily.
- View with the right eye and hold the ophthalmoscope in the right hand to examine the patient's right eye, and vice versa.
- Hold the ophthalmoscope with the index finger on the flywheel and the middle finger at the top of the base.
- Find the red reflex and follow it in toward the pupil. *Get VERY close—your middle finger should be touching the patient's cheek.* (Failure to get close to the patient is the most frequent cause of inability to see the fundus.)
- Change the angle of the ophthalmoscope (and your body) to view the optic nerve and surrounding retina. The optic nerve will take up most of the field of view (the view will not look like the panoramic illustrations in the textbooks).
- Don't be afraid to use dilating drops (see the Tips and Tricks box in the section on "Angle-closure glaucoma").
- Ask a colleague from ophthalmology for help if you do not get a good view or if there is any question about subtle findings.

Neuroimaging fails to show a mass lesion, and the ventricular size is normal for age. Subtle findings reflecting increased cerebrospinal fluid (CSF) pressure on MRI include a Chiari malformation, an empty sella, distention of the subarachnoid space within the optic nerve sheaths, flattening of the posterior sclera, and protrusion of the optic papilla into the vitreous humor [12]. A brain CT scan will be normal. Lumbar puncture (LP) in children and adults discloses an opening pressure ≥250 mm of CSF in most cases. The headache may improve following LP, but failure to improve after removing CSF does not exclude the diagnosis. An ophthalmologic examination, including perimetry, is needed to document and follow visual function.

✋ CAUTION!

A brain CT scan is inadequate to exclude increased intracranial pressure. The opening pressure of the LP, measured with the patient in the lateral decubitus position with the legs relaxed, is required for the diagnosis. While it is tempting to sedate the patient for the LP, the associated hypoventilation and hypercapnea increase CSF pressure and may lead to an erroneous diagnosis, particularly in patients without papilledema.

Subtypes

The two major subtypes are IIH and intracranial hypertension without ventriculomegaly from a secondary cause. Secondary causes include exogenous agents, obstruction to cerebral venous outflow, endocrinologic disorders, and other medical disorders.

Pathophysiology

The pathophysiology of IIH is unknown. Several models have been proposed to explain the increase in intracranial pressure and lack of ventriculomegaly or cerebral edema that characterize the disorder. Walter Dandy, whose 1937 case series described the typical diagnostic features of the disorder, was the first to comment on the contribution of vasomotor control to the development of IIH [13]. CSF is continuously produced by the choroid plexus, and is reabsorbed via both the arachnoid villi (into the cerebral veins) and the olfactory lymphatics. While there is general agreement that the defect is on the absorption side of the equation (i.e., there is not an overproduction of CSF), the lack of ventricular dilation is not explained by dysfunction of the arachnoid villi. Cerebral venous hypertension is a key occurrence in IIH, although it is not clear whether it is the initiating factor or a consequence of high intracranial pressure. Cerebral venous pressure must be higher than CSF pressure in order to maintain the directionality of CSF absorption. However, numerous studies have shown that venous sinus stenosis commonly reverses after the volume of CSF is reduced, suggesting that radiographic stenosis is the consequence, rather than the cause, of IIH. Obesity is the best established risk factor for IIH, but no distinctive hormonal or genetic fingerprint has yet been discovered. There are several reports of familial cases; obesity and a shared environment may be confounding factors.

Comorbidities

IIH is associated with obesity and recent weight gain [14]. The syndrome of intracranial hypertension without ventriculomegaly may be caused by a number of exogenous agents. Many case reports exist, but the best established associations are with tetracycline, minocycline, doxycycline, vitamin A and isotretinoin, human growth hormone, corticosteroid withdrawal, nalidixic acid, chlordecone, and lithium. Any condition impeding venous outflow from the brain, such as cerebral or jugular venous thrombosis, produces a similar clinical condition. Pseudotumor cerebri may be comorbid with polycystic ovarian syndrome, obstructive sleep apnea, iron deficiency anemia, renal failure, antiphospholipid antibody syndrome, orthostatic edema, and Turner syndrome. There is no increased risk of developing IIH during pregnancy, and pregnancy is not contraindicated in women with known IIH [15].

Progression and prognosis

The course of IIH is quite variable. Some patients present with asymptomatic optic nerve edema that resolves spontaneously. Symptomatic relief and recovery may occur after the diagnostic LP, while other patients may have persistent symptoms and intracranial hypertension for years. Many patients will experience headaches after their papilledema has resolved and the disease appears otherwise to be in remission [16]. Permanent visual field loss, as assessed by standard perimetric testing, occurs in up to 50% of affected patients [17]. Profound visual loss occurs in approximately 5% of patients, with legal or complete blindness. Factors associated with a poor visual prognosis include systemic anemia, renal failure, high grade of papilledema, visual loss at presentation, and onset during the teenage years.

There are few long-term natural history data, but some patients seem to have a very prolonged course of illness [18]. Patients frequently continue to experience headaches following other successful treatment of IIH, and the condition may relapse years later with weight gain [16].

Management

There are no randomized, controlled clinical trials to provide evidence-based treatment strategies for IIH. The goal of treatment is to preserve vision, which generally requires a team approach among neurologists, ophthalmologists, neurosurgeons, and primary care physicians. The neurologist (or neuro-ophthalmologist, if available) generally takes the lead in patient management, incorporating data regarding visual status (including perimetry, acuity and optic nerve appearance) from the ophthalmologist. Thus, good communication among providers is essential. Acute treatment options include therapeutic LP, CSF diversion procedures, optic nerve sheath fenestration (ONSF), carbonic anhydrase inhibitors, and other diuretics. Chronic management incorporates weight loss and dietary sodium restriction. Venous sinus stenting has been recently employed, with variable results. The use of corticosteroids is controversial, but they may be helpful acutely to stabilize or improve vision while arranging surgical intervention. However, the side effects of corticosteroids are counterproductive in the long term, and they are not indicated for maintenance therapy. Preventive medications for headache management, such as topiramate and tricyclic antidepressants, are often needed.

LP offers the advantage of immediately lowering the CSF pressure. Its effectiveness is often short-lived, as new CSF is produced continuously. The procedure may be technically difficult with obese patients, necessitating the use of fluoroscopic guidance, which adds the risk of radiation exposure. Although generally disliked by both patients and practitioners, repeated LPs may be appropriate when there is a need to acutely lower the CSF pressure, and during pregnancy (avoiding fluoroscopy) when therapeutic options are limited. ONSF frequently halts or reverses visual loss both ipsilateral and contralateral to the surgical site [19]. Approximately 50% of patients also benefit from improved headaches following ONSF, although the procedure is only recommended if papilledema and visual loss are present. Its advantage is the lack of implanted hardware, although there is a small risk of visual worsening from the procedure. Shunting (ventriculoperitoneal and lumboperitoneal) offers the benefit of "treating the disease" by lowering CSF pressure, but incorporates hardware that frequently fails [20].

Acetazolamide is the mainstay of medical treatment, and a clinical trial (the Idiopathic Intracranial Hypertension Treatment Trial) is currently underway to evaluate the effectiveness of acetazolamide and a supervised weight loss program compared to placebo and dietary management. Other diuretics that inhibit CSF secretion, such as methazolamide and furosemide, are also used. Several prospective case series indicate that a loss of approximately 6% of body weight in obese patients is associated with a reduction in papilledema and improved vision [21]. Bariatric surgery may be considered in morbidly obese patients, and confers the potential advantage of reducing cardiovascular risk factors and promoting other long-term general health benefits.

IIH in children is managed similarly to IIH in adults. A secondary cause is often identified in young children, such as mastoiditis or a medication. Although boys and girls are equally affected prior to puberty, the disease is very similar to the presentation in adults after age 12 years.

IIH during pregnancy may be treated with serial LPs or surgery if needed. Acetazolamide has been used without untoward sequelae after the first trimester [22].

The psychosocial aspects of IIH have not been well studied. Patients with IIH are more likely to be depressed or anxious than their obese peers without IIH [23]. As the condition commonly occurs in obese women, patients are frequently blamed for their disease and find it difficult to cope in the absence of outward signs of disability. It is not uncommon for patients to be misdiagnosed by numerous providers before ophthalmoscopy is finally performed. Significant visual loss is uncommon but life-altering.

> ★ TIPS AND TRICKS
>
> Intracranial hypertension from any cause is a diagnostic consideration in all patients being evaluated for headache. Ophthalmoscopy should be routinely performed in the examination of such patients, particularly those with new or worsening headaches. Other key features of IIH such as female gender, obesity, pulsatile tinnitus, and transient obscurations of vision raise the suspicion for IIH. Tetracycline antibiotics and systemic retinoids for the treatment of acne in teenagers and young adults are common secondary causes.

Cerebral venous sinus thrombosis

Diagnosis

Cerebral venous sinus thrombosis (CVST) accounts for only 1% of all strokes, affecting primarily young adults and children [24]. The signs and symptoms are varied and often subtle or nonspecific [25]. The most common presenting symptom is headache (70%–90% of cases), often described as "the worst headache of my life." One-third to three-quarters of patients have focal neurologic deficits, impaired level of consciousness, or papilledema. Seizures are the initial manifestation in 30%–50% of cases. The symptoms usually evolve over days to weeks, but CVST is in the differential diagnosis of a thunderclap headache. Superior sagittal sinus thrombosis may produce bilateral or alternating deficits with or without seizures. Painful ophthalmoplegia with proptosis and conjunctival chemosis characterizes cavernous sinus thrombosis.

The diagnosis requires a high index of suspicion, as CVST may mimic a tumor, IIH, brain abscess, encephalitis, or arterial stroke [26]. A CT scan is often employed as the first diagnostic test in the emergency department. Noncontrast CT is normal in up to 50% of cases, but may reveal generalized edema or areas of hemorrhagic infarction, visualization of a hyperdense thrombosed cortical vein [24]. The classic "empty delta" sign with contrast enhancement is only present in 10%–20% of cases. This finding consists of a low-attenuating thrombus surrounded by a high-intensity triangle of contrast enhancement within the superior sagittal sinus. Magnetic resonance venography and CT venography are the imaging tests of choice. Both tests show the thrombosis and offer the advantage of viewing changes in the brain parenchyma such as ischemia, hemorrhage, and cerebral edema. Catheter angiography is sometimes necessary to confirm the diagnosis. LP is performed in the appropriate clinical context to exclude meningitis or subarachnoid hemorrhage (SAH), as well as in patients who have a clinical picture of pseudotumor cerebri. Tests for underlying thrombophilia include factor V Leiden mutation, resistance to activated protein C, proteins C and S, anti-thrombin III, plasminogen, fibrinogen and anticardiolipin antibodies, and hyperhomocysteinemia [27]. Investigations for malignancy and connective tissue disease may be warranted in some circumstances.

Pathophysiology

The superior sagittal sinus and lateral sinuses are most frequently affected. More than one sinus is involved in 30%–40% of cases, sometimes in concert with cerebral or cerebellar vein thrombosis [25]. Ongoing thrombosis and thrombolysis contribute to the slow growth of the thrombus and gradual onset of symptoms, with the development of collateral venous drainage vessels in most cases. Hemorrhagic infarction occurs in 10%–15% of cases.

There are two proposed theories regarding the pathogenesis of CVST [28]. One theory postulates that venous thrombosis results in intracranial hypertension. The increased venous pressure reduces capillary perfusion pressure and blood volume. Although collateral pathways are recruited, the high intracranial pressure disrupts the blood–brain barrier, leading to vasogenic edema. Decreased cerebral perfusion pressure and cerebral blood flow disrupt the intracellular water content, producing cytotoxic edema. Both vasogenic and cytotoxic edema are associated with CVST.

The second theory accounts for thrombosis of the major venous sinuses, such as the superior sagittal sinus. The high pressure in the thrombosed sinus impedes CSF absorption, causing intracranial hypertension.

Comorbidities

Once a common cause, infections (mastoiditis, meningitis, ear infections, tonsillitis, or sinusitis) are identified as a predisposing factor in about 8% of cases of CVST. The cavernous sinus is frequently affected by infections. Connective tissue disorders, anemia, granulomatous and inflammatory bowel disease, sarcoidosis, and malignancies are common. CVST occurs more frequently in the puerperium than during pregnancy. Oral contraceptives and coagulation disorders are frequent associations in women; use of oral contraceptive increases the risk of CVST by over 10-fold. Protein C, protein S, and antithrombin III deficiency, factor V Leiden, and prothrombin G20210A gene mutations account for a large percentage of children and 10%–15% of adults with CVST. More than one risk factor may be implicated in an individual patient.

Progression and prognosis

The mortality rate from CVST has declined from up to 50% to less than 15%, largely as a consequence of modern imaging [28]. Poor prognosis is associated with age over 37 years, male sex, initial presentation with coma, seizures, altered mental status, or neurologic deficits, associated deep cerebral venous thrombosis, intracranial hemorrhage, posterior fossa lesions, cancer, and infection. Patients with isolated intracranial hypertension have the best prognosis. The most common cause of death is transtentorial herniation in the presence of a large cerebral hemorrhage.

> **⚡ CAUTION!**
>
> Patients with CVST and focal deficits may deteriorate rapidly! Any deterioration in their level of consciousness requires urgent attention.

Management

Current therapies include the use of anticoagulants, thrombolysis, control of seizures, and control of intracranial pressure. The presence of intracranial hemorrhages has provoked considerable debate regarding the use of anticoagulation, although anticoagulants are effective in treating the thrombosis. Adequately powered randomized controlled trials have not been performed due to the large sample size required (approximately 300 patients). One small randomized trial of intravenous heparin showed improved recovery with no fatality in the heparin group compared to the placebo group, including those with pre-treatment hemorrhage, and one death from pulmonary embolism in the placebo group [29]. A second trial of 60 patients performed with low molecular weight heparin rather than unfractionated heparin also showed a trend toward improved outcomes in the treatment group [30]. Meta-analyses by the Cochrane Collaboration, and the European Federation of Neurological Societies concluded that anticoagulation was safe and was associated with a nonsignificant, yet potentially important, improvement in outcome [31].

Systemic and local thrombolysis have been employed in clinical practice. Most patients treated with recombinant tissue plasminogen activator (rtTPA) achieve complete recanalization of the thrombosed sinus, albeit with an increased risk of hemorrhage [30, 31]. Thrombolysis may be considered in patients who have a poor prognosis (i.e., patients who are comatose or who have hemorrhagic infarctions). Mechanical thrombectomy (balloon angioplasty, stenting, clot maceration, or rheolytic thrombectomy) is an alternative to thrombolysis and may be a useful adjunctive therapy in some patients. Surgical decompression is limited to patients with refractory increased intracranial pressure. Other therapeutic measures include steroids, antiepileptics, carbonic anhydrase inhibitors, diuretics (except osmotic diuretics), shunting procedures, and hyperventilation.

Giant cell arteritis

Diagnosis

Giant cell arteritis (GCA) is a systemic vasculitis with many manifestations. It is a disorder that one never wants to miss, but the diagnosis may be elusive because of the variability of presentations. The symptoms of GCA may lead patients to see a variety of providers, including internists, rheumatologists, dentists, neurologists, dermatologists, and ophthalmologists. GCA must always be considered in the differential diagnosis of headaches developing in individuals over the age of 50 years, only rarely occurring in younger persons. The prevalence of GCA ranges from 20/100,000 in the sixth decade to 1100/100,000 in the ninth decade of life [32]. It is more common among white individuals than other racial or ethnic populations. Thus, the greatest risk factor is age, the most common presenting symptom is headache, and the most significant consequence is blindness.

Headaches are the most common symptom, occurring in 65%–75% of patients. The headache of GCA is nonspecific. It may be unilateral or bilateral, aching or throbbing, and is often severe enough to interfere with sleep. The headache features may suggest new daily persistent headache, migraine without aura, tension-type headache, or hemicrania continua. Visual symptoms include amaurosis fugax, visual loss, diplopia, and eye pain, with findings of ocular ischemic lesions such as anterior ischemic optic neuropathy, central retinal artery occlusion, cilioretinal artery occlusion, ocular ischemic syndrome, and posterior ischemic optic neuropathy. Approximately one-third of patients have "occult" GCA, experiencing only the visual complications with no systemic symptoms [33].

The presence of jaw claudication is highly specific for diagnosing GCA. Other symptoms include malaise, fever, weight loss, scalp tenderness, symptoms of polymyalgia rheumatica (PMR), arthralgias, depression, necrotic lesions of the skin or tongue, mental status changes, transient ischemic attacks, peripheral neuropathies, stroke, and cardiac manifestations [34].

Laboratory evaluation includes a Westergren erythrocyte sedimentation rate (ESR), complete blood count with platelet count, C-reactive protein, and fibrinogen level. The diagnosis may be difficult to prove, as no test is 100% sensitive. A markedly elevated ESR, an elevated C-reactive protein level, anemia of chronic disease, thrombocytosis, and elevated fibrinogen levels support the diagnosis. However, patients with GCA may have a normal ESR, particular if they are not anemic. Temporal artery biopsy, the "gold standard" for diagnosis, is abnormal approximately 95% of the time. Patients with initial negative biopsies who were later diagnosed with GCA accounted for 19% of all negative biopsies in one series; older age, headache, and thrombocytosis were more common in that group [35]. As patients with GCA will be treated with corticosteroids for a prolonged period of time, confirmation of the diagnosis with a biopsy is always recommended. If the suspicion of GCA remains high in the setting of a negative biopsy, imaging of the aorta and the proximal arterial tree may be fruitful [34]. The branches of the aortic arch are involved in 10%–15% of cases, and thoracic aortic aneurysm is 17 times as likely in patients with GCA as in those without the disease [36].

Pathophysiology

GCA is an inflammatory vasculopathy of the medium and large arteries. Although frequently termed "temporal arteritis," it is a systemic disease. The inflammation is most pronounced in the intima and internal elastic lamina. Noncontiguous involvement produces "skip lesions" that must be accounted for in the acquisition of the surgical specimen and the pathologic examination [32]. The pathologic hallmark, the multinucleated giant cell, is caused by T cells and macrophages (Figure 3.2). Giant cells are not universally present, nor are they required for the diagnosis. Other pathologic findings include disruption of the elastic lamina and inflammatory cells in the arterial wall, particularly the media. Pro-inflammatory cytokines are likely involved in the generation of the systemic symptoms of the disease, and elevated levels of interleukin-6 are often found in active GCA. A viral cause has never been confirmed. Studies of GCA and PMR show a significant association with human leukocyte antigen (HLA)-DR4 [32]. A sequence polymorphism within the second hypervariable region of the HLA-DRB1 gene was identified in both GCA and PMR.

Comorbidities

Symptoms of PMR are present in about 40% of patients with GCA, and there is a pathologic and clinical continuum between PMR and GCA. The symptoms of PMR include hip and shoulder pain, muscle aches, neck pain and stiffness, fever, malaise, weight loss, fever, and fatigue. The ESR

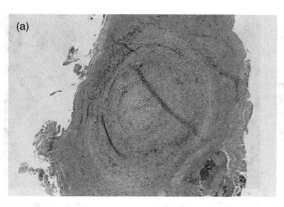
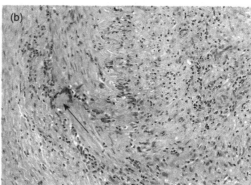

Figure 3.2. (a) Low-power magnification of a temporal artery biopsy specimen showing a marked inflammatory response with obliteration of the arterial lumen. (b) Multinucleated giant cell (arrow). (Photographs courtesy of M. Tariq Bhatti, MD.)

is usually elevated, and patients with PMR are often anemic.

Progression and prognosis

The most feared complication of GCA is blindness. Visual loss is usually attributed to ischemic optic neuropathy which produces sudden, generally severe, visual impairment. There may be simultaneous involvement of both eyes, or the disease may affect the two eyes in rapid succession. The loss of vision in GCA is permanent, and there is little or no improvement in most patients, even with treatment. Visual loss occurs in about 20% of patients with GCA and may be the sole presenting symptom.

Most patients note a dramatic improvement in their systemic symptoms within days of starting corticosteroids. Aside from visual loss, the prognosis of treated disease is generally favorable, although the side effects of corticosteroids may be quite problematic in the affected age group. Osteopenia, fracture, ulcer, skin bruising, and weight gain are common. Relapses may occur in up to 50% of patients, but are less likely when the prednisone is tapered, incorporating a slow taper to a maintenance dose of at least 7.5 mg daily (a higher dose may be needed in patients with visual loss).

Management

High-dose corticosteroid treatment (intravenous methylprednisolone or oral prednisone 100 mg daily) must be initiated immediately, especially if the patient has amaurosis fugax or evidence of visual loss. The eyes are often involved sequentially, and prompt treatment usually prevents involvement of the second eye. The biopsy should be performed within a week to increase the likelihood of finding the typical pathologic changes of GCA. The systemic features generally respond quickly to prednisone treatment, although vision loss may not improve. Treatment with prednisone is continued for at least a year, with close monitoring of laboratory parameters and clinical symptoms. Supplementation with vitamin D, calcium, and bisphosphonates is prudent. Methotrexate and other immunosuppressant medications have been used as adjunctive therapy, but prednisone remains the most effective primary treatment of GCA.

★ TIPS AND TRICKS

When GCA is suspected, one should "treat now and ask questions later." Intravenous corticosteroid treatment is recommended for patients with visual loss to try and prevent second eye involvement, although progression may occur despite this measure. *Always perform a biopsy before committing the patient to long-term corticosteroid treatment.* The biopsy should be performed within a week, and the steroids may be discontinued if there is no evidence to support the diagnosis; bilateral biopsies do not significantly increase the diagnostic yield.

Rehabilitation

Bilateral optic neuropathy from GCA has devastating consequences for patients and their caregivers. Patients may be rendered legally or completely blind at a time in their life when they are least able to cope with it physically, socially, or psychologically. Assistance from local agencies for the blind and visually handicapped is invaluable for such patients.

Cervical artery dissections

Diagnosis

Dissections of the cervical arteries are one of the most frequent causes of stroke in young adults, accounting for 8%–25% of strokes in this age group [37].

Internal carotid artery dissection is suspected in patients with a new onset of unilateral head or neck pain and an ipsilateral Horner syndrome until proven otherwise. The spectrum of carotid dissection ranges from transient monocular visual loss to stroke and death, necessitating prompt diagnosis and treatment. Neuro-ophthalmic symptoms and signs are common, most frequently amaurosis fugax, a painful Horner syndrome, or visual scintillations [38]. Permanent visual loss from ischemic optic neuropathy and ocular motor nerve palsies are infrequent. Other neurologic manifestations include contralateral hemiparesis, pulsatile tinnitus, dysguesia, dysphagia, palatal weakness, hoarseness, and hemilingual paralysis [37, 39, 40]. Headache is present in the majority of cases [37]. The headache or neck pain may precede the ischemic symptoms by days or weeks. The pain is characteristically over the ipsilateral carotid artery, in the jaw or upper face.

Vertebral artery dissection typically presents with pain in the posterior neck or head followed by posterior circulation ischemia. The headache is most commonly occipital, which may be unilateral or bilateral, throbbing, steady, or sharp. The headache is often mistaken for a migraine, particularly in patients with a history of migraine headaches [41]. Ischemic symptoms generally appear within 15 hours of the headache, although there may be an interval of 2 weeks between the development of neck pain and the neurologic symptoms. The ischemic manifestations affect the lateral medulla, thalamus, and cerebral or cer-

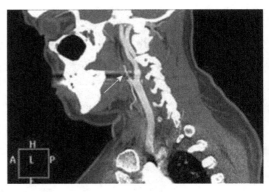

Figure 3.3. Computed tomography angiography demonstrates a dissection of the internal carotid artery with a "string sign" (arrow). (Photograph courtesy of Per-Lennart Westesson, MD, DDS, PhD.)

ebellar peduncles. Isolated cervical spinal cord ischemia and transient ischemic attacks are rare.

The diagnosis is made using MRI, which reveals an abnormal intravascular signal from stagnant blood flow on axial images. Ultrasound, magnetic resonance angiography (MRA), CT angiography (CTA; Figure 3.3) and conventional angiography may be employed. Although the sensitivity for ultrasound detection for cervical artery dissection is high, intramural hematomas may be missed using this modality [42].

> **⚠ CAUTION!**
>
> The presentation of a unilateral head/neck ache and an ipsilateral Horner syndrome is a carotid dissection until proven otherwise.

Pathophysiology

Dissections may be traumatic or spontaneous. "Spontaneous" dissections are often associated with physical activity, including seemingly trivial exertion. They generally occur at locations where the arteries are mobile, such as the pharyngeal portion of the internal carotid arteries. The tear in the media produces bleeding within the arterial wall, which dissects longitudinally. Expansion of the arterial blood through the intima may enter the arterial lumen, causing compression of the lumen and thrombus formation. Dissections may also originate from the intimal surface and dissect into the media, creating true and false lumens separated by an intimal flap. Aneurysmal and pseudoaneurysmal dilatation may occur [41].

Comorbidities

Dissection is associated with Ehlers–Danlos syndrome, Marfan syndrome, autosomal dominant polycystic kidney disease, osteogenesis imperfecta type 1, and fibromuscular dysplasia, but an underlying connective tissue disorder is not found in most patients. Approximately 5% of patients with a spontaneous dissection have at least one family member who has had a dissection of the aorta or its main branches, suggesting a genetic predisposition. No specific genetic defect has been identified.

Progression and prognosis

The prognosis is related to the severity of the ischemia. Death occurs in less than 5% of patients. The headache generally resolves but sometimes persists for years following a dissection. Some patients have recanalization of the artery, and pseudoaneurysm formation is not uncommon. The formation of thrombi at the edge of hematoma may produce intracranial emboli. The rate of recurrent dissection in an unaffected artery is about 2% in the first month, and then about 1% yearly.

Management

The treatment is controversial; anticoagulation, antiplatelet therapy, and interventional vascular techniques have been employed in various circumstances. Patients with a Horner syndrome or minimal neurologic deficits several weeks after the acute event are usually treated with daily aspirin. There have been no randomized trials, and the low recurrence rate would require over 1000 patients per treatment arm to support therapeutic guidelines [43].

Cerebrospinal fluid hypovolemia and "low-pressure" headaches

Spontaneous intracranial hypotension

Diagnosis

Orthostatic headache is the most common presentation of a low-pressure headache syndrome.

Spontaneous intracranial hypotension (SIH) is caused by one or more spinal CSF leaks. It affects women more commonly than men, with an estimated annual incidence of 5 per 100,000 [44]. SIH is part of the differential diagnosis of new daily persistent headache. While most patients with SIH experience headaches that worsen in the upright posture and improve or remit when recumbent, others have chronic daily headaches with only vague orthostatic features [45]. The positional headache generally occurs within 15 minutes of commencing the upright posture but may occur hours later in some patients; 15–30 minutes of recumbency generally provides relief. Some patients report exertional headaches, and rare patients describe headaches that paradoxically worsen when supine.

The location of the headache is nonspecific, although most patients describe suboccipital or occipital pain. The pain may be throbbing or non-throbbing in character, and is sometimes described as pulling. Relief of headache pain with the patient in the Trendelenburg position is useful for diagnosing patients with SIH [46]. Associated symptoms include neck stiffness, tinnitus, hypacusia (echoing or like "being under water"), photophobia, imbalance, and lower cranial nerve involvement. Neuro-ophthalmic manifestations may be similar to those of increased intracranial pressure, including diplopia from sixth nerve paresis, transient visual obscurations, blurred vision, visual field defects, photophobia, and nystagmus [47]. SIH is part of the differential diagnosis of stupor and coma, subdural hematoma, parkinsonism, cerebellar hemorrhage, and cognitive decline.

The characteristic imaging findings on cranial MRI are subdural fluid collections, pachymeningeal enhancement, engorgement of venous structures, pituitary hyperemia, and sagging of the brain [44]. The subdural fluid collections are present in approximately 50% of patients and generally cause no mass effect. Subdural hematomas are not uncommon and rarely require surgical evacuation. The pachymeningeal enhancement is diffuse, nodular, and both supratentorial and infratentorial, and spares the leptomeninges. Twenty percent of patients with SIH do not exhibit pachymeningeal enhancement. Brain sagging is characterized by effacement of the perichiasmatic cisterns with bowing of the optic chiasm over the

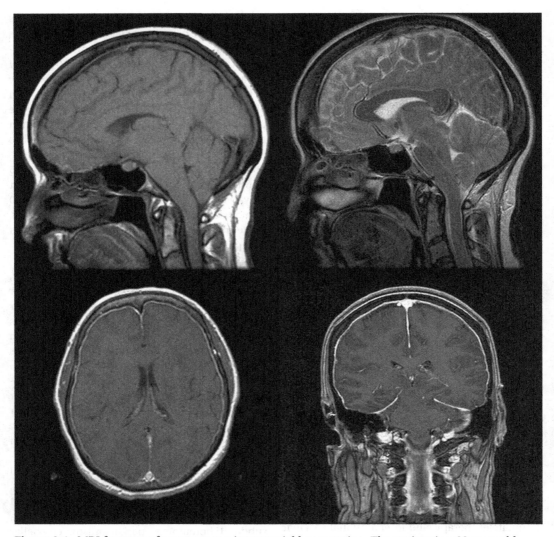

Figure 3.4. MRI features of spontaneous intracranial hypotension. The patient is a 60-year-old woman with postural headaches exacerbated by coughing, sneezing, and straining. There is brain sag with descent of the cerebellar tonsils beyond the foramen magnum and flattening of the anterior pons against the clivus on sagittal images. The axial and coronal views show characteristic pachymeningeal enhancement. (Photograph courtesy of Henry Wang, MD.)

pituitary fossa, flattening of the pons against the clivus, and descent of the cerebellar tonsils (acquired Chiari I malformation) (Figure 3.4).

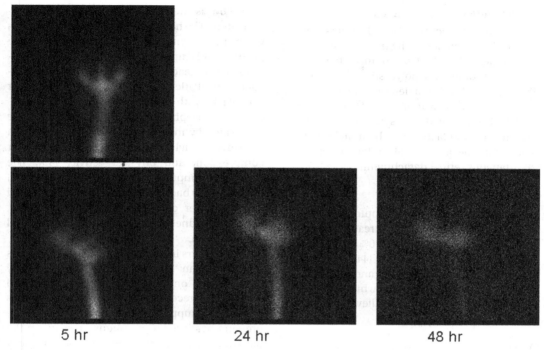

| 5 hr | 24 hr | 48 hr |

Figure 3.5. Radionuclide cisternogram revealing failure of the tracer to reach the cerebral convexity at 48 hours in a patient with spontaneous intracranial hypotension. (Photograph courtesy of Henry Wang, MD.)

Radionuclide cisternography is most useful when the diagnosis is in doubt since its low resolution often fails to show the site of the CSF leak. Typical findings include early accumulation of tracer in the kidneys and bladder with slow ascent along the spinal axis and a paucity over the cerebral convexities [44] (Figure 3.5). LP shows an opening pressure of less than 60 mm CSF in most cases, but the pressure may be unmeasurable, negative, or normal. A lymphocytic pleocytosis, elevated protein content, and xanthochromia are often present.

Localizing the CSF leak is challenging. Conventional spinal MRI shows indirect signs, such as dilated epidural or intradural veins, dural enhancement, meningeal diverticulae, extrathecal CSF collections, and retrospinal C1–C2 fluid collections. CT myelography and heavily T2-weighted magnetic resonance myelography are useful for localizing the CSF leak prior to a targeted epidural blood patch or neurosurgical intervention [48].

Pathophysiology
Spinal fluid leaks may be provoked by trauma or an underlying structural weakness of the spinal meninges. The dural defects allow CSF to leak into the epidural space where the CSF is ultimately resorbed into the epidural venous plexus or paraspinal soft tissues. CSF hypovolemia and an altered distribution of craniospinal elasticity from spinal loss of CSF are postulated in the mechanism underlying SIH. The headache is attributed to downward traction on pain-sensitive structures when the patient is upright. The loss of buoyancy resulting from CSF hypovolemia, and subsequent brain sag, creates tension on the meninges and other pain-sensitive structures such as the arteries and nerves [49]. Altered mental status occurs with sagging of the pons against the clivus. The loss of CSF volume must be compensated for by an increase in intravascular volume in order to maintain homeostasis; the secondary arterial and venous dilatation may contribute to the headache.

Comorbidities

Numerous connective tissue disorders are described in association with SIH, including Marfan syndrome, Ehler–Danlos syndrome type II, and autosomal dominant polycystic kidney disease. Patients with SIH often demonstrate joint hypermobility with or without facial thinning, and skeletal features of Marfan syndrome, such as tall stature, arachnodactyly, or a high-arched palate. There may be a personal or family history of spontaneous retinal detachment.

Progression and prognosis

The headaches and other symptoms of SIH are often disabling. Nonsurgical treatment is effective in most patients, with a 10% likelihood of a recurrent spinal leak over time [44]. Patients with abnormal brain MRI findings and a focal spinal leak have the best prognosis, while those with a normal MRI and diffuse, multilevel leaks have a poor prognosis [50].

Management

There are no randomized clinical trials upon which to base treatment decisions. Bed rest, oral hydration, caffeine intake, and an abdominal binder may be effective. The mainstay of treatment is an autologous blood patch into the spinal epidural space, which may produce an immediate relief of symptoms. A volume of 10–20 mL of blood is used initially; if unsuccessful, a high-volume patch using 20–100 mL of blood may be injected into the thoracolumbar area and lower lumbar area. High-volume blood patches are often limited by back pain. A directed epidural blood patch or percutaneous fibrin sealant is often effective if the site of leakage is known. Surgical treatment is reserved for refractory cases. Rebound intracranial hypertension may occur.

Postdural puncture headache

Diagnosis

Postdural puncture headache (PDPH) is characterized by a postural headache following an LP, myelogram, spinal anesthesia, or cranial surgery. It also occurs following accidental dural puncture during epidural anesthesia. About 90% of patients experience PDPH within 72 hours of the puncture, and 66% have the onset of headache within 48 hours. In rare circumstances, the onset of headache is delayed until 5–14 days post-procedure. The headache is produced or worsens when the patient moves to a sitting or standing posture, and improves while lying flat. The features of the headache vary, but it may be incapacitating. Patients may describe occipital or frontal pain with radiation to the neck and shoulders, or holocephalic pain. The headache may be aggravated by movements of the head, Valsalva maneuver, coughing, sneezing, straining, ocular compression, and physical activity [49]. The associated symptoms are similar to those of SIH, including low back pain, vertigo, tinnitus, altered hearing, lower cranial nerve palsies, diplopia, cortical blindness, nausea, photophobia, and phonophobia.

PDPH occurs in approximately 20% of patients undergoing an LP. The diagnosis is generally made based on the patient's symptoms and history of preceding dural puncture. Various maneuvers support the diagnosis of a low-pressure headache. Continuous pressure on the patient's abdomen by the examiner's hand may relieve the headache within 30 seconds. Putting the patient in the Trendelenburg position for 1–2 minutes may also produce relief. MRI shows changes similar to those seen in SIH in some patients, but is frequently normal and generally unnecessary in the typical clinical setting.

Several serious conditions can mimic PDPH, including meningitis, subdural hematoma, SAH, brain tumor, cerebral venous thrombosis, and posterior leukoencephalopathy.

Pathophysiology

The pathophysiology is similar to that of SIH. Risk factors include female sex, a history of PDPH from a prior procedure, a history of chronic headaches prior to the procedure, and slim body habitus. PDPH is more likely to occur using a beveled Quincke needle than a blunt Sprotte needle. A larger bore needle, the orientation of the bevel during needle insertion, stylet replacement, and operator experience are also contributory factors.

Prevention

Several of the risk factors for developing PDPH are modifiable. Measures to prevent PDPH incorporate needle selection, technique, experience of the clinician, and other procedural factors. The size and shape of the spinal needle are perhaps the most important determinants of PDPH. The incidence of PDPH using a Quincke cutting needle is 36% with a 22-gauge needle, 25% with a 25-gauge needle, 2%–12% with a 26-gauge needle, and less than 2% with a needle of 29-gauge or more [51]. However, using a needle smaller than 22-gauge prolongs the LP and may yield a less accurate CSF pressure measurement. Numerous studies have shown that atraumatic needles, such as Sprotte and Whitacre needles, are less likely to produce PDPH [52, 53]. These needles are designed to separate the dural fibers rather than tear them, minimizing damage to the dura. However, they are more difficult to use and more expensive than cutting needles, which are included on a standard LP tray.

PDPH is less common if the bevel of a cutting spinal needle is inserted and removed while oriented parallel to the long axis of the spine. Stylet reinsertion prior to withdrawing the needle also lowers the incidence of PDPH, possibly because it prevents inadvertent pulling of strands of arachnoid. PDPH is less common in the hands of a more experienced clinician, particularly in epidural anesthesia [51].

Factors that are often implicated but never proven to be associated with PDPH include bed rest following the procedure, patient position during the puncture, hydration status, volume of CSF removed, number of attempts required, and pre-treatment with oral or intramuscular caffeine. Pre-treatment with intravenous caffeine or oral frovatriptan may be helpful.

Prognosis

Most patients have relief of PDPH within a week using conservative treatment (rest, hydration, and pain medication). Rare patients have persistent symptoms for weeks, months, or years.

Management

Conservative treatment consists of bed rest, hydration, abdominal binders, analgesics, and antiemetics. If these are not effective after a few days, intravenous methylxanthines (caffeine or theophylline), occipital nerve blocks, intravenous adrenocorticotropic hormone, gapapentin, mirtazapine, methergine, or epidural morphine may be employed. Epidural blood patches are widely used, with some evidence of efficacy from randomized trials [54]. Percutaneous injection of fibrin glue and surgery are used as the last resort.

Aneurysm and subarachnoid hemorrhage (SAH)

Aneurysmal SAH affects 30,000 patients in North America annually, and 1 in 100 headache patients presenting to the emergency department has an SAH [55]. The typical headache of SAH falls into the general category of "thunderclap headache," an acute and severe headache that is maximally intense at onset. SAH is the most common cause of secondary thunderclap headache [56]. Of patients presenting with severe, abrupt-onset headache and a normal neurologic examination, 10% have an SAH. In general, SAH accounts for up to 25% of patients with thunderclap headache [56]. Rupture of an intracranial aneurysm accounts for 85% of SAHs, nonaneuysmal perimesencephalic hemorrhages account for 10%, and other rare disorders (e.g., transmural arterial dissection, cerebral arteriovenous malformation, dural arteriovenous fistula, mycotic aneurysm, and cocaine abuse) account for the remaining 5% of cases.

Up to half of patients experiencing an SAH relate a history of a sentinel or warning headache days to weeks prior to aneurysm rupture. The sentinel headache may also be thunderclap in nature although not accompanied by symptoms of meningismus, altered level of consciousness, or focal neurologic manifestations [56]. Usually, there is only one sentinel headache, lasting minutes to days, that is unilateral or occipital and may radiate to the neck [57]. Because of its nonspecific nature, patients often disregard the sentinel headache, or they are misdiagnosed at this stage.

The headache of SAH may occur in isolation or with other symptoms. The typical headache of SAH lasts a few days and may be preceded by physical exertion or sexual intercourse. One-third of patients have loss of consciousness. Other symptoms include seizures, altered mental status, stroke, visual disturbances, photophobia, nausea, vomiting, dizziness, and neck stiffness. The physical examination is often unrevealing, although retinal hemorrhages occur in 20%–40% of patients.

Neuro-ophthalmic manifestations are common [58]. Aneurysms of the posterior communicating artery, the location of 30% of all intracranial aneurysms, generally produce an oculomotor nerve palsy and ipsilateral headache. Ptosis is generally the earliest manifestation, progressing over hours to involve the pupil and other ocular muscles innervated by the third nerve. A third nerve palsy may also reflect uncal herniation. An internal carotid artery aneurysm within the cavernous sinus may produce an abducens palsy and ipsilateral Horner syndrome. The oculomotor and trochlear nerves may become involved as the aneurysm enlarges, although cavernous aneurysms do not commonly rupture. Aneurysms of the internal carotid artery near the origin of the ophthalmic artery or the superior hypophyseal artery produce slowly progressive visual loss, usually without rupture. Papilledema occurs in 10%–24% of patients with SAH.

Noncontrast CT of the brain is the first diagnostic test of choice when evaluating patients for suspected SAH (Figure 3.6a). The sensitivity of CT nears 100% within the first 12 hours of the event but declines thereafter. Many factors contribute to the failure to diagnosis SAH by CT scanning, including the volume of blood present, the expertise of the physician reading the scan, low hematocrit, and technical factors (the resolution of the scanner, motion, and metal artifact) [55]. LP with spectrophotometry retains a high sensitivity for the detection of SAH after the first 12 hours. Xanthochromia is reliably present 12 hours after the hemorrhage [59]. Rare patients with SAH have negative CT and CSF findings [60]. Although the resolution of CTA is quite good, catheter cerebral angiography remains the test of choice for diagnosis (Figure 3.6b and 3.6c).

Comorbidities and risk factors

Intracranial aneurysms are associated with connective tissue disorders such as autosomal dominant polycystic kidney disease, Ehlers–Danlos syndrome type IV, neurofibromatosis type I, and Marfan syndrome [61]. The familial aggregation of aneurysms has been borne out in multiple studies. Among the first-degree relatives of patients with aneurysmal SAH, the risk of an unruptured aneurysm is four times higher than the risk in the general population. Aneurysms are rare in children, and the mean age of rupture is around 50 years. Cigarette smoking increases the risk of SAH by 3–10 times, possibly related to a decreased level of alpha-1-antitrypsin. Hyper-

tension may be a risk for SAH, although the data are less consistent than for cigarette smoking. A moderate to high level of alcohol consumption and binge-drinking increase the risk of SAH. Before the fifth decade, aneurysmal SAH is more frequent in men; there is a female predominance after age 50 years.

> ### SCIENCE REVISITED
>
> Alpha-1-antitrypsin is a protease inhibitor, protecting tissues from the enzymes of inflammatory cells. In its absence, elastase is free to break down into elastin. Cigarette smoking can lead to oxidation of the methionine 358 of alpha-1-antitrypsin, a residue essential for binding elastase, thus producing chronic tissue breakdown.

Pathophysiology

About 2% of individuals harbor intracranial aneurysms, 85% of which are located in the anterior circulation. Approximately 25% of cases have multiple aneurysms. Aneurysms are located at the bifurcations of major cerebral arteries. The wall of the aneurysm is composed primarily of intima and adventitia, with little to no tunica media and an absent or fragmented internal elastic lamina [61]. Ruptured aneurysms tend to have variable wall thickness and one or more daughter sacs. The point of rupture is generally at the dome of the aneurysm. All aneurysms are unique, and attempts to identify structural risk factors have failed to yield uniform recommendations.

The risk of rupture depends on the size and location of the aneurysm. The International Study of Unruptured Intracranial Aneurysms revealed a 0.05% per year rate of rupture for aneurysms less than 10 mm in size in the anterior circulation, compared to close to 1% for aneurysms over 10 mm in size [62]. While no size is "safe," the mean size of most unruptured aneurysms is between 4 and 6 mm, and most ruptured aneurysms are between 5 and 8 mm. Posterior circulation aneurysms carry a higher risk of rupture than anterior circulation aneurysms, with multilobulated posterior circulation aneurysm portending the highest risk. A high aspect ratio (size : neck ratio), an irregular surface, the

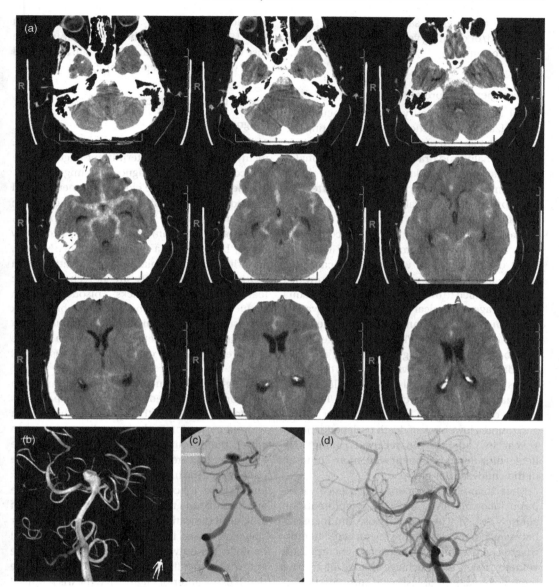

Figure 3.6. SAH. (a) Noncontrast CT scan of the brain in a 51-year-old man presenting to the emergency department with an acute, severe headache. There is a massive SAH with blood in the basal cisterns, quadrigeminal cistern, suprasellar cisterns, and interhemispheric fissure, and tracking along the right temporal lobe, right Sylvian fissure, bilateral frontal lobes, and third and fourth ventricles. (b) CTA reveals a large aneurysm at the top of the basilar artery. (c) Catheter angiography confirms the CTA findings. (d) A catheter angiogram shows successful coiling of the aneurysm. (Photographs courtesy of Babak Jahromi, MD.)

presence of daughter sacs, and a small parent artery and/or draining vessels appear to increase the risk of rupture.

Management and prognosis

Initial care of an aneurysmal SAH focuses on recognizing complications and preventing rebleeding [59]. Acute complications include hydrocephalus and brain edema. Hydrocephalus responds to ventricular drainage, but brain edema may be difficult to control and portends a poor prognosis. The calcium channel blocker nimodipine is effective in delaying ischemic damage and improving functional outcome, possibly related to neuroprotection, as it has no effect on angiographic vasospasm. Nicardipine reduces angiographic vasospasm but controlled trials have failed to demonstrate delayed ischemia with this agent. Surgical clipping and endovascular coiling exclude the aneurysm from the circulation (Figure 3.6d). Wide-necked aneurysms or those with branching vessels are generally approached surgically, while basilar tip aneurysms are best treated endovascularly. The International Subarachnoid Aneurysm Trial randomized 2143 patients to craniotomy or coiling and found a lower risk of death or dependency at 1 year in patients who received coiling [63]. Rebleeding and retreatment were more common in the endovascular group.

More than 60% of patients experience vasospasm following SAH, which is symptomatic in about 30% [59]. The risk of vasospasm increases between 3 and 7 days following an acute hemorrhage. The treatment of vasospasm incorporates volume repletion to achieve a state of relative hypervolemia. Anigoplasty and intra-arterial infusion of vasodilating agents may be employed in patients who are refractory to medical therapy or in whom volume expansion poses a medical risk. Numerous medical complications following SAH pose challenges at all phases of recovery, including fever, hyperglycemia, neurogenic pulmonary edema, cardiomyopathy, hyponatremia, and the syndrome of inadequate secretion of antidiuretic hormone and venous thromboembolism.

Despite significant advances in neurosurgical technique, interventional radiology, and critical care treatment, SAH remains a disorder of high morbidity and mortality. Sudden death occurs in 10%–15% of patients at the time of rupture. The case fatality rate is about 50% overall, and a third of survivors remain dependent [56].

Angle-closure glaucoma

Diagnosis

Although not a common cause of headaches, recurrent episodes of intermittent angle-closure glaucoma may be misdiagnosed as migraine [64]. The head pain of angle closure is generally mild to moderate in intensity, and located around the ipsilateral eye or the ipsilateral side of the head. The attacks last from several minutes to a few hours, briefer than a typical migraine. Nausea, vomiting, photophobia, and aggravation with routine physical activity are not characteristic features of subacute attacks. Episodes range in frequency from occasional to daily. A high index of suspicion and gonioscopy (examination of the anatomic angle between the cornea and the iris) are required to make the diagnosis at this stage.

Angle-closure glaucoma is more common in hyperopic (far-sighted) patients. If the patient is unsure of their refractive state (i.e., their vision without correction is clearer at distance than up close), the examiner may be able to determine whether they are hyperopic by observing the patient wearing his or her spectacles. The convex lenses used to correct hyperopia magnify the appearance of the eyes. Additionally, when looking at the patient's cheekbones through their spectacle lenses, the edge of the cheekbones will be deflected outward. Further evaluation of the eye with a penlight can help to estimate the depth of the anterior chamber. If the iris is bowed forward, producing a narrow anterior chamber, a light source projected from the lateral aspect of the eye will cast a shadow on the nasal side of the iris, making it appear darker than the temporal iris [65].

Typical symptoms of complete angle closure are ocular pain, headache, nausea, and vomiting. The attack is often accompanied by blurry vision, and patients often complain of seeing halos around lights. However, unlike migraine patients, patients with acute angle closure will typically demonstrate the following ocular signs [66]:

- *Elevated intraocular pressures* (typically >30 mmHg). When tonometry is unavailable, the affected eye may be palpated under closed lids using the thumb pad. A hard, unyielding globe indicates an elevated pressure.
- *. Conjunctival injection.* The eye is typically red, and there is often a ring of vascular congestion surrounding the corneal-scleral junction.
- *A shallow anterior chamber.* The iris is commonly rotated forward towards the back side of the cornea, making the anterior chamber shallower.
- *A mid-dilated pupil.* The pupil is usually dilated and either fixed or sluggishly reactive. The combination of pain and dilated pupil angle closure may be mistaken for a third cranial nerve palsy, but the elevated pressure and the lack of ptosis or ocular motor palsy excludes that diagnosis.
- *Corneal edema.* The cornea may appear edematous or cloudy.

★ TIPS AND TRICKS

Many physicians are reluctant to incorporate pupillary dilation in their routine office examinations for fear of precipitating angle-closure glaucoma. The penlight test (described in the text) will help to screen for susceptible patients. The risk of producing angle closure using mydriatic drops is less than 1 in 5000, and is negligible using phenylephrine alone. Moreover, the rare patient who develops angle closure as the mydriatic drops wear off can be easily and effectively treated with laser peripheral iridotomy, preventing any further attacks.

Pathophysiology and comorbidities

Acute angle-closure glaucoma occurs when intraocular pressure rapidly rises as a result of closure or blockage of the drainage angle of the eye, the site of aqueous outflow. It may occur in any situation associated with pupillary dilation, which causes the iris to move anteriorly (e.g., when emerging from a darkened movie theater).

Risk factors include advancing age, a strong family history of glaucoma, a history of ocular trauma, Asian ethnicity, hyperopia, and pseudoexfoliation of the lens [67]. Medications, such as topical anticholinergic or sympathomimetic dilating drops, tricyclic antidepressants, monoamine oxidase inhibitors, antihistamines, antiparkinsonian drugs, antipsychotic medications, antispasmolytic agents, sulfonamide drugs and topiramate, are associated with angle-closure glaucoma [68].

Prognosis

The prognosis is excellent if the condition is detected early and treated. Permanent angle scarring, glaucomatous optic neuropathy, and visual field loss occur with repeated attacks.

Management

Whereas the pain associated with angle closure may improve using analgesics, it quickly subsides once the intraocular pressure has been controlled. Intraocular pressure control is usually achieved using cholinergic agents such as pilocarpine to constrict the pupil and open the angle. When the intraocular pressure is very elevated (>45 mmHg), topical medications such as beta-blockers and alpha-2-adrenergic agonists, as well as intravenous mannitol and carbonic anhydrase inhibitors, may be needed. Laser peripheral iridotomy is a definitive therapy in nearly all cases. A trabeculectomy is seldom required.

Chiari type I malformation

Diagnosis

A Chiari type I malformation is characterized by elongation of the cerebellar tonsils and medial lobules both descending with the medulla into the spinal canal with minimal or no lengthening or alteration of the fourth ventricle [69]. It is best visualized on a midsagittal view on brain and cervical MRI. Small (<5 mm) Chiari type I malformations are often detected as incidental findings in asymptomatic patients, or in those with poorly defined symptoms, presenting a quandary regarding their relevance to the patient's complaints or the appropriate management. Symptoms are generally proportional to the degree of tonsillar descent and the extent of posterior fossa deformity.

Headache is the most common symptom reported by both adults and children [70]. It is generally posteriorly located and precipitated or exacerbated by neck movement. The pain may radiate anteriorly or into the neck and shoulders unilaterally. The character of the pain may be dull, throbbing, or lancinating. Precipitating movements include neck flexion, coughing, sexual activity, or other forms of exertion or Valsalva maneuver [69, 71]. The headaches last from minutes to hours and may simulate migraine or tension-type headaches. Other symptoms include dizziness, vertigo, positive or negative sensory symptoms in the upper extremities, ataxia, diplopia, blurred vision, visual obscurations, oscillopsia, limb weakness, torticollis, hearing loss, hoarseness, central sleep apnea, and tremor. The examination may reveal downbeat nystagmus, periodic alternating nystagmus, or horizontal, torsional, and other types of nystagmus. Weakness, sensory deficits, long tract signs, cerebellar signs, and lower cranial nerve palsies may be present [72].

Cine phase-contrast analysis of CSF flow shows pulsatile downward motion of the tonsils that further occludes a restricted subarachnoid space at the level of the foramen magnum [69].

Pathophysiology and comorbidities

The normal flow supratentorially and in the spinal canal caudal to the malformation creates a pressure gradient, causing transient increased intracranial pressure with Valsalva maneuver and the associated increase in venous pressure and volume. The hindbrain-supporting structures, such as the occipital dura, occipital bone, first cervical vertebra, and rectus capitis posterior minor muscle, are innervated by the upper cervical nerves. Mechanical changes and traction at the skull base likely contribute to head pain with nociceptive input into the trigeminal nucleus caudalis.

Syringomyelia, scoliosis, hydrocephalus, fused cervical vertebrae, platybasia, Klippel–Feil syndrome, cervicomedullary kinking, and atlantooccipital assimilation may co-exist [70, 72]. There is an increased incidence of Chiari malformations in patients with neurofibromatosis type I and IIH. Acquired Chiari-like malformations arise with overshunting from lumboperitoneal shunts.

Prognosis

A study examining headaches and CSF flow dynamics in children with Chiari type I malformations found that patients with frontal or generalized headaches were 10-fold less likely to demonstrate obstructed CSF flow and eightfold less likely to have tonsillar descent of greater than 7 mm compared to children with occipital headaches [70]. Following surgical decompression, none of the 10 patients experiencing occipital headaches had recurrent symptoms at 12 months, compared to 57% of (4 of 7) patients with frontal headaches. Decompressive surgery failed to improve headaches in patients with nonobstructive flow.

Management

The headaches may respond to medications such as nonsteroidal anti-inflammatory drugs, triptans, tricyclic antidepressants, acetazolamide, or other analgesics. Surgical options include CSF diversion procedures, suboccipital craniectomy, duraplasty, and resection of the arch of the atlas.

Rhinosinusitis

Diagnosis

Acute sinusitis accounts for over 3 million physician visits annually [73]. The diagnosis of "sinus headache" is made frequently by practitioners and sufferers, and considerable controversy exists regarding the diagnosis. Headaches attributed to rhinosinusitis are associated with facial pain and pressure. The overlapping clinical features between tension-type headaches, migraine headaches, and sinus headaches lead to misdiagnosis and incorrect management.

Diagnostic criteria for sinus headache have been proposed by the American Academy of Otolaryngology-Head and Neck Surgery (AAO-HNS) and the International Headache Society [74]. Headache alone is not sufficient for diagnosis in either classification system. The AAO-HNS criteria include major factors (purulence in the nasal cavity; facial pain, pressure, congestion, and fullness; nasal obstruction, blockage, discharge, and purulence; fever in acute sinusitis; and hyposmia and anosmia) and minor factors (headache, fever, halitosis, fatigue, dental pain, cough, ear pain, and fullness). A diagnosis of rhinosinusitis requires the presence of at least two major factors or at least one major and two minor factors.

The International Classification of Headache Disorders-2 (ICHD-2) criteria require clinical, nasal endoscopic, CT and/or imaging, and/or laboratory evidence of acute or acute-on-chronic rhinosinusitis. Clinical evidence consists of purulence in the nasal cavity, nasal obstruction, hyposmia, anosmia, and/or fever. The headache is frontal accompanied by pain in one or more regions of the face, ears, or teeth. The headache and facial pain must develop simultaneously with the onset or acute exacerbation of rhinosinusitis, and resolve within 7 days after the remission or successful treatment of acute or acute-on-chronic rhinosinusitis. Headache attributable to chronic sinusitis is not recognized in the ICHD-2.

A pilot study evaluating 47 patients with self-diagnosed sinus headache found that 90% met the diagnostic criteria for migraine and responded to subsequent treatment with sumatriptan [75]. Features of migraine contributing to the misdiagnosis of sinus headache included sinus pressure, sinus pain, lacrimation, eyelid edema, rhinorrhea, and nasal congestion. Migraine triggers suggesting sinus disease included weather changes, exposure to allergen, seasonal variation, and change in altitude [76]. A larger study of patients with sinus headache via self-report or physician diagnosis found that a large percentage of subjects experienced typical migraine symptoms such as moderate to severe pain, pulsatile pain, photophobia and phonophobia, aura, and vomiting [77]. Similarly, the Sinus, Allergy and Migraine Study evaluated 100 consecutive patients with self-reported sinus headache and found that 52% had migraine with or without aura, 23% had probable migraine, 11% had medication overuse headache, 3% had rhinosinusitis, 9% had unclassifiable headaches, and 2% had a trigeminal autonomic cephalalgia [76]. Seventy-six percent of individuals with migraine described pain in the distribution of the maxillary nerve, and 62% had bilateral forehead and maxillary pain.

True sinus pain tends to be pressure-like, dull, usually bilateral, and periorbital. The pain is generally worse in the morning and improves as the day progresses, owing to turbinate, sinus, and nasal congestion that worsens with recumbency and is relieved with sinus medication taken in the morning. Sinus-related pain is associated with nasal obstruction or congestion, lasts for days at a time, and is not associated with nausea, vomiting, or visual disturbances [74]. Pain induced by sinus percussion is less reliable for diagnosing acute sinusitis than focal pain while bending over [78].

Most patients with sinusitis are diagnosed by history and physical examination. Plain sinus radiographs have a sensitivity of 87% and specificity of 89%, but cannot reliably distinguish viral from bacterial sinusitis. The occipitomental (Waters) view is the optimal view for visualizing the paranasal sinuses, and most commonly demonstrates sinus fluid or opacity. There may be mucous membrane thickening. Ultrasonography is less useful. CT is more sensitive than radiography but has a high false-positive rate in acute sinusitis and requires a much higher dose of radiation [78].

Comorbidities

Sinus disease is associated with a septal deviation or concha bullosa (enlargement of the middle turbinate) in some cases. As sinus disease, migraine, and allergic rhinitis are fairly common entities, comorbidity is likely based on the prevalence of these conditions. Risk factors for acute sinusitis include age (being more common in young children and older adults), smoke and air pollutants, air travel and changes in atmospheric pressure, swimming, and dental disease. Persons with chronic nasal congestion, particularly those with allergies and asthma, may be predisposed to developing acute sinusitis [73]. Immunocompromised individuals, such as patients with AIDS, poorly controlled diabetes, or autoimmune disorders (Wegener granulomatosis), and patients with cystic fibrosis, Kartagener syndrome (bronchiectasis, sinusitis, and dextrocardia), facial injuries, nasal polyps, and a deviated septum are at higher risk for contracting sinus infections.

Pathophysiology

The trigeminal afferents convey nociceptive sensory input from the pain-sensitive structures of the head, including the meninges, dural blood vessels, temporomandibular joints, neck, and gingival, nasal, and sinus mucosa. Migraine attacks may be accompanied by autonomic symptoms arising from activation of the cranial parasympathetic pathways: conjunctival injection, lacrimation, nasal congestion, and rhinorrhea are symptoms common to migraine, cluster headache, sinusitis, and allergic rhinitis. Parasympathetic efferents form the superior salivatory nucleus synapse in the sphenopalatine, otic and carotid mini-ganglia. The vasomotor efferents travel with the ethmoidal nerve to innervate the cerebral blood vessels. The innervation of the sinuses and facial structures helps to explain why migraine pain is often misperceived as originating from the sinuses. It also explains why inflammation or infection of the sinus mucosa leads to headaches or triggers migraine in susceptible individuals [74].

Management and prognosis

Most sinusitis is viral, and 80% of patients recover within 2 weeks without treatment [73]. The risk for bacterial sinusitis increases after 7–10 days. Nonpharmacologic therapy includes steam inhalation, hydration, and sinus irrigation. Widespread prescribing of antibiotics for suspected sinusitis promotes drug-resistant strains of common respiratory pathogens without proven benefit. A Cochrane review concluded that the use of antibiotics in the treatment of acute bacterial sinusitis reduced the risk of clinical failure at 7–15 days but was associated with significant side effects [78]. If treatment is required, amoxicillin is generally used as a first-line agent, substituting with trimethoprim-sulfamethoxazole in penicillin-allergic patients. Second-line treatments include amoxicillin-clavunate, second- or third-generation cephalosporins, doxycycline, macrolides, and fluoroquinolones. Other nonantibiotic treatments may be helpful, such as oral antihistamines, nasal decongestions, and mucolytic agents.

★ TIPS AND TRICKS

Rhinosinusitis does not present with headache as the sole manifestation; recurring "sinus headaches" most likely represent migraine. Phonophobia, photophobia, nausea, vomiting, and aggravation with routine physical activity are features that help to distinguish migraine from sinus disease. Most acute sinusitis is viral, and antibiotics are not considered until at least a week after symptom onset.

Conclusion: key practice points

The vast majority of patients seeking medical attention for headaches have a primary headache disorder. There is a difficult balance between being overly cautious and performing unnecessarily diagnostic tests and risking a diagnosis of medical or surgical importance. Because headache is subjective, the provider relies greatly on the patient's history and physical examination. Key symptoms, "red flags," and examination findings that raise the suspicion for a secondary cause of headache are summarized in Table 3.1. The importance of ophthalmoscopy cannot be overemphasized as a key component of the physical examination.

Table 3.1. Evaluation of suspected secondary headaches

Symptoms and signs	Differential diagnosis	Preferred imaging tests	Other tests to consider
First or worst headache	SAH Intracerebral hematoma Abscess Meningitis Venous thrombosis Intracranial hypertension Tumor	CT without and with contrast MRA/CTA/catheter angiogram if suspected aneurysm	LP with opening pressure for unconfirmed SAH, meningitis, leptomeningeal metastasis Pseudotumor cerebri
Headache with focal neurologic symptoms and signs	Cervical dissection Stroke SAH Subdural, epidural, or intracerebral hematoma Pituitary apoplexy Abscess Venous thrombosis Tumor Arteriovenous malformation Carcinomatous or infectious meningitis Intracranial hypertension (VIth cranial nerve palsy)	MRI without and with contrast Consider MRA or CTA MRV or CTA for suspected venous thrombosis	LP for suspected carcinomatous or infectious meningitis LP with opening pressure for suspected pseudotumor cerebri
History of cancer or HIV	Metastatic disease Abscess Meningitis	MRI with contrast	
Headache and altered mental status	Carcinomatous or infectious meningitis Subdural hematoma Epidural hematoma Vasculitis Infectious encephalopathy	MR with contrast CT with contrast for subdural hematoma Arteriogram for vasculitis	LP with PCR for suspected herpes
Headache onset over age 50 years	Tumor Brain metastasis GCA	MRI with contrast	ESR, C-reactive protein, CBC, temporal artery biopsy for suspected GCA
Escalation in previously stable headache pattern	Brain tumor Arteriovenous malformation Abscess Intracranial hypertension	MRI with contrast	LP with opening pressure measurement
Postural headache	Spontaneous intracranial hypotension Post-LP headache	MRI with contrast	Spinal CT or MRI Radionucleide cisternography LP

(Continued)

Table 3.1. (*Continued*)

Symptoms and signs	Differential diagnosis	Preferred imaging tests	Other tests to consider
Headache in obese female of childbearing age	Intracranial hypertension	MRI	LP with opening pressure Ophthalmic examination
Headache and transient vision loss	Intracranial hypertension GCA Glaucoma Venous sinus thrombosis Carotid dissection	MRI MRV for suspected venous sinus thrombosis	Ophthalmic examination ESR, C-reactive protein, CBC, temporal artery biopsy for suspected GCA
Headache and enduring vision loss	GCA Intracranial hypertension Optic neuritis Glaucoma Occipital ischemia Pituitary tumor Pituitary apoplexy Venous sinus thrombosis	MRI for suspected intracranial hypertension, tumor, and occipital ischemia MRV for suspected venous sinus thrombosis	Ophthalmic examination LP with opening pressure for suspected intracranial hypertension ESR, C-reactive protein, CBC, temporal artery biopsy for suspected GCA
Headache and diplopia	Aneurysm Microvascular cranial neuropathy Intracranial hypertension Tolosa–Hunt syndrome Tumor Vasculitis Carcinomatous or infectious meningitis Intracranial hypotension GCA Cavernous sinus thrombosis	MRI with contrast MRA/CTA/angiogram for suspected aneurysm or vasculitis MRV for suspected sinus thrombosis	ESR, C-reactive protein, CBC, temporal artery biopsy for suspected GCA HgbA1c, cholesterol, lipid panel for microvascular cranial neuropathy

CBC, complete blood count; HgbA1c, hemoglobin A1c; MRV, magnetic resonance venography; PCR, polymerase chain reaction.

References

1. Buckner JC, Brown PD, O'Neill BP, Meyer FB, Wetmore CJ, Uhm JH. Central nervous system tumors. *Mayo Clin Proc* 2007;**82**:1271–86.
2. Goffaux P, Fortin D. Brain tumor headaches: from bedside to bench. *Neurosurgery* 2010; **67**:459–66.
3. Schankin CJ, Ferrari U, Reinisch VM, Birnbaum T, Goldbrunner R, Straube A. Characteristics of brain tumour-associated headache. *Cephalalgia* 2007;**27**:904–11.
4. Reulecke BC, Erker CG, Fiedler BJ, Niederstadt T-U, Kurlemann G. Brain tumors in children: initial symptoms and their influence

on the time span between symptom onset and diagnosis. *J Child Neurol* 2008;**23**: 178–83.

5. Forsyth PA, Posner JB. Headaches in patients with brain tumors: a study of 111 patients. *Neurology* 1993;**43**:1678–83.

6. Frishberg BM. The utility of neuroimaging in the evaluation of headache in patients with a normal neurologic examination. *Neurology* 1994;**44**:1191–7.

7. Wang SJ, Hung CW, Fuh JL, Limg JF, Hwu CM. Cranial autonomic symptoms in patients with pituitary adenoma presenting with headaches. *Acta Neurol Taiwan* 2009;**18**: 104–12.

8. Wilbrink LA, Ferrari MD, Kruit MC, Haan J. Neuroimaging in trigeminal autonomic cephalalgias: when, how and of what? *Curr Opin Neurol* 2009;**22**:247–53.

9. Levy MJ, Matharu M, Goadsby PJ. Chronic headache and pituitary tumors. *Curr Pain Headache Rep* 2008;**12**:74–8.

10. Bosco D, Belfiore A, Fava A, et al. Relationship between high prolactin levels and migraine attacks in patients with microprolactinoma. *J Headache Pain* 2008;**9**:103–7.

11. Friedman DI. Pseudotumor cerebri presenting as headache. *Expert Rev Neurotherap* 2008;**8**:397–407.

12. Brodsky MC, Vaphiades M. Magnetic resonance imaging in pseudotumor cerebri. *Ophthalmology* 1998;**105**:1686–93.

13. Dandy W. Intracranial pressure without brain tumor: diagnosis and treatment. *Ann Surg* 1937;**106**:492–513.

14. Ireland B, Corbett JJ. The search for causes of idiopathic intracranial hypertension. *Arch Neurol* 1990;**47**:315–20.

15. Digre KB, Varner MV, Corbett JJ. Pseudotumor cerebri and pregnancy. *Neurology* 1984;**34**:721–9.

16. Friedman DI, Rausch EA. Headache diagnoses in patients with treated idiopathic intracranial hypertension. *Neurology* 2002; **58**:1551–3.

17. Wall M, George D. Visual loss in pseudotumor cerebri: incidence and defects related to visual field strategy. *Arch Neurol* 1987;**44**: 170–5.

18. Shah VA, Kardon RH, Lee AG, Corbett JJ, Wall M. Long-term follow-up of idiopathic intrac-

ranial hypertension. The Iowa experience. *Neurology* 2008;**70**:634–40.

19. Chandrasekaran S, McCluskey P, Minassian D, Assaad N. Visual outcome for optic nerve sheath fenestration in pseudotumor cerebri and related conditions. *Clin Exp Ophthalmol* 2006;**34**:661–5.

20. McGirt MJ, Woodworth G, Thomas G, Miller NR, Williams M, Rigamonti D. Cerebrospinal fluid shunt placement for pseudotumor cerebri-associated intractable headache: predictors of treatment response and analysis of long term outcomes. *J Neurosurg* 2004;**101**:627–32.

21. Kupersmith MJ, Gamell L, Turbin R, Spiegel P, Wall M. Effects of weight loss on the course of idiopathic intracranial hypertension in women. *Neurology* 1998;**50**:1094–8.

22. Lee AG, Pless M, Falardeau J, Capazzoli T, Wall M, Kardon RH. The use of acetazolamide in idiopathic intracranial hypertension during pregnancy. *Am J Ophthalmol* 2005; **139**:855–9.

23. Kleinschmidt JJ, Digre KB, Hanover R. Idiopathic intracranial hypertension. Relationship to depression, anxiety, and quality of life. *Neurology* 2000;**54**:319–24.

24. Fischer C, Goldstein JM, Edlow JA. Cerebral venous sinus thrombosis in the emergency department: retrospective analysis of 17 cases and review of the literature. *J Emerg Med* 2009;**38**:140–7.

25. Cohen JE, Boitsova S, Itshayek E. Cerebral venous sinus thrombosis. *Isr Med Assoc J* 2009;**11**:685–8.

26. Bentley JN, Figueroa RE, Vender JR. From presentation to follow-up: diagnosis and treatment of cerebral venous thrombosis. *Neurosurg Focus* 2009;**27**:E4.

27. McBane RD, 2nd, Tafur A, Wysokinski WE. Acquired and congenital risk factors associated with cerebral venous sinus thrombosis. *Thromb Res* 2010;**126**:81–7.

28. Filippidis A, Kapsalaki E, Patramani G, Fountas KM. Cerebral venous sinus thrombosis: review of demographics, pathophysiology, current diagnosis, and treatment. *Neurosurg Focus* 2009;**27**:E3.

29. Stam J, Lensing AW, Vermeulen M, Tijssen JG. Heparin treatment for cerebral venous and sinus thrombosis. *Lancet* 1991;**338**:1154.

30. Medel R, Montieth SJ, Crowley W, Dumont AS. A review of therapeutic strategies for the management of cerebral venous sinus thrombosis. *Neurosurg Focus* 2009;**27**:E6.

31. Einhäupel K, Stam J, Bousser M-G, et al. EFNS guideline on the treatment of cerebral venous and sinus thrombosis in adults. *Eur J Neurol* 2010;**17**:1229–35.

32. Schwedt TJ, Dodick DW, Caselli RJ. Giant cell arteritis. *Curr Pain Headache Rep* 2006;**10**:415–20.

33. Hayreh SS, Podhajsky PA, Zimmerman B. Occult giant cell arteritis: ocular manifestations. *Am J Ophthalmol* 1998;**125**:521–6.

34. Melson MR, Weyland CM, Newman NJ, Biousse V. The diagnosis of giant cell arteritis. *Rev Neurol Dis* 2007;**4**:128–42.

35. Breuer GS, Nesher R, Nesher G. Negative temporal artery biopsies: eventual diagnoses and features of patients with biopsy-negative giant cell arteritis compared to patients without arteritis. *Clin Exp Rheumatol* 2008;**26**:1103–6.

36. Salvarani C, Cantini F, Bioiardi L, Hunder GG. Polymyalgia rheumatica and giant-cell arteritis. *New Engl J Med* 2002;**347**:261–71.

37. Schwartz NE, Vertinsky AT, Hirsch KG, Albers GW. Clinical and radiographic natural history of cervical artery dissections. *J Stroke Cerebrovasc Dis* 2009;**18**:416–23.

38. Biousse V, Touboul P-J, D'Anglejan-Chatillon J, Lévy C, Shciason M, Bousser M-G. Ophthalmologic manifestations of internal carotid artery dissection. *Am J Ophthalmol* 1998;**126**:565–77.

39. Caplan LR. Dissections of brain-supplying arteries. *Nat Clin Pract Neurol* 2008;**4**:34–42.

40. Caplan LR, Biousse V. Cervicocranial arterial dissections. *J Neuro-ophthalmol* 2004;**24**:299–305.

41. Schievink WI. Spontaneous dissection of the carotid and vertebral arteries. *N Engl J Med* 2001;**344**:898–906.

42. Nebelsieck J, Sengelhoff C, Nassenstein I, et al. Sensitivity of neurovascular ultrasound for the detection of spontaneous cervical artery dissection. *J Clin Neurosci* 2009;**16**:79–82.

43. Lyrer P, Engelter S. Antithrombotic drugs for carotid artery dissection. In: *Cochrane Database Syst Rev* 2003;(3):CD000255.

44. Schievink WI. Spontaneous spinal cerebrospinal fluid leaks and intracranial hypotension. *JAMA* 2006;**295**:2286–96.

45. Mokri B. Spontaneous cerebrospinal fluid leaks: from intracranial hypotension to cerebrospinal fluid hypovolemia—evolution of a concept. *Mayo Clin Proc* 1999;**74**:1113–23.

46. Rozen TD, Swiden S, Hamel R, Saper JR. Trendelenburg position: a tool to screen for the presence of a low CSF pressure syndrome in daily headache patients. *Headache* 2008;**48**:1366–71.

47. Horton JC, Fishman RA. Neurovisual findings in the syndrome of spontaneous intracranial hypotension from dural cerebrospinal fluid leak. *Ophthalmology* 1994;**101**:244–51.

48. Wang Y-F, Lirng J-F, Fuh J-L, Hseu S-S, Wang S-J. Heavily T2-weighted MR myelography vs CT myelography in spontaneous intracranial hypotension. *Neurology* 2009;**73**:1982–9.

49. Bezov D, Lipton RB, Ashina S. Post-dural puncture headache. I. Diagnosis, epidemiology, etiology and pathophysiology. *Headache* 2010;**50**:1144–52.

50. Schievink WI, Maya MM, Louy C. Cranial MRI predicts outcome of spontaneous intracranial hypotension. *Neurology* 2005;**64**:1282–4.

51. Turnbull DK, Shepherd DB. Post-dural puncture headache: pathogenesis, prevention and treatment. *Br J Anaesth* 2003;**91**:718–21.

52. Bezov D, Ashina S, Lipton RB. Post-dural puncture headache. II. Prevention, management and prognosis. *Headache* 2010;**50**:1482–98.

53. Kleyweg RP, Hertzberger LI, Carbaat PA. Significant reduction in post-lumbar puncture headache using an atraumatic needle. A double-blind, controlled trial. *Cephalalgia* 1998;**18**:635–7.

54. van Kooten F, Oedit R, Bakker SLM, Dippel DWJ. Epidural blood patch in post dural puncture headache: a randomised, observer-blind, controlled clinical trial. *J Neurol Neurosurg Psychiatry* 2007;**79**:553–8.

55. Edlow JA, Malek AM, Ogilby CS. Aneurysmal subarachnoid hemorrhage: update for emergency physicians. *J Emerg Med* 2007;**34**:237–51.

56. Schwedt TJ, Matharu MS, Dodick DW. Thunderclap headache. *Lancet Neurol* 2006;**5**: 621–31.

57. Verweij RD, Wijdicks FM, van Gihn J. Warning headache in aneurysmal subarachnoid hemorrhage: a case-control study. *Arch Neurol* 1988;**45**:1019–20.

58. Purvin VA. Neuro-ophthalmic aspects of aneurysms. *Int Ophthalmol Clin* 2009;**49**: 119–32.

59. Rabinstein AA, Lanzino G, Wijidicjks EFM. Multidisciplinary management and emerging therapeutic strategies in aneurysmal subarachnoid hemorrhage. *Lancet Neurol* 2010;**9**:504–19.

60. Eggers C, Liu W, Brinker G, Fink GR, Burghaus L. Do negative CCT and CSF findings exclude a subarachnoid haemorrhage? A retrospective analysis of 220 patients with subarachnoid hemorrhage. *Eur J Neurol* 2011;**18**: 300–5.

61. Schievink WI. Intracranial aneurysms. *N Engl J Med* 1997;**336**:28–40.

62. Lall RR, Eddleman CS, Bendok BR, Batjer HH. Unruptured intracranial aneurysms and the assessment of rupture risk based on anatomical and morphological factors: sifting through the sands of data. *Neurosurg Focus* 2009;**26**.E2.

63. Molyneux AJ, Kerr RS, Yu LM, et al. International subarachnoid aneurysm trial (ISAT) of neurosurgical clipping versus endovascular coiling in 2143 patients with ruptured intracranial aneurysms: a randomised comparison of effects on survival, dependency, seizures, rebleeding, subgroups, and aneurysm occlusion. *Lancet* 2005;**366**:809–17.

64. Shindler KS, Sankar PS, Volpe NJ, Piltz-Seymour JR. Intermittent headaches as the presenting sign of subacute angle-closure glaucoma. *Neurology* 2005;**65**:757–8.

65. Nesher R, Hering-Hanit R, Nesher G. Subacute glaucoma masquerading as migraine. *Postgrad Med* 2006;**119**:70–3.

66. Ang LP, Ang LP. Current understanding of the treatment and outcome of acute primary angle-closure glaucoma: an Asian perspective. *Ann Acad Med Singapore* 2008;**37**: 210–15.

67. Lee DA, Higginbotham EJ. Glaucoma and its treatment: a review. *Am J Health Syst Pharm* 2005;**62**:691–9.

68. Fraunfelder FW, Fraunfelder FT, Keates EU. Topiramate-associated acute, bilateral secondary angle-closure glaucoma. *Ophthalmology* 2004;**111**:109–11.

69. Arnett BC. Tonsillar ectopia and headaches. *Neurol Clin N Am* 2004;**22**:229–36.

70. McGirt MJ, Nimjee SM, Floyd J, Bulsara KR, George TM. Correlation of cerebrospinal fluid flow dynamics and headache in Chiari I malformations. *Neurosurgery* 2005;**56**: 716–21.

71. Martins HA, Ribas VR, Lima MD, et al. Headache precipitated by Valsalva maneuvers in patients with congenital Chiari I malformation. *Arq Neuropsiquiatr* 2010;**68**:406–9.

72. Steinbok P. Clinical features of Chiari I malformation. *Childs Nerv Syst* 2004;**20**:329–31.

73. Wilson JF. In the clinic: Acute sinusitis. *Ann Intern Med* 2010;**153**:ITC31-15.

74. Cady RK, Dodick DW, Levine HL, et al. Sinus headache: a neurology, otolaryngology, allergy, and primary care consensus on diagnosis and treatment. *Mayo Clin Proc* 2005; **80**:908–16.

75. Cady RK, Wendt JK, Kirchner JR, Sargent JD, Rothrock JF, Skaggs H, Jr. Treatment of acute migraine with subcutaneous sumatriptan. *JAMA* 1991;**265**:2831–5.

76. Eross EJ, Dodick DW, Eross M. The sinus, allergy and migraine study (SAMS). *Headache* 2007;**47**:213–24.

77. Schreiber CP, Hutchinson S, Webster CJ, Ames M, Richardson MS, Powers C. Prevalence of migraine in patients with a history of self-reported or physician-diagnosed "sinus" headache. *Arch Int Med* 2004;**164**:1769–72.

78. Ahovou-Saloranta A, Borisenko OV, Kovanen N, et al. Antibiotics for acute maxillary sinusitis. *Cochrane Database Syst Rev* 2008;(**2**): CD000243.

Part II

Migraine

Diagnosis and Subtypes of Migraine

Seymour Solomon and Brian M. Grosberg

Albert Einstein College of Medicine, Bronx, NY, USA

Introduction

Although tension-type headache is the most prevalent type of headache, migraine is the most commonly seen in doctors' offices. It affects 12% of the population. The diagnostic criteria for migraine are now well established in the first and second editions of the International Classification of Headache Disorders (ICHD) [1]. The specific criteria have enabled many randomized-controlled trials of agents to treat the acute attacks and establish prophylactic measures. Nevertheless, migraine is greatly underdiagnosed and suboptimally treated.

Migraine may begin at any age, but the onset is usually in adolescence or young adult life. Before puberty, the female:male ratio is 1:1. After puberty, however, the female:male ratio is 3:1; migraine affects approximately 18% of women and 6% of men [2].

Clinical features of migraine

The two major types of migraine are migraine without aura (the majority of cases) and migraine with aura (representing about 20% of the total). The diagnostic criteria are listed in Table 4.1. The full-blown attack has four phases: premonitory, aura, headache, and postdrome. Most patients do not experience all four phases.

The *premonitory symptoms* occur hours or days before the headache and may be psychological, neurologic, or systemic [3, 4]. Depression, elation, irritability, apathy, hyperactivity, and drowsiness are examples of the psychological symptoms. Neurologic symptoms include photophobia, phonophobia, difficulty concentrating, and yawning. Examples of the many potential systemic symptoms are stiffness, coldness, thirst, food cravings, increased or decreased urination, and diarrhea or constipation.

The *aura* may arise from any area of the brain, and virtually any neurologic symptom may be the aura of migraine. It may precede or, less likely, accompany the headache. Typically, the aura evolves slowly over 5–20 minutes and lasts for 15–20 minutes but not more than 1 hour. Ninety percent of the time the aura is a positive visual phenomenon, such as an arc of scintillating lights or fortification spectra within homonymous visual fields. Other visual auras may be photopsias (flashes of light) or shimmering of vision (like heat waves) [5, 6].

Sensory phenomena are the next most common type of aura, manifested by paresthesias ascending from the hand up the arm to the face. Unusual auras are weakness, dysphasia, ataxia, dysarthria, and impaired consciousness. These unusual auras will be discussed later in the chapter in the

Headache, First Edition. Edited by Matthew S. Robbins, Brian M. Grosberg, and Richard B. Lipton.
© 2013 John Wiley & Sons, Ltd. Published 2013 by John Wiley & Sons, Ltd.

Table 4.1. ICHD diagnostic criteria for migraine

A. At least 5 attacks fulfilling criteria B–D
B. Headache attacks lasting 4–72 hours (untreated or unsuccessfully treated)
C. Headache has at least 2 of the following characteristics:
   1. Unilateral location
   2. Pulsating quality
   3. Moderate or severe pain intensity
   4. Aggravation by or causing avoidance of routine physical activity (e.g., walking or climbing stairs)
D. During headache, at least 1 of the following:
   1. Nausea and/or vomiting
   2. Photophobia and phonophobia
E. Not attributed to another disorder

section on familial hemiplegic migraine (FHM) and basilar-type migraine. Altered visual perceptions such as metamorphopsia, macropsia, or micropsia are most common in children and lead to the label of Alice in Wonderland syndrome. Sometimes a visual aura will fade away as the sensory aura develops [7, 8].

The ICHD criteria for migraine with aura focuses on the qualities of the aura rather than the headache. Typically, the headache has the characteristics of migraine without aura. However, auras have also been reported with cluster headache and other primary headache disorders [9–11]. Auras may also occur without headache. The latter phenomena most often occur in older individuals and have been called "late-life migrainous accompaniments." Repeated and stereotyped bouts of scintillating scotoma, which last for 15–25 minutes and occur without other focal symptoms, are almost pathognomonic for migraine with aura [12–14]. However, other symptoms must be differentiated from transient ischemic attacks (TIAs) or, less likely, focal seizures.

★ TIPS AND TRICKS

In contrast to TIAs and seizures, typical auras evolve slowly, last less than 1 hour, and manifest as positive features rather than negative ones (e.g., visual and sensory symptoms consist of bright spots instead of visual loss, and tingling rather than numbness or sensory loss).

Nevertheless imaging and other studies may be warranted to make the differentiation, especially when the symptoms first occur after age 40 years, when negative features are predominant, or when the aura is of atypical duration [15].

The *headache* of migraine is typically unilateral, throbbing, and moderate or severe in intensity. It is usually aggravated by physical activity. Its duration ranges from a few hours to all day (the ICHD criteria allowing 4–72 hours in an adult, and 1–72 hours in children). As the ICHD criteria note, only two of the four headache qualities need be present [1]. For example, in 40% of migraineurs the headache is bilateral. Usually, the headache varies from one side to the other during an attack or with subsequent attacks, but in 20% the headache is "locked" to the same side on repeated attacks [16]. Usually, the pain affects the temporal areas, but it often radiates to adjacent areas and even down the neck to the shoulder.

★ TIPS AND TRICKS

People with migraine may experience jabs or jolts of icepick-like head pain, lasting for seconds, independent of the migraine headaches. Labeled primary stabbing headache, these jabs and jolts of pain occur in about 40% of migraineurs [17].

In other patients, the initial phase of the headache may fulfill the criteria for episodic tension-type headache, but then the symptoms can evolve into migraine. Because these initial tension-type headaches respond to the triptans, they probably represent a *forme fruste* of migraine. When headache sufferers experience symptoms that meet all but one of the features listed in the ICHD criteria for migraine, their headaches are classified as "probable migraine." Recent studies have shown that the 1-year period prevalence of probable migraine is 4.5%, and more than 20% of these patients are severely disabled [18].

Associated phenomena

To fulfill the ICHD criteria, migraine attacks must be accompanied by nausea with or without vomiting, or hypersensitivity to light and sound (photophobia and phonophobia). Most patients experience all of these phenomena and more. Gastroparesis, or less frequently diarrhea, contributes to gastrointestinal distress and poor absorption of oral medication [19]. Blurred vision may occur. Hypersensitivity to odors (osmophobia) and touch (allodynia) are common. Dizziness may range from lightheadedness to vertigo. Any of the premonitory symptoms may extend into the headache phase; mood and mental changes are almost universal. There may be pallor or redness of the face. Sensations of heat or cold may also occur. Sometimes fluid retention is seen as periorbital edema.

> ✋ **CAUTION!**
>
> Pain or pressure over the paranasal sinuses, accompanied by nasal congestion, often leads to the false diagnosis of sinusitis and is followed by inappropriate therapy.

The associated symptoms, particularly nausea and vomiting, add to and may be the major cause of disability. A Migraine Disability Assessment (MIDAS) score is a useful measurement of the impact of migraine on patients' lives [20].

Postdromal phase

After the headache, the patient may feel "washed out" and experience any of the symptoms of the premonitory phase. This phase may last for hours or days.

Aggravating and ameliorating factors

The attack is often aggravated by external stimuli and ameliorated by their absence. Aggravation by normal physical activity such as climbing stairs is one of the ICHD criteria for migraine. Migraine is often made worse by menstruation. It may be triggered or aggravated by emotional stress, too much or too little sleep, changes in the weather, alcoholic beverages, and nitrate-containing foods such as hot dogs, chocolate, citrus fruits, and hard cheeses. During an attack, the migraine sufferer instinctively prefers to lie immobile in a quiet dark room. The patient should list present and past medications. Prompting may be necessary to include over-the-counter agents and birth control pills. A diary may help the patient to identify unrecognized triggers and then help to avoid them.

Basilar-type migraine and hemiplegic migraine

Two specific types of migraine with aura are basilar-type migraine and hemiplegic migraine. In basilar-type migraine, the aura arises in the posterior fossa region of the brain. The features may include dysarthria, ataxia, vertigo, tinnitus, hearing impairment, double vision, visual impairment in the nasal or temporal fields of both eyes (i.e., not homonymously), bilateral paresthesias, and a reduced level of consciousness.

Hemiplegic migraine is rare and is usually familial rather than sporadic. As the name implies, the aura is manifested by hemiparesis. Hemisensory impairment may also occur as well as symptoms of basilar-type migraine. Cerebellar ataxia occurs in 20% of patients with hemiplegic migraine. In contrast to typical auras, the motor defects often last more than 1 hour and as long as 24 hours. At least one first-degree relative has had similar attacks [21]. FHM is the first migraine type that has been linked to a set of specific genetic polymorphisms. The three known loci for FHM lie on chromosomes 1, 2, and 19 [22–26].

Childhood periodic syndromes that are commonly precursors of migraine

The common features of these disorders, which predominantly affect children and adolescents, are their recurrent, periodic nature and the co-association with migraine or a family history of migraine.

Cyclic vomiting occurs in infants and children, and rarely in adolescents or later in life. It is characterized by repeated and stereotyped episodes of nausea and vomiting, lasting from 1 hour to 5 days; these bouts may lead to dehydration. Between bouts, these children are healthy. Intermittent bowel obstruction, metabolic disease, and systemic disease must be ruled out before assigning a diagnosis of cyclic vomiting. General treatment measures include hydration and antiemetics [27].

Abdominal migraine affects children and is manifested by recurrent bouts of midline abdominal pain lasting from 1 hour to 3 days. Like migraine, the pain is moderate to severe in intensity and is often associated with anorexia, nausea, vomiting, and pallor, but occurs without headache or head pain. Gastrointestinal and renal disease need to be excluded before this diagnosis can be made [28].

Benign paroxysmal vertigo of childhood more often occurs in younger rather than older children. Rarely, this condition can occur in adults. It is characterized by recurrent attacks of sudden unsteadiness or vertigo, with no alteration in the affected individual's level of consciousness. Vomiting may or may not occur, and nystagmus may be noted on examination. The symptoms usually last a few minutes, and afterwards the child is normal and will resume play or want to sleep. The episodes often occur in clusters over days to weeks and then subside. The most common triggering factor for benign paroxysmal vertigo is fatigue. Neurologic examination and audiometric and vestibular functions are all normal between attacks. Benign recurrent vertigo often coexists with migraine and is a comorbid condition [29].

Retinal migraine

Retinal migraine is a rare and poorly understood disorder manifested by recurrent attacks of fully reversible monocular visual impairment occurring before or during migraine headache. The visual symptoms may be a positive scintillation or negative visual loss. The patient should be asked to cover one eye and then the other during the attacks to differentiate the monocular defect from the much more common homonymous symptom of migraine with aura. Other causes of monocular visual loss must be considered, including optic neuritis, retinal detachment, and TIAs. A recent review suggests that a high percentage of patients with retinal migraine may develop a permanent residual visual field defect [30, 31].

Complications of migraine

Several possible complications of migraine include chronic migraine, status migrainosus, persistent aura without infarction, migrainous infarction, and migraine-triggered seizure.

The most common complication of migraine is *chronic migraine*, a disorder defined by headaches of more than 4 hours' duration occurring on 15 or more days per month for at least 3 months. Episodic migraine often increases in frequency to become a daily or almost daily headache. This transformation usually occurs over 3 or more months. As migraine episodes increase in frequency, they often lose many of the characteristics of migraine and take on the features of tension-type headache. However, to be classified as chronic migraine, they should have evolved from episodic migraine, with 8 or more days of headache per month fulfilling the criteria for migraine without aura. Other daily or almost daily primary and secondary headaches must be excluded.

To complicate matters, the evolution of episodic migraine or tension-type headache to a daily or almost daily headache is usually associated with overuse of medication(s) designed to treat acute attacks. Medication overuse headache is defined as a headache that is present on 15 or more days per month, occurring in the setting of regular overuse of one or more acute symptomatic treatment drugs for more than 3 months. These include acute antimigraine drugs and/or opioids or combination analgesics taken on more than 10 days a month, or simple over-the-counter analgesics taken on more than 15 days a month.

> ✋ **CAUTION!**
>
> Before assigning a diagnosis of chronic migraine, medication overuse headache must be excluded [32, 33].

Status migrainosus is the term used when an attack of migraine lasts for more than 72 hours and the intensity or disability continues to be severe. Patients with status migrainosus require aggressive treatment, which may include fluid and electrolyte replacement, drug detoxification, intravenous pharmacotherapy to control pain, treatment of nausea and vomiting, and concurrent implementation of migraine prophylaxis (if indicated) [34].

Persistent aura without infarction is diagnosed when aura symptoms, otherwise typical for the patient, persist for more than 1 week without radiographic or physical evidence of infarction.

Persisting aura symptoms are rare. They are often bilateral and may last for months or years. There is currently insufficient clinical information to support specific recommendations for the medical therapy of persistent aura without infarction, although acetazolamide and valproic acid have helped in a few cases [35–37].

Migrainous infarction fortunately is a rare occurrence. In this situation, an otherwise typical aura lasts for more than 1 hour, and neurologic examination with neuroimaging reveals a brain infarct. The neurologic deficit develops during the course of an otherwise typical attack of migraine with aura, and mimics the aura of previous attacks. Other causes of stroke should be excluded [38].

Migraine and epilepsy are comorbid, but *migraine-triggered seizures* are a rare occurrence. The seizure occurs during the migraine attack or within 1 hour after the end of the aura. This phenomenon, sometimes referred to as migralepsy, has been described in patients with migraine with aura [39].

Comorbidities of migraine

Comorbidity refers to the association in the same individual of two conditions whose occurrence is greater than coincidental chance. Table 4.2 outlines a list of the conditions that can occur comorbidly with migraine.

Table 4.2. Comorbidities of migraine

Neurologic
Epilepsy
Stroke
Psychiatric
Depression
Bipolar disease
Anxiety disorders
Panic disorder
Cardiac
Myocardial infarction
Angina
Patent foramen ovale
Other
Raynaud's syndrome
Irritable bowel syndrome
Asthma
Other pain disorders

The relationship of migraine to vascular disease is particularly troublesome. Ischemic stroke occurs one and one half times more commonly in women with aura than in matched controls. The risk rises in women who have migraine with aura and become pregnant, and the incidence is especially high in those who smoke [40]. These figures are alarming at first glance, but the absolute number of strokes in women with migraine is very small. On the other hand, subclinical cerebellar infarcts as seen on MRI scanning occur much more often in people with migraine than in a control group. This is especially so in those who have auras and more than one attack per month [41]. Similarly, white matter abnormalities on the MRI are seen four times more often in people with migraine than in a control population. These are probably of vascular origin but appear to be clinically insignificant [42].

In spite of all of the above, people with migraine can be assured that they should have a normal, long and healthy life.

References

1. Headache Classification Committee of the International Headache Society. The International Classification of Headache Disorders. *Cephalalgia* 2004;**24**:1–160.
2. Stewart WF, Simon D, Shechter A, Lipton RB. Population variation in migraine prevalence: a meta-analysis. *J Clin Epidemiol* 1995;**48**: 269–80.
3. Giffin NJ, Ruggiero L, Lipton RB. Premonitory symptoms in migraine: an electronic diary study. *Neurology* 2003;**60**(6):935–40.
4. Schoonman GG, Evers DJ, Terwindt GM, van Dijk JG, Ferrari MD. The prevalence of premonitory symptoms in migraine: a questionnaire study in 461 patients. *Cephalalgia* 2006;**26**(10):1209–13.
5. Silberstein SD, Young WB. Migraine aura and prodrome. *Semin Neurol* 1995;**45**:175–82.

6. Klee A, Willanger R. Disturbances of visual perception in migraine. *Acta Neurol Scand* 1966;**42**:400–14.

7. Russel MB, Olesen J. A nosographic analysis of the migraine aura in a general population. *Brain* 1996;**119**:355–61.

8. Hosking G. Special forms: variants of migraine in childhood. In Hockday JM (ed.), *Migraine in Childhood*. Boston, MA: Butterworth; 1988: pp. 35–53.

9. Matharu MJ, Goadsby PJ. Post-traumatic chronic paroxysmal hemicrania (CPH) with aura. *Neurology* 2001;**56**:273–5.

10. Peres MF, Siow HC, Rozen TD. Hemicrania continua with aura. *Cephalalgia* 2002;**22**: 246–8.

11. Silberstein SD, Niknam R, Rozen TD, et al. Cluster headache with aura. *Neurology* 2000;**54**:219–21.

12. Whitty CVM. Migraine without headache. *Lancet* 1967;**ii**:283–5.

13. Willey RG. The scintillating scotoma without headache. *Ann Ophthalmol* 1979;**11**:581–5.

14. Ziegler DK, Hanassein RS. Specific headache phenomena: their frequency and coincidence. *Headache* 1990;**30**:152–60.

15. Fisher CM. Late-life migraine accompaniments as a cause of unexplained transient ischemic attacks. *Can J Neurol Sci* 1980; **7**:9–17.

16. Selby G, Lance JW. Observations on 500 cases of migraine and allied vascular headaches. *J Neurol Neurosurg Psychiatry* 1960;**23**:23–32.

17. Raskin NH, Schwartz RK. Icepick-like pain. *Neurology* 1980;**30**:203–5.

18. Silberstein S, Loder E, Diamond S, Reed ML, Bigal ME, Lipton RB; AMPP Advisory Group. Probable migraine in the United States: results of the American Migraine Prevalence and Prevention (AMPP) study. *Cephalalgia* 2007;**27**(3):220–34.

19. Boyle R, Behan PO, Sutton JA. A correlation between severity of migraine and delayed gastric emptying measured by an epigastric impedance method. *Br J Clin Pharmacol* 1990;**30**:405–9.

20. Lipton RB, Stewart WF, Sawyer J, Edmeads JG. Clinical utility of an instrument assessing migraine disability: the Migraine Disability Assessment (MIDAS) questionnaire. *Headache* 2001;**41**(9):854–61.

21. Staehelin-Jensen T, Olivarius B, Kraft M, Hansen H. Familial hemiplegic migraine. A reappraisal and long-term follow up study. *Cephalalgia* 1981;**1**:33–9.

22. Carrera P, Stenirri S, Ferrari M, Battistini S. Familial hemiplegic migraine: an ion channel disorder. *Brain Res Bull* 2001;**56**:239–41.

23. De Fusco M, Marconi R, Silvestri L, et al. Haploinsufficiency of ATP1A2 encoding the Na$^+$/K$^+$ pump alpha2 subunit associated with familial hemiplegic migraine type 2. *Nat Genet* 2003;**33**:192–6.

24. Ducros A, Denier C, Joutel A, et al. The clinical spectrum of familial hemiplegic migraine associated with mutations in a neuronal calcium channel. *N Engl J Med* 2001;**345**:17–24.

25. Ophoff RA, Terwindt GM, Vergouwe MN, et al. Familial hemiplegic migraine and episodic ataxia type-2 are caused by mutations in the Ca2+ channel gene CACNL1A4. *Cell* 1996;**87**:543–52.

26. Ophoff RA, Terwindt GM, Vergouwe MN, et al. Wolff Award 1997. Involvement of a Ca2+ channel gene in familial hemiplegic migraine and migraine with and without aura. Dutch Migraine Genetics Research Group. *Headache* 1997;**37**:479–85.

27. Li BU. Cyclic vomiting syndrome. *Curr Treat Options Gastroenterol* 2000;**3**(5):395–402.

28. Catto-Smith AG, Ranuh R. Abdominal migraine and cyclical vomiting. *Semin Pediatr Surg* 2003;**12**(4):254–8.

29. Drigo P, Carli G, Laverda AM. Benign paroxysmal vertigo of childhood. *Brain Dev* 2001; **23**:38–41.

30. Grosberg BM, Solomon S, Lipton RB. Retinal migraine. *Curr Pain Headache Rep* 2005;**9**: 268–71.

31. Grosberg BM, Solomon S, Friedman DI, Lipton RB. Retinal migraine reappraised. *Cephalalgia* 2006;**26**:1275–86.

32. Silberstein SD, Lipton RB, Saper JR. Chronic daily headache including transformed migraine, chronic tension-type headache, and medication overuse headache. In Silberstein SD, Lipton RB, Dodick DW (eds.), *Wolff's Headache and Other Head Pain*. New York: Oxford University Press; 2008: pp. 315–77.

33. Katsarava Z, Fritsche G, Muessig M, Diener HC, Limmroth V. Clinical features of with-

drawn headache following overuse of triptans and other headache drugs. *Neurology* 2001; **57**:1694–8.

34. Silberstein SD, Freitag FG, Bigal ME. Migraine treatment. In Silberstein SD, Lipton RB, Dodick DW (eds.), *Wolff's Headache and Other Head Pain.* New York: Oxford University Press; 2008: pp. 177–292.

35. Haas DC. Prolonged migraine aura status. *Ann Neurology* 1982;**11**:197–9.

36. Haan J, Sluis P, Sluis IH, Ferrari MD. Acetazolamide treatment for migraine aura status. *Neurology* 2000;**55**:1588–9.

37. Rothrock JF. Successful treatment of persistent migraine aura with divalproex sodium. *Neurology* 1997;**48**:261–2.

38. Rothrock JF, Walicke P, Swenson MR, et al. Migrainous stroke. *Arch Neurol* 1988;**45**: 63–7.

39. Marks DA, Ehrenberg BL. Migraine-related seizures in adults with epilepsy, with EEG correlation. *Neurology* 1993;**43**:2476–83.

40. Welch KM. Stroke and migraine – the spectrum of cause and effect. *Funct Neurology* 2003;**18**:121–6.

41. Kruit MC, van Buchem MA, Hofman PA, et al. Migraine as a risk factor for subclinical brain lesions. *JAMA* 2004;**291**(4):427–34.

42. Swartz RH, Kern RZ. Migraine is associated with MRI white matter abnormalities: a meta-analysis. *Arch Neurol* 2004;**61**:1366–8.

Epidemiology, Progression, Prognosis, and Comorbidity of Migraine

Richard B. Lipton[1,2], C. Mark Sollars[2], and Dawn C. Buse[1,2]

[1]Albert Einstein College of Medicine, Bronx, NY, USA
[2]Montefiore Headache Center, Bronx, NY, USA

Introduction

Understanding the epidemiology of migraine is important for a number of reasons. Epidemiologic data define the scope and distribution of the public health problem imposed by migraine. This will facilitate planning to meet the needs of persons with migraine and to remediate the burden of the disorder. Epidemiologic studies provide information about the rates and risk factors for the onset, progression, and remission of migraine.

Clinical observation and longitudinal population studies demonstrate that a small subgroup of persons with episodic migraine (EM) progress to chronic migraine (CM) every year. Because only a minority progress, understanding the risk factors, particularly the remedial risk factors associated with progression, provides a first step toward clarifying mechanisms and developing preventive interventions. Transitions are bidirectional as both EM and CM may remit.

Migraine can be disabling and burdensome and often affects individuals' occupational, academic, social, family and personal functioning [1, 2, 3]. The burden of migraine occurs both during and between attacks [4, 5]. In this chapter, we review the epidemiology, burden, and common comorbidities of EM and CM. Next, we consider the prognosis of EM and factors that may contribute to the development of CM. We close with a brief discussion of the clinical implications of these data.

🔬 SCIENCE REVISITED

The American Migraine Prevalence and Prevention (AMPP) is a longitudinal US population-based study. In 2004, surveys were mailed to a sample of 120,000 US households selected to represent the population according to census data for age, sex, race, income, and region of the country. Surveys were returned by 77,879 households (a 64.9% response rate), yielding data for 162,756 household members aged 12 years or older. There were 30,721 respondents who reported experiencing "severe headache." Usable data were obtained from 30,291 individuals, of whom 28,261 reported having experienced "severe headache" in the preceding year.

Stratified by gender, 17.37% of females and 5.7% of males had EM, and 0.91% met

Headache, First Edition. Edited by Matthew S. Robbins, Brian M. Grosberg, and Richard B. Lipton.
© 2013 John Wiley & Sons, Ltd. Published 2013 by John Wiley & Sons, Ltd.

criteria for CM (1.29% of females, and 0.48% of males) [6, 7]. Follow-up surveys were administered annually from 2005 to 2009 to 24,000 of the respondents to the 2004 survey who reported experiencing "severe" headache. Data including headache frequency, symptoms, sociodemographics, and headache-related disability, comorbidities, medication use, healthcare resource utilization, and related costs have been collected and analyzed.

Epidemiology of migraine

A review of migraine epidemiology can be approached by evaluating various factors in both EM and CM.

Episodic migraine: prevalence and incidence

Prevalence by age and gender

Estimates of the 1-year prevalence of migraine have remained remarkably stable across different populations and time points. Three large-scale population studies in the USA conducted over a 15-year period demonstrate this consistency with prevalence estimates of 12% overall, 18% in females, and 6% in males (Table 5.1). Migraine is significantly more common in females, but the female:male gender prevalence ratio varies with age. A recent analysis from the AMPP study found that the adjusted female:male prevalence ratios for migraine ranged from 1.5 to 1 for those aged 12–17 years, to 3.25 to 1 for those 18–29 years old [8]. Migraine was not only more common in females than in males, but was also more severe. For example, females were more likely to have aura, to experience most migraine-related symptoms, to use prescription medications and emergency department/urgent care clinics for headache, and to have greater

headache-related impairment. Despite higher rates of migraine diagnosis, females with migraine were not more likely than males to be using preventive pharmacologic treatment for headache.

Prior to puberty, migraine may be more common in boys than girls. After puberty, the prevalence of migraine rises gradually in males and much more rapidly in females. In the AMPP, the prevalence of migraine in individuals aged 12–19 years was 6.3% (boys 5.0%, girls 7.7%) [9]. Throughout adolescence, the prevalence in boys (adjusted for socioeconomic factors) increased from 2.9% to 4.1% The adjusted prevalence in girls peaked at age 17 at 9.8%.

Prevalence by socioeconomic status and race

North American studies consistently find an inverse relationship between the prevalence of migraine and socioeconomic status, as measured by income or education. European studies have conflicting findings. The American Migraine Study I (AMS-I), AMS-II, and AMPP have examined prevalence in a large population of Americans and found correlations between declining household income and increasing prevalence of migraine [5, 10, 11]. These findings were confirmed by a study from the UK. In contrast, studies from the Netherlands, Denmark, and Canada do not support this inverse relationship [12, 13, 14].

Researchers propose two hypotheses to account for the inverse relationship between migraine prevalence and socioeconomic status. The social causation hypothesis suggests that a factor associated with low income, such as a stressful lifestyle or poor diet, may increase the rate of migraine onset. The social selection hypothesis states that illness itself interferes with social or occupational function and causes low income. As discussed below, persons from low-income households have a higher incidence of migraine, supporting the social causation hypothesis [15].

Table 5.1. Comparison of three US population studies of migraine prevalence

Study	Survey year	Subjects	Migraine prevalence (%)		
			Overall	Males	Females
AMS-I [123]	1989	20,468	12.1	5.7	17.6
AMS-II [11]	1999	29,727	12.6	6.5	18.2
AMPP [124]	2004	162,576	11.7	5.6	17.1

Table 5.2. Comparison of migraine point prevalence worldwide

Region	Male prevalence (number of studies)	Female prevalence (number of studies)	Overall prevalence (number of studies)
Global	6% (41)	14% (43)	11% (41)
Africa	3% (4)	6% (4)	5% (5)
Asia	6% (8)	11% (8)	9% (8)
Australia	–	22% (1)	–
Europe	7% (13)	18% (14)	15% (14)
North America	6% (7)	18% (7)	13% (9)
Central/South America	4% (10)	12% (10)	9% (10)

Reproduced from Stovner LJ, Hagen K, Jensen R et al. *Cephalalgia* 27(3): 2007 [18]. Reprinted with permission of SAGE.

After adjusting for socioeconomic status, migraine prevalence varies by race in the USA [17]. The prevalence is highest in white females and males (20.4% and 8.6%, respectively), intermediate in African-American females and males (16.2% and 7.2%, respectively), and lowest in Asian-American females and males (9.2%, 4.2%, respectively) [10]. A meta-analysis of studies conducted using the International Criteria for Headache Disorders (ICHD) [1, 16] criteria for migraine showed that the prevalence of migraine was highest in North America and Europe and lower in Asia and Africa, supporting these differences by race (Table 5.2) [2].

> **SCIENCE REVISITED**
>
> Lifting the Burden: The Global Campaign Against Headache, developed in concert with the World Health Organization, undertook a major initiative to determine the prevalence of migraine around the world. They found that migraine prevalence was highest in Europe, and lowest in Africa [18]. These differences by region of the world and race could be explained by genetic differences, environmental differences, or both. Results of the study, patient education and handouts, questionnaires, and other useful information are available in print and online at http://www.who.int/mental_health/neurology/headache/en/index.html.

Incidence of episodic migraine

Incidence refers to the rate of onset of new cases of a disease in a defined population over a given period of time, and is usually expressed as new cases per 1000 person–years of follow-up. To determine incidence, one common approach is to screen the population of interest to identify current cases of migraine. The migraine-free population is then followed to identify new cases. This approach was taken by the Copenhagen group in a 12-year longitudinal study. The incidence of migraine was 8.1 per 1000 person–years, with a female:male ratio of 6.2:1 [19]. No significant differences in age or gender were found when comparing migraine with aura (MA) and migraine without aura (MO). Incidence declined with age, peaking in 25- to 34-year-old females at 23 per 1000 person–years, and in males at about 10 per 1000 person–years. In the 55–64 years of age group, the incidence was less than 5 per 1000 person–years.

Recently, migraine incidence was estimated in the AMPP study [20]. This study used reported age of onset among prevalent cases to model age incidence profiles using the reconstructed cohort method. The incidence of migraine peaked in the 20- to 24-year age group in females (18.2 per 1000 person–years), and in the 15- to 19-year-old age group in males (6.2 per 1000 person–years). Broadly, these findings agree with the results of the Copenhagen study. The median age of onset was 25 years in females and 24 years in males, and the cumulative lifetime incidence was 43% in females and 18% in males.

These values are far higher than the 1-year period prevalence of migraine in the same population, probably indicating a high rate of migraine remission. Earlier studies using reconstructed cohort methods found an earlier age of migraine onset [21]; the study sample may have been too young (12–29 years). A follow-up analysis in the AMPP assessed the influence of income on incidence of migraine: migraine incidence was highest in persons from low-income households, supporting the social causation hypothesis.

Chronic migraine: prevalence and incidence

Prevalence of chronic migraine

Global estimates of the prevalence of CM typically range from 1.4% to 2.2% depending on a number of factors [22]. A recent systematic review examined the influence of diagnostic criteria on prevalence estimates for CM, using various definitions and criteria [23]. The prevalence of transformed migraine (a term that was previously used for a condition similar to CM) ranged from 0.86% to 5.1%, whereas the prevalence of CM was generally lower, ranging from 0% to 0.7%. When the studies were pooled together, transformed migraine or CM was more prevalent in Europe, followed by the Western Pacific and then the Americas. The prevalence of CM in adolescents was estimated at 0.76% (confidence interval [CI] 0.05%–1.48%), with a gradual rise with increasing age through the teenage years. The prevalence was higher in teenage girls than boys (1.39% versus 0.15%).

A recent analysis of US population data from the AMPP study found a prevalence of 0.91% overall (1.29% of females, and 0.48% of males) [5]. Modified Silberstein–Lipton criteria were used to classify CM (meeting the ICHD-2 criteria for migraine with a headache frequency of ≥15 days over the preceding 3 months) [23]. Relative to 12- to 17-year-olds, the age- and sex-specific prevalence for CM peaked in the 40s at 1.89% for females and 0.79% for males (prevalence ratio 3.35, 95% CI 1.99–5.63). The gender prevalence ratio was 4.57 (95% CI 3.13–6.67). As discussed for migraine, the prevalence of CM was inversely related to household income. CM represented 7.7% of migraine cases overall (excluding proba-

ble migraine), and the proportion generally increased with age.

Incidence of chronic migraine

Few data are available on the incidence of CM in the population, as CM usually progresses from EM. An analysis of data from 8219 individuals with EM from the AMPP database in 2005 found that 2.5% developed CM in 2006 [24]. The incidence of CM in the general population requires further study. Risk factors for onset of CM in persons with EM are presented in Table 5.3.

Burden of migraine

Migraine is a highly burdensome condition for individual sufferers, families, and society. The 2001 World Health Organization report cited 135 health conditions, particularly mental and neurologic disorders, that accounted for nearly 40% of all years lived with disability worldwide. Migraine was cited as the 19th leading cause of years lived with disability overall, and is the 12th leading cause of years lived with disability among females of all ages [25]. Migraine can impact the function of the individual in multiple roles and settings including occupational, academic, social, familial, and personal [1, 2, 3]. The societal burden is magnified in that migraine prevalence is highest in the second, third, fourth, and fifth decades of life, when productivity is often at its peak.

The burden of migraine occurs both during (ictal) and between (interictal) attacks [4, 26]. The ictal burden is related to head pain, nausea, vomiting, and sensitivity to environmental stimuli, all of which limit function during attacks. The interictal burden is related to difficulty in planning and fear of the next attack, among other factors. Anxiety in anticipation of the next migraine attack (i.e., interictal anxiety) may lead migraineurs to use acute pain medications before any symptoms of an attack occur, ultimately resulting in the overuse of these medications. Avoidance of activities because of fear of headache (i.e., cephalalgiaphobia) is a contributor to the interictal burden of migraine. Cephalalgiaphobia may also decrease the threshold for initiating the consumption of analgesics, leading to medication overuse [27].

Table 5.3. Risk factors for progression from EM to CM or CDH, and recommended interventions

Variable	Modifiable status	Recommended intervention(s)
Younger age [77]	Non-modifiable	N/A
Low education/ socioeconomic status [77]	Non-modifiable	N/A
Head or neck injury [79]	Non-modifiable	N/A
White race [77]	Non-modifiable	N/A
Medical comorbidities (e.g., arthritis, diabetes) [77]	Potentially modifiable	Assess, treat (or refer for treatment) medical conditions with appropriate pharmacologic and behavioral interventions
Headache/attack frequency [24, 77, 125]	Potentially modifiable	Treat headache disorder with appropriate migraine-specific acute medications, consider adding preventive medications and behavioral interventions
Obesity [77]	Modifiable	Treat (or refer for treatment) obesity with appropriate pharmacologic and behavioral interventions including education, diet, and exercise. Consider use of headache diary and cognitive behavioral therapy. Avoid preventive medications that lead to weight gain, consider use of preventive medications that may lead to weight loss
Snoring/sleep apnea [78]	Modifiable	Treat snoring/sleep apnea (or refer for treatment) with appropriate pharmacologic and behavioral interventions
Medication overuse [24]	Modifiable	Monitor medication misuse or overuse, modify treatment regime, consider migraine-specific acute medications, preventive medications, and behavioral interventions, follow detoxification protocols
Caffeine intake [82]	Modifiable	Monitor and reduce caffeine intake. Consider use of patient diary. Teach patient about all sources of caffeine including medication and dietary
Major life changes/SLEs [83]	Modifiable	Assess and monitor stress, refer to psychologist for treatment with cognitive behavioral therapy to teach stress management, cognitive restructuring, coping skills, biofeedback and relaxation techniques
Comorbid pain syndromes (e.g., neck pain) [43, 126]	Modifiable	Assess, treat (or refer for treatment) pain conditions with appropriate pharmacologic and behavioral interventions. Consider prophylactic treatments that may simultaneously improve migraine and comorbid syndrome. Consider physical and occupational therapy

Table 5.3. (*Continued*)

Variable	Modifiable status	Recommended intervention(s)
Psychiatric comorbidities (e.g., depression [102], anxiety [105])	Modifiable	Assess and monitor psychiatric conditions with validated instruments (e.g., PHQ-9, GAD-7), refer for treatment as appropriate for medication (psychiatry) and cognitive behavioral therapy to teach stress management, cognitive restructuring, coping skills, biofeedback, and relaxation techniques (psychology)
Allodynia and central sensitization [88]	Modifiable	Treat headache disorder with appropriate migraine-specific acute and preventive medications and behavioral interventions. Avoid medications that potentiate allodynia, particularly opiates. Educate patient to treat attacks early

GAD, generalized anxiety disorder; N/A, not applicable.
Reproduced from Lipton RB, Bigal ME. Migraine: epidemiology, impact and risk factors for progression. *Headache* 2005; 45(Suppl. 1): S1–S13 [75].

★ TIPS AND TRICKS

Effective communication between healthcare providers and patients is an integral to achieving good outcomes [28]. Asking about headache-related disability improves outcomes by helping healthcare providers to develop treatment plans that are matched to the severity of illness [29].

Several validated instruments are available to add in the assessment of headache-related disability and headache impact. The Migraine Disability Assessment (MIDAS) scale is a well-validated, brief tool that can be used to assess and track disability and is available free of charge [30]. MIDAS is scored in units of lost days due to headache over 3 months in the domains of work and school, household work and chores, and family, social, and leisure activities. Scores range from 0 to 270. Responses are summed and coded into four grades of headache-related disability: Grade I, little or no disability (0–5); Grade II, mild disability (6–10); Grade III, moderate disability (11–20); Grade IV: severe disability (≥21). A large percentage of MIDAS sum scores for persons with CM fall into Grade IV, which limits the ability of the MIDAS score to differentiate severity of headache-related disability among persons with CM. To address this issue, researchers have subdivided Grade IV into two categories: Grade IV-A, severe disability (21–40); and Grade IV-B, very severe disability (41–270) [31]. The Headache Impact Test (HIT-6) [32] is a shorter version of a longer Web-based adaptive test and assesses activity limitations in several domains as well as pain severity, fatigue, frustration, and difficulty with concentration.

Alternatively, studies have shown that the simple statement "Tell me about your headaches and how they affect your life" opens a dialogue about headache that improves healthcare provider and patient satisfaction and appropriate treatment while shortening visit length [33].

The health-related quality of life (HRQoL) burden of EM is high, comparable to other chronic illnesses such as hypertension, diabetes, and congestive heart failure [34]. Researchers compared HRQoL among individuals with and without migraine in a population-based, case–control study of the residents of Greater London [35]. They conducted a telephone survey with 200 randomly selected migraineurs and 200 matched nonmigraineur participants. The migraineurs scored significantly lower than the controls on HRQoL, which was found to be inversely related to headache-related disability.

Indirect costs make up most of the economic burden of migraine, which largely take the form of lost productive time. The indirect cost (i.e., excluding direct medical costs) of migraine to US employers is enormous and is estimated at $13 billion annually [36]. In a survey of lost productive time due to common pain conditions in the US workforce over a 2-week period, Stewart and colleagues found that headache was the most commonly reported pain condition (followed by back pain and arthritis), leading to a loss of productive time of 3.5 ± 0.1 hours per week [37]. Using a large employer database, Hawkins and colleagues determined that employees with recognized migraine each cost the employer approximately $2800 more annually than employees without migraine, because of absenteeism, short-term disability, and workers' compensation claims [36].

Both clinic- and population-based studies have demonstrated that, in comparison to those with EM, persons with CM have greater headache-related disability [5, 38, 39] and impact of headache [32], lower socioeconomic status [7], decrements in HRQoL [40], higher rates of comorbid medical and psychiatric conditions [7, 41], increased healthcare resource utilization [39], and higher direct and indirect costs [42]. An analysis of 24,000 individuals with "severe" headache who responded to the 2005 AMPP survey identified 655 respondents with CM and 11,249 respondents with EM. Respondents with CM (relative to EM) had statistically significantly lower levels of household income, were less likely to be employed full time, and were more likely to be occupationally disabled [7]. In addition, persons with CM (relative to EM) had much higher rates of headache-related disability (assessed with MIDAS). Among persons with CM, 24.8% had MIDAS scores that were in MIDAS Grade IV-B ("very severe" headache-related disability), in comparison with just 3.2% of those in the EM group. After adjusting for sociodemographic covariates, the odds of increased headache-related disability among persons with CM (relative to EM) were nearly four times greater (odds ratio [OR] 3.90, 95% CI 3.54–4.31; $P < 0.001$). Headache-related disability was highest among females. Among females with CM, 26.3% had "very severe" headache-related disability, compared to only 3.4% of those with EM. Among males with CM, 20.3% had "very severe" headache-related disability, compared to 2.7% of those with EM.

An analysis of the HIT-6 from the AMPP study revealed a similar pattern [32]. Individuals with CM were significantly more likely to experience "severe" impact of headache (72.9% versus 42.3% of those with EM), as were individuals who were younger, experienced more migraine symptoms (other than pain) and at greater intensity, reported more severe head pain, and met the criteria for depression.

This same pattern was seen in the International Burden of Illness Study, a Web-based survey of nearly 20,000 participants from nine countries [31]. CM participants had significantly greater headache-related disability (mean MIDAS sum scores) than EM participants. In addition, those with CM also reported greater healthcare resource utilization, including twice as many primary care visits, three times as many neurologist visits, and 1.5 times as many emergency department visits using the EM group for comparison.

Comorbidities of migraine

Comorbidity is defined as the greater than chance association of two or more disorders in the same individual. Medical disorders comorbid with migraine include asthma, myocardial infarction, obstructive sleep apnea, Raynaud's phenomenon, systemic lupus erythematosus, and nonheadache pain disorders, including temporomandibular disorder (TMD) and fibromyalgia [43, 44, 45]. Neurologic comorbidities include epilepsy, stroke, restless legs syndrome, and multiple sclerosis. Psychiatric comorbidities include depression, anxiety, and bipolar disease, among others. Although all of these conditions are, evidence from rigorous population studies is variable.

Cardiovascular disease

Many studies show that migraine is a risk factor for cardiovascular disease (CVD). Prior to 2004, 11 case–control studies, three cohort studies, and one cross-sectional study examined this link. A subsequent meta-analysis suggested that both MA and MO might be associated with ischemic stroke, and that this risk seemed higher in females, oral contraceptive users, and adults younger than age 45 years [46]. Data from the Atherosclerotic Risk in Communities study showed an association between MA and transient ischemic attack or stroke symptoms and verified ischemic stroke; however, this study did not adjust for risk factors for CVD at the time of the headache history [47]. Scher et al. demonstrated that migraineurs (especially those with MA) have a higher CVD risk profile than people without migraine [48].

Two large-scale, prospective, cohort population studies examined migraine as an independent risk factor for CVD. In the Women's Health Study, Kurth et al. examined the 385 strokes that occurred in a population of nearly 40,000 female healthcare professionals aged 45 or older, all of whom lacked a history of CVD, cancer, or any other major illness [49]. MA was defined as a "warning" of impending headache, a definition that may include premonitory features. Migraineurs overall, as well as participants reporting MO, had no increased stroke risk (of any type), but persons with MA had an increased risk of total and ischemic stroke. Investigators then evaluated the association between MA and MO and the subsequent risk of ischemic CVD events in a 10-year mean follow-up period, which included a cohort of patients with active migraine (3610 females) [50]. Females with active MA had a doubling of their risk for major CVD, ischemic stroke, nonfatal myocardial infarction, coronary revascularization, angina, and death. Females reporting active MO had no increased risk of any of the above CVD outcomes. Females having MA

with the fewest conventional CVD risk factors (Framingham score) may be disproportionately at risk for an adverse CVD event [51]. A parallel analysis from the Physicians' Health Study assessed male physicians aged 40 or older lacking a history of CVD, cancer, or other major illnesses [52]. Males with migraine were at increased risk of major CVD and myocardial infarction. This study did not differentiate between MA and MO.

MA is a risk factor for brain lesions. These lesions include deep white matter lesions, subtentorial white matter lesions, and stroke-like posterior circulation areas. A large population study of persons with MA, MO, and controls showed that posterior circulation stroke-like lesions were more likely in the MA group and more common in those with more attacks of MA [53]. The adjusted OR for MA was 13.7 (95% CI 1.7–112), with an even higher figure for MA patients with more than one attack per month, who had an OR of 15.8 (95% CI 1.8–140).

A recent follow-up study reimaged the same patients at an average interval of 9 years. Comparison with the baseline images revealed a statistically significant increase in the number of deep white matter lesions, particularly in the group of females reporting MO. Although there was not a statistically significant increased risk for posterior circulation stroke or cognitive decline, there was a nonsignificant trend in the direction of more difficulty for the MA group [54].

A meta-analysis of the migraine stroke data showed that the risk for ischemic stroke was doubled for migraineurs. However, the increased risk was carried entirely by those with MA versus those with MO. Further, the meta-analysis indicated that females were twice as susceptible to ischemic stroke as males [55].

A meta-analysis of the relationship between migraine and patent foramen ovale (PFO), was conducted by Schwedt et al. [56]. The overall association between PFO and migraine was validated, with an OR of 5.13 (95% CI 4.67–5.59). The association was weaker for PFO and MA, with an OR of 3.21 (95% CI 2.38–4.17). Evidence that closure of PFO had a beneficial impact on migraine was deemed low grade, and insufficient to draw any conclusions [57].

Epilepsy

Migraine and epilepsy are both chronic disorders with episodic manifestations related to neuronal hyperexcitability [58]. Using the Epilepsy Family Study of Columbia University, the comorbidity of these neurologic disorders was demonstrated, with a twofold bidirectional risk [59]. This association may be due to shared genetic susceptibility in some individuals and shared environmental risk factors in others [60].

Psychiatric condition

Migraine occurs comorbidly with several psychiatric disorders including depression, anxiety disorders, bipolar disorder, post-traumatic stress disorder, personality disorders, and suicide attempts. In a large health plan-based study, the prevalence of major depression was highest in subjects with ICHD-2-defined migraine, at 29.1%; the prevalence in probable migraine and nonmigraine controls was 19.5% and 10.3%, respectively [61]. A large Norwegian population study assessed depression and anxiety disorders in more than 50,000 persons with migraine, other nonmigraine headache, and headache-free controls. The comorbidity estimates for depression and anxiety were adjusted for the prevalence of the other psychiatric comorbidities [62]. Relative to the headache-free controls, the adjusted ORs for depression and anxiety in persons with migraine were 1.9 (95% CI 1.6–2.3) and 2.7 (95% CI 2.4–3.1), respectively. When the subjects were classified by tertiles of headache frequency, the adjusted OR of both depression and anxiety increased linearly. Specifically, subjects reporting 15 or more days of migraine per month had an adjusted OR of 6.4 (95% CI 4.4–9.3) for depression and 6.9 (95% CI 5.1–9.4) for anxiety.

The prevalence of several psychiatric disorders was determined in a sample of over 36,000 subjects in a Canadian population-based cohort [63]. Major depression, bipolar disorder, panic disorder, and social phobia were all at least twice as prevalent in migraine subjects, and were independent of demographic and socioeconomic variables. Persons with migraine and one of the psychiatric comorbidities had a lower HRQoL than those having either disorder alone. A small but interesting study conducted at a tertiary headache center suggested that post-traumatic stress disorder is more common in patients with CM relative to patients with EM, Thus, post-traumatic stress disorder may be a risk factor for migraine progression [64].

Depression, panic disorder, and generalized anxiety disorder have been associated with migraine and other chronic pain conditions [65]. In fact, research has shown elevated odd ORs for migraine, arthritis, and back pain in subjects with the three baseline psychiatric diagnoses. All three pain conditions were most strongly associated with the anxiety disorders.

Comorbidities of chronic migraine

Both clinic- and population-based studies have demonstrated higher rates of comorbid medical and psychiatric conditions in persons with CM (relative to EM) [7, 41]. An analysis of 24,000 individuals with "severe" headache from the 2005 AMPP survey identified 655 respondents with CM and 11,249 respondents with EM [7]. Relative to those with EM, respondents with CM were approximately twice as likely to have depression, anxiety, and chronic pain. Respiratory disorders including asthma, bronchitis and chronic obstructive pulmonary disease, and cardiac risk factors including hypertension, diabetes, high cholesterol level, and obesity, were also significantly more likely to be reported by those with CM.

The International Burden of Illness study revealed a similar pattern [67]. Data were collected on comorbid medical and psychiatric conditions. Participants were asked, "Have you been told by a doctor or any other health professional that you have any of the following health problems?" Conditions were divided into five categories: psychiatric, pain, vascular risk factors, vascular disease events, and other. In a comparison of study respondents with migraine in the USA (n = 1204) and Canada (n = 681), approximately one-half (USA 49.0%, Canada 50.9%) of CM participants reported pain-related comorbidities, compared to only 26.7% and 25.2% of EM participants in the USA and Canada, respectively ($P < 0.0001$ for all comparisons). Canadian CM participants were significantly more likely than EM participants to have a vascular disease event (12.7% versus 4.8%; $P = 0.017$). Almost one-half (45.2%) of US CM participants reported a psychiatric disorder, compared to approximately one-third (29.0%) of EM participants ($P = 0.003$).

Comorbidity profiles were also examined among patients with EM and CM in the Taiwan National Health Insurance Research Database [41]. Compared with patients with "other migraines" (n = 2226), patients with CM (n = 681) had a higher risk of medical comorbidities—hyperlipidemia (relative risk [RR] = 1.32; $P = 0.041$), asthma (RR = 1.77; $P = 0.007$); and psychiatric comorbidities—depression (RR = 1.88; $P \leq 0.0001$), bipolar disorder (RR = 1.81; $P = 0.022$), and anxiety disorders (RR = 1.48; $P \leq 0.0001$). Compared with patients without migraine (n = 3790), patients with CM (n = 948) had significantly increased risks (1.6- to 3.9-fold) of CVD, sinusitis, asthma, gastrointestinal ulcers, vertigo, and psychiatric disorders.

The natural history of migraine

Clinical trajectories

Longitudinal population studies as well as clinic-based observational studies have improved our understanding of the natural history and the prognosis of migraine [68, 69]. Researchers posit four partially overlapping clinical trajectories in persons with EM: complete remission, partial remission, persistence, and progression. Individuals with migraine (EM or CM) may achieve complete clinical remission, becoming symptom-free for prolonged periods of time. Some individuals may experience partial clinical remission whereby migraine attacks are less frequent and less severe, and exhibit fewer typical migraine features. Those with CM may revert to EM and those with high-frequency EM (HFEM) may revert to low-frequency EM (LFEM). These individuals may also be reclassified with probable migraine or tension-type headache. Another group of individuals may persist without major changes in frequency, severity, or symptom profiles. Finally, some individuals may experience progression (also referred to as chronification in the case of progression to CM). In these individuals, the frequency of migraine attacks may increase from LFEM to HFEM or CM (Figure 5.1). In addition, symptom profiles and headache-related disability may increase. Clinical progression is often associated with the experience of cutaneous allodynia and sensitization at the level of the trigeminal nucleus caudalis (i.e., physiologic progression.) Moreover, anatomic correlates of attack frequency, including stroke and deep white matter lesions (i.e., anatomic progression), might manifest [70].

Course of episodic migraine

An analysis of AMPP data over the course of 2 years provides insight into the natural course of EM. Of 24,000 individuals with "severe" headache surveyed in 2005, 16,573 returned completed surveys; of these, 8219 had EM and returned completed surveys in 2006 (Figure 5.2). A review of these individuals found that 82.8% still had

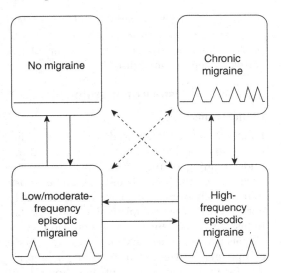

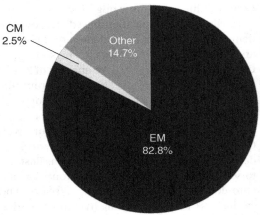

Figure 5.2. One-year follow-up of persons with EM in the population: outcomes. Data from the AMPP study questionnaires in 2005 and 2006. A total of 8219 respondents had EM (ICHD-2-defined migraine with <15 headache days per month) and returned completed surveys in 2006. (Reproduced from Bigal ME, Serrano D, Buse D, Scher A, Stewart WF, Lipton RB. Acute migraine medications and evolution from episodic to chronic migraine: longitudinal population-based study. *Headache* 2008; 48: 58–66 [74].)

Figure 5.1. Possible clinical trajectories. Clinical possibilities for persons with migraine include complete remission, partial remission, persistence, and progression. It is most common for individuals to move between adjacent frequency states; however, although rare, individuals may also move from no migraine to a new daily persistent headache or from CM to complete clinical remission. Changes between adjacent states are more common and may occur in both directions. The rate of progression from EM to CM is 2.5%, and there are known risk factors for progression. (Reproduced from Bigal ME, Lipton RB. Clinical course in migraine: conceptualizing migraine transformation. *Neurology* 2008; 71: 848–55 [68].)

EM, 2.5% had developed CM, and 14.0% had other outcomes (e.g., remission, probable migraine, or tension-type headache.) Both a higher frequency of headache days in 2005 and certain classes of acute medication use (i.e., use of barbiturates or opioids) were associated with progression to CM. Frequency of headache days interacted with medication use. This finding is discussed further in the section "Risk factors for onset of chronic migraine."

Course of chronic migraine

Researchers analyzed AMPP data to determine the natural course of CM. Of 24,000 respondents with headache surveyed in 2005, 18,514 returned completed questionnaires, including 383 individuals with CM who contributed data in 2006 and 2007 (Figure 5.3). Of individuals with CM in 2005, 238 had CM in at least 1 year of follow-up, and 292 had either CM or HFEM in at least 1 year of follow-up. Almost 34% ($n = 130$) had CM in all 3 years (i.e., persistent CM), whereas 26.1% ($n = 100$) had CM in 2005 but had other headache conditions (e.g., LFEM, no headache, probable migraine, episodic tension-type headache, or other episodic headache) in both 2006 and 2007 (i.e., they had remitted CM). Multivariate models found that predictors of remission included a lower baseline frequency of headache days per month (15–19 days/month versus 25–31 headache days/month; OR 0.29, 95% CI 0.11–0.75) and the absence of cutaneous allodynia (OR 0.45, 95% CI 0.23–0.89). Surprisingly, use of preventive medication was associated with lower remission rates (OR 0.41, 95% CI 0.23–0.75), but this effect

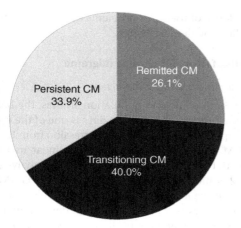

Figure 5.3. One-year follow-up of persons with CM in the population: outcomes. Data from the AMPP study. Of 383 individuals with CM in 2005, 33.9% (n = 130) had CM in all 3 years (i.e., persistent CM). A total of 26.1% (n = 100) had CM in 2005 but had other headache conditions (i.e., remitted CM; e.g., outcomes included LFEM, no headache, probable migraine, episodic tension-type headache, or other episodic headache) in 2006 and 2007. In addition, 33.9% (n = 153) had CM at baseline but did not meet the criteria for persistent or remitted CM in both 2006 and 2007 and were labeled "transitioning CM." (Reproduced from Manack A, Buse D, Serrano D, Turkel C, Lipton RB. Rates, predictors, and consequences of remission from chronic migraine to episodic migraine. *Neurology* 2011; 76: 711–18 [71].)

lost significance when frequency of headache days was included. This finding may represent confounding in that individuals with the most severe disease may be more likely to take preventive medication. Not surprisingly, over the 2 years of observation, participants with persistent CM demonstrated increased headache-related disability, whereas those with remitted CM had decreased headache-related disability.

Course of migraine in adolescents

A 3-year observational study of 209 adolescents (seventh through ninth grade) with ICHD-2-defined migraine in Thailand showed an improvement in 12% of boys and 16% of girls, no

improvement in 1% of both boys and girls, and a deterioration in 3% of boys and 7% of girls [72]. An voidance of precipitating causes or unknown reasons/spontaneous remission accounted for the majority of improvement seen. Stress-related daily school activities and inadequate rest were reported as common precipitating factors among students with non-improving or worsening outcomes.

Wang and colleagues [73] evaluated the outcome of adolescents aged 12–14 with chronic daily headache (CDH). Baseline data were collected in 2000, with final follow-up in 2008. At the 8-year follow-up, only 12% still had CDH. CDH in 2008 was predicted by the onset of CDH prior to 13 years of age. In addition, 64% of the cohort reported some or a substantial improvement in headache intensity, whereas 20% reported no change, and 16% reported worsening. A total of 68% of the cohort reported some or a substantial improvement in headache frequency, whereas 20% reported no change, and 12% reported worsening. The presence of CDH for more than 2 years, onset prior to 13 years of age, presence of CDH at the 2001 follow-up, and migraine with and without aura all significantly predicted worsening of headache frequency at the 8-year follow-up.

Risk factors for migraine

Risk factors for onset of chronic migraine

The majority of individuals with EM in the population do not develop CM; however, it is estimated that 2.5% experience chronification [24]. This subset of individuals who progress to CM may provide important clues into the mechanisms of progression [74, 75, 76]. Researchers have identified a set of potential markers or risk factors for the new onset of CM. These risk factors can be divided into nonmodifiable, modifiable, and putative risk factors (see Table 5.3) [74]. Non-modifiable risk factors include older age, female gender, white race (in a US sample), low educational level, lower socioeconomic status, and genetic factors. Modifiable factors are important because they provide targets for intervention and include attack frequency, obesity, medication overuse, snoring, stressful life events (SLE), depression, and anxiety. Putative factors, or factors currently being investigated, include pro-inflammatory states and pro-thrombotic states.

Risk factors for chronic daily headache conditions

Several studies have examined progression using CDH as an outcome. CDH is defined as headaches that occur on 15 days or more per month, for at least 3 months. The condition comprises CM, chronic tension-type headache, new daily persistent headache, and hemicrania continua. Although studies using CDH include conditions in addition to CM, they still provide insight into factors predicting the onset of frequent headache.

In the Frequent Headache Epidemiology Study, Scher et al. studied 1134 individuals with CDH and non-CDH headache participants (defined as 2–104 headaches per year) to identify factors that predicted the onset or remission of CDH [77]. At follow-up, 3% of the non-CDH headache participants reported 180 or more headaches per year. Higher baseline headache frequency and obesity were significantly associated with new-onset CDH. Individuals with three or more monthly attacks were at risk for incident CDH, and the risk increased exponentially with rising attack frequency. Remission was associated with non-white race, being married, higher levels of educational achievement, and diabetes.

Research has implicated obesity as a risk factor for incident CDH. In the Frequent Headache Epidemiology Study, overweight (adjusted OR 1.97, 95% CI 0.4–9.0) and obese (adjusted OR 5.28, 95% CI 1.3–21.1) individuals were at increased risk for CDH relative to those of normal weight. The Frequent Headache Epidemiology Study has also shown that habitual snoring, which was associated with CDH independently of obesity [78], as well as head or neck injury, was related to CDH onset [79]. Comorbid pain disorders (especially arthritis and musculoskeletal pain) have been identified as a risk factor for the development of CDH [80].

Habitual high daily caffeine consumption has long been associated with CDH [81] and may particularly induce CDH in females younger than 40 years of age [82]. In individuals aged 40 and older, a recent SLE (e.g., marital separation, divorce, relocation, occupational change, the death of a relative or friend, or problems with children) predicts incident CDH [83].

Risk factors for chronic migraine

Baseline headache frequency

In both clinic and population studies, the baseline number of headache days is one of the most important risk factors for progression from EM to CM. The risk increases in a nonlinear manner with baseline headache frequency. An analysis of 8219 individuals with EM from the 2005 AMPP database found that baseline frequency of headache days was predictive of the development of CM, even when controlling for the monthly use of acute pain medication [24].

There are several explanations for the longitudinal influence of headache frequency on the transition from EM to CM. Headache frequency may be a marker of headache evolution, a consequence of a biologic process and not the cause of the process that leads to CM. Alternatively, repetitive episodes of pain may lead to central sensitization with the generation of free radicals and anatomic changes in the areas that control pain, with a consequent higher predisposition to further pain [84]. Last, an increased headache frequency may reflect an inherent predisposition to pain.

Acute medication use

Symptomatic medication overuse has long been associated with poor outcomes in persons with migraine [60]. Several clinic-based studies have suggested that medication overuse is a risk factor for headache transformation [85]. The results of these studies suggest that, in persons with migraine, an excessive use of analgesics for any reason (e.g., headache relief or relief of non-headache pain) is associated with an increased risk for developing CM. An analysis of 8219 individuals with EM from the 2005 AMPP database found that several classes of acute medication commonly used for migraine were associated with progression from EM to CM [24]. Using acetaminophen as the reference group and adjusting for sex, frequency and severity of headaches, and preventive medication use, the risk of developing CM from EM was approximately twofold among those using barbiturate-containing compounds (OR 2.06, 95% CI 1.3–3.1) and opioids (OR 1.98, 95% CI 1.4–2.2) [24]. The use of triptans (OR 1.25, 95% CI 0.9–1.7) and nonsteroidal anti-inflammatory drugs (NSAIDs; OR 0.85, 95% CI 0.63–1.17) was not identified as a risk factor, although the results varied when the participants were stratified by the frequency of headaches day per month.

Barbiturates and opiates could be used in patients at increased risk for transformation due to frequent or disabling attacks. To disentangle these influences, researchers ran a series of adjusted models including monthly days of headache, preventive medication use, as well as headache severity and disability in the entire sample and in sex-defined subgroups. In these adjusted analyses, although the effects of medications were attenuated, barbiturates (OR 1.73, 95% CI 1.1–2.7) or opioids (OR 1.4, 95% CI 1.1–2.1) remained significant predictors of the new onset of CM at follow-up. For both opioids and barbiturates, a dose–response curve was demonstrated indicating that an increasing number of days of use was associated with an increased risk of CM onset [67]. In the entire study population, those using triptans (OR 1.05, 95% CI 0.8–1.6) or NSAIDs (OR 0.97, 95% CI 0.7–1.34) were not at increased risk, although there are complex interactions with headache frequency and days of dosing.

The odds of transition to CM increased with elevated monthly barbiturate exposure (OR 1.25, 95% CI 1.1–1.4), controlling for the effects of gender and monthly frequency of headaches. The risk seemed to increase at values of 5 days per month and greater. The barbiturate effect was stronger in females. The findings were similar for opioids (OR 1.44, 95% CI 1.1–1.8). The risk seemed to increase at doses of 8 days per month or more, and opioid effects were more pronounced in males. NSAID use at low to moderate monthly frequency of headache days was protective against the development of CM, whereas use in individuals with 10–14 days of headache per month was associated with an increased risk of CM onset. The study authors hypothesized that anti-inflammatory medications might directly treat migraine-related inflammation in LFEM, but in HFEM central sensitization may be more persistent, rendering NSAIDs less effective.

☝ CAUTION!

Opioid and barbiturate use is associated with an increased risk of CM onset among persons with EM, especially among those patients with a higher headache frequency [24]. It is also related to worse outcomes [86]. Therefore, exercise caution when using these medications and instead use migraine-specific acute medications and consider adding preventive pharmacologic treatments and empirically supported behavioral interventions when appropriate.

Cutaneous allodynia

Cutaneous allodynia, or the perception of pain associated with ordinarily nonpainful stimuli, has been identified as a predictor of onset of new CM. In EM, allodynia is an ictal state phenomenon. Clinic- and population-based studies show that about two-thirds of individuals with migraine develop cutaneous allodynia [87, 88, 89]. In the AMPP study, the population prevalence of cutaneous allodynia was significantly higher among persons with CM (68.3%) than those with EM (63.2%, $P < 0.01$), and higher in both of these groups compared to persons with other headache types [89]. In CM, allodynia persists between attacks. An analysis of the AMPP data found that the presence of cutaneous allodynia was a risk factor for the onset of CM [90].

⚖ SCIENCE REVISITED

Cutaneous allodynia is a clinical marker of sensitization of the trigeminal pathways in the brain. Sensitization in the trigeminocervical complex produces allodynia in the distribution of the trigeminal nerve [91, 92]. Extracephalic allodynia likely arises from sensitization of the thalamic neurons. Researchers hypothesize that recurrent severe headaches lead to persistent sensitization and other alterations in the nociceptive pathways. According to this hypothesis, repeated attacks of persistent pain may alter the threshold for activation of the pain pathways (both primary pain pathways and modulatory pathways), potentially leading to a pain-prone state marked by cutaneous allodynia and sensitization.

Medical comorbidities and concomitant illnesses as risk factors for progression

Obesity

The link between obesity and the frequency of primary headaches has been demonstrated in several population studies. In the Frequent Headache Epidemiology Study, Scher et al. found that relative odds of CDH were five times higher in individuals with a body mass index (BMI) $\geq 30 \, kg/m^2$ and three times higher among "overweight" individuals compared to individuals of "normal" weight [77]. BMI is also associated with the frequency of headache attacks in migraineurs [93]. In the "normal" BMI group, just 4.4% of individuals with migraine had 10–14 headache days per month, compared to 5.8% of the "overweight" group (OR 1.3, 95% CI 0.6–2.8), 13.6% of the "obese" group (OR 2.9, 95% CI 1.9–4.4), and 20.7% of the "severely obese" (OR 5.7, 95% CI 3.6–8.8). Obesity was found to be a risk factor for transformed migraine (i.e., CM), but not chronic tension-type headache. When analyzed by BMI category, the prevalence of CM ranged from 0.9% of the "normal" weight BMI (reference) group to 2.5% of the "severely obese" group (OR 2.2, 95% CI 1.5–3.2) [94]. An analysis of the AMPP data also showed that obesity was an exacerbating factor for migraine but not other headache types [95].

SCIENCE REVISITED

Researchers hypothesize that several of the inflammatory mediators that are increased in obese individuals are important in migraine pathophysiology, including interleukins and calcitonin gene-related peptide [96]. Both migraine and obesity are pro-thrombotic states. Substances that are important in metabolic control (e.g., adiponectin) are nociceptive at lower levels.

Hypothalamic dysfunction in the orexin pathways seems to be a risk factor for both conditions. Finally, the metabolic syndrome and autonomic dysfunction may also participate in the relationship between obesity and migraine progression. It is important to emphasize that several remediable cardiovascular risk factors (i.e., the metabolic syndrome, hyperlipidemia, and hypertension) may influence migraine progression by mediating the effects of obesity [97].

Snoring and sleep apnea

The relationship between headache progression and snoring has been studied in both case–control and population studies. A large, cross-sectional study of 3323 Danish men found that snoring was associated with any form of headache (independent of weight, age, gender, hypertension, and other sleep disturbances, including cases secondary to caffeine consumption) [98]. Another population-based case–control study found that individuals with CDH were more likely to be habitual or daily snorers than were controls [78]. The mechanisms of the relationship between obstructive sleep apnea and migraine progression are not fully understood but may involve intracranial and arterial pressure fluctuations during snore in an individual susceptible to pain progression, hypoxia, hypercapnia, sleep fragmentation and disruptions, and increased muscle activation during awakenings.

Temporomandibular disorders

TMDs includes a range of disorders characterized by alterations or dysfunction of the masticatory muscles, the temporomandibular joint, and its associated structures [99]. Population studies show that headache is more common in persons with TMD than in those free of TMD ($P = 0.000$). Using the no-headache group as the reference, incremental TMD symptoms yielded increased relative odds of all other headaches [100].

Head trauma and traumatic brain injury

Head injury can cause de novo post-traumatic headache. In addition, trauma can be a factor exacerbating migraine and sometimes leading to CDH [79]. In the Frequent Headache Epidemiology Study, patients with CDH and a comparison group with episodic headache (2–102 days with headache per year) were asked about the occurrence of headache or neck injuries. Any headache or neck injury was associated with a 15% increased risk of CDH. The attributable risk was 15%. The odds of CDH increased with the number of lifetime injuries in all groups ($P < 0.05$ for trend).

⚗ SCIENCE REVISITED

TMD is associated with cutaneous allodynia. In a clinic study, individuals with EM and TMD were more likely to have moderate or severe cutaneous allodynia associated with their headaches compared with those with EM without TMD, even after adjusting for aura, gender, and age [101]. Using quantitative sensory testing, thresholds for heat and mechanical nociception were also significantly lower interictally in individuals with TMD. TMDs were also associated with changes in extracephalic pain thresholds. These findings are of interest because cutaneous allodynia is an important risk factor for migraine progression. As a pro-allodynic comorbidity, TMD is a candidate risk factor for the onset of CM in persons with EM.

Psychiatric comorbidities as risk factors for migraine progression

Both clinic and population studies around the world show that, in cross-section, CM is associated with increased rates of several psychiatric comorbidities. Several studies have examined the role of psychiatric comorbidities as predictors of CM onset. The increased risk of depression and anxiety in persons with CM could arise in several ways. First, depression or anxiety could emerge as a consequence of increasing headache frequency. Second depression or anxiety could be a risk factor for migraine progression. Third, depression or anxiety could be associated with some other factor that was primarily responsible for driving the increased risk of CM (i.e., a confounding factor).

Researchers examined 6657 AMPP study participants with EM in 2005 and found that 160 (2.4%) developed CM in 2006 and 144 (2.2%) developed CM in 2007 [102]. Depression was a significant predictor of CM onset (OR 1.65, 95% CI 1.12–2.45), after adjusting for sociodemographic variables and headache characteristics. Additionally, there was a depression–dose effect. Relative to study respondents with no or mild depression, those with moderate (OR 1.77, 95% CI 1.25–2.52), moderately severe (OR 2.35, 95% CI 1.53–3.62), and severe (OR 2.53, 95% CI 1.52–4.21) depression were at increased risk for the onset of CM at increasingly higher rates.

A study of 122 adolescent patients with CDH in Taiwan reported that major depression was an independent predictor of the persistence of CDH at 2 years in multivariate analyses. In univariate analyses, panic disorder, social phobia, and obsessive-compulsive disorder were also risk factors [103]. A recent review by Smitherman et al. highlights the probability that anxiety disorders, rather than depression, contribute more to migraine progression, and that possible mechanisms include shared dysfunction of the serotonergic system, medication overuse derived from a lack of appropriate coping behaviors, and an inherent ideology that magnifies pain and unpleasant associated features [104]. Anxiety was also identified as a risk factor for progression in the AMPP study [105].

★ TIPS AND TRICKS

Longitudinal studies have revealed that depression is a risk factor for the onset of CM among persons with EM. Although it is has not been empirically demonstrated, this suggests that monitoring and treating depression is a wise clinical decision to reduce the risk of chronification. Treating either migraine or depression separately will likely lead to global improvements, and some pharmacologic agents target both conditions. However, outcomes are often better when the migraine and the psychiatric comorbidity are separately addressed with both appropriate pharmacologic and nonpharmacologic treatments.

Major life events and stressful life events

An analysis of AMPP data demonstrated that major life events (MLEs) and SLEs are more common among persons with CM than those with EM [106]. MLEs assessed included change of residence, employment status, marital status, changes related to their children, the deaths of relatives or close friends, and "extremely stressful" ongoing situations. Study participants were asked to rate the level of stress associated with each event, identifying the MLEs that were also SLEs. Because cross-sectional designs precluded the possibility of determining directionality, it remains unclear whether the event or the CM was the primary event in the AMPP cross-sectional analysis. However, the Frequent Headache Epidemiology Study assessed the role of MLEs as risk factors for the new onset of CDH using a case–control design [83]. CDH and control cases were asked about the same SLEs as used in the AMPP analysis. Compared with controls with episodic headache, CDH cases had had more major life changes in the prior or current year. After adjusting for age, gender, headache type, and year of event, the odds of frequent headaches increased additionally with each antecedent MLE (OR 1.20, 95% 1.1–1.3; $P < 0.001$), but not with subsequent events (OR 0.94, 95% CI 0.8–1.1; $P < 0.4$). The specificity of association for events preceding but not following the onset of CDH supports the possibility of a causal relationship.

Genetic and perinatal factors

Twin studies and family studies suggest that genetic factors account for about half of the risk for developing EM [107, 108, 109]. Emerging evidence shows that, in addition to contributing to the risk of EM, familial and genetic factors may contribute to the onset of CM as well [110]. The prevalence of CM is elevated in the first-degree relatives of probands with CM. Although this is best explained by a heritable biologic predisposition, other explanations are possible [67]. Family aggregation also increases with illness severity [111, 112].

The Attention Brazil Project investigated the influence of parental headache history on headache characteristics in the offspring [113]. In this study, the offspring of parents with a negative history of headache were compared with the offspring of parents with any headache history. The offspring of parents with any headache history were at increased risk of episodic headache (OR 1.6, 95% CI 1.3–1.8) and of CDH (OR 6.6, 95% CI 1.4–28.4). The frequency of headaches in the mother predicted the frequency of headaches in the children. When the mothers had a low frequency of headaches, the children had an increased chance of low or intermediate headache frequency (RR 1.4, CI 1.2–1.6) but not CDHs. When the mother had CDH, the risk of CDH was increased by almost 13-fold, but the risk of infrequent headaches was not increased. In multivariate models, frequency of headaches in the children was independently predicted by frequency of headaches in the mother after adjustments, suggesting that headache frequency (and not only headache status) aggregates in the family.

This study also highlighted the enormous susceptibility of the pain pathways during early development. The odds of CDH were significantly higher when maternal tobacco use was reported. For active tobacco use, the OR for CDH was markedly elevated (OR 4.2, 95% CI 2.1–8.5). Alcohol use in pregnancy more than doubled the risk of CDH in the offspring, from 11% in unexposed individuals to 24% in those exposed (OR 2.3, 95% CI 1.2–4.7). The risk remained significantly elevated after adjusting for family income, parental headache status and medical care during pregnancy, hypertension during pregnancy, and use of illegal drugs.

> ### ⚖ SCIENCE REVISITED
>
> Distinct genetic factors may contribute to the onset and progression of migraine. A number of genes associated with chronic pain have been identified, although their role in progression of migraine remains to be determined [114, 115]. In particular, functional variants in the genes that code for enzymes involved in catecholamine systems have been implicated in chronic pain. These enzymes include catechol-O-methyl transferase and dopamine beta hydroxylase among others.

Effects of modifying risk factors in persons with chronic migraine

A few studies have examined outcomes among persons with CM when they intervened with risk factors. Bond et al. assessed 24 "severely obese" patients with migraine before and 6 months after bariatric surgery. The mean number of headache days was reduced from an average of 11.1 preoperatively to 6.7 postoperatively ($P < 0.05$), after a mean percent excess weight loss of 49.4%. They also observed a reduction in severity of headache pain and in the number of patients reporting moderate to severe disability [116]. Calhoun and Ford tested the effects of a cognitive-behavioral intervention designed to improve sleep on CM status [117]. In a randomized, placebo-controlled study, they tested whether behavioral sleep modification would result in an improvement in headache frequency and intensity, and in remission from CM to EM in 43 females with transformed migraine (i.e., CM). Compared to the control group, the behavioral sleep modification group reported statistically significant reductions in headache frequency and headache intensity, and were more likely to remit to EM. By the end of the study, 48.5% of those who participated in behavioral sleep modification had reverted to EM.

Conversely, researchers tested whether reducing headache days from CM to EM would improve risk factors and related outcomes [118]. Thirty-two outpatients (age > 18 years) with CM and comorbid depressive disorders were recruited from three outpatient centers. Participants were treated with OnabotulinumtoxinA. At 24 weeks, treatment of CM with OnabotulinumtoxinA was associated with reductions in headache and migraine frequency as well as reductions in depression, anxiety, headache-related disability, and impact, and an improvement in HRQoL. As OnabotulinumtoxinA has no known direct effect on mood, the improvements seen may be attributable to an improvement in headache. Additional blinded studies with larger samples are necessary to fully explore the results seen in all of these studies. Additionally, intervention in other risk factors for CM should be tested to determine if progression to CM can be avoided, and if the treatment of risk factors can lead to remission from CM to EM or no migraine.

> ### ☆ TIPS AND TRICKS
>
> Treatment plans should be tailored based on migraine severity and associated symptoms, comorbidities, and patient preference [119, 120]. Mild migraine may require little more than reassurance, education, and an over-the-counter acute treatment. Disabling migraine may require a comprehensive treatment plan, including both acute and preventive pharmacologic treatments and empirically supported behavioral therapies [119, 121]. Several validated instruments aid in the assessment of the variables necessary for effective treatment planning. For a review, see Buse et al., 2012) [122].

Summary: clinical implications and future directions

Migraine is a common and often disabling neurologic condition. CM is less frequent but is much more burdensome and disabling, as seen on multiple types of outcomes. Approximately 2.5% of persons with EM progress to CM over the course of 1 year. Several variables have been associated with the progression to CM, including nonmodifiable, modifiable, and putative risk factors. Modifiable factors are important because they provide targets for intervention and include attack frequency, obesity, medication overuse, snoring, SLEs, depression, and anxiety. Putative factors, or factors currently being investigated, include pro-inflammatory states and pro-thrombotic states. Because only a subset of episodic individuals with migraine progress to CM in any given year, progression likely occurs as a function of genetic and environmental risk factors. Understanding the risk factors that differentiate individuals with migraine who progress to CM from those who do not may provide insights into the mechanisms, prevention, and treatment of CM. Future work should include the systematic testing of interventions of modifiable risk factors to determine if progression can be prevented. Conversely, it would also be useful to test whether modifying these risk factors once CM has developed would increase rates of remission.

Acknowledgment

The authors would like to thank Michael T. Lynch, BS for his assistance with figures and artwork.

References

1. Leonardi M, Steiner TJ, Scher AT, Lipton RB. The global burden of migraine: measuring disability in headache disorders with WHO's classification of functioning, disability and health (ICF). *J Headache Pain* 2005;**6**: 429–40.

2. Terwindt GM, Ferrari MD, Tijhuis M, Groenen SMA, Picavet HSJ, Launer LJ. The impact of migraine on quality of life in the general population. The GEM Study. *Neurology* 2000;**55**:429–40.

3. Lipton RB, Hemelsky SW, Kolodner KN, Steiner TJ, Stewart WF. Migraine, quality of life and depression. A population-based case-control study. *Neurology* 2000;**55**: 629–35.

4. Dahlof CGH, Dimenäs E. Migraine patients experience poorer subjective well-being/ quality of life even between attacks. *Cephalalgia* 1995;**15**:31–6.

5. Buse DC, Manack AN, Fanning K, et al. Chronic migraine prevalence, disability, and sociodemographic factors: results from the American Migraine Prevalence and Prevention Study. *Headache* 2012;**52**:1456–70.

6. Lipton RB, Bigal ME, Diamond M, Freitag F, Reed ML, Stewart WF. Migraine prevalence, disease burden, and the need for preventive therapy. *Neurology* 2007;**68**;343–9.

7. Buse DC, Manack A, Serrano D, Turkel C, Lipton RB. Sociodemographic and comorbidity profiles of chronic migraine and episodic migraine sufferers. *J Neurol Neurosurg Psychiatry* 2010;**81**:428–32.

8. Buse DC, Loder E, Gorman JA, Stewart WF, Reed ML, Lipton RB. Sex differences in prevalence, symptoms, and other features of migraine, probable migraine and other severe headache: results of the American Migraine Prevalence and Prevention Study. *Headache* 2013; in press.

9. Bigal ME, Lipton RB, Winner P, Reed ML, Diamond S, Stewart WF, on behalf of the AMPP advisory group. Migraine in adolescents: association with socioeconomic status and family history. *Neurology* 2007; **69**:16–25.

10. Stewart WF, Lipton RB, Liberman J. Variation in migraine prevalence by race. *Neurology* 1996;**47**:52–9.

11. Lipton RB, Stewart WF, Diamond S, Diamond M, Reed ML. Prevalence and burden of migraine in the United States: data from the American Migraine Study II. *Headache* 2001;**41**:646–57.

12. Launer LJ, Terwindt GM, Ferrari MD. The prevalence and characteristics of migraine in a population-based cohort: the GEM study. *Neurology* 1999;**53**:537–42.

13. Rasmussen BK. Migraine and tension-type headache in a general population: psychosocial factors. *Int J Epidemiol* 1992;**21**: 1138–43.

14. O'Brien B, Goeree R, Streiner D. Prevalence of migraine headache in Canada: a population-based survey. *Int J Epidemiol* 1994;**23**:1020–6.

15. Stewart WF, Lipton RB, Celentano DD, Reed ML. Prevalence of migraine headache in the United States: relation to age, income, race, and other sociodemographic factors. *JAMA* 1992;**267**:64–9.

16. Headache Classification Committee of the International Headache Society. Classification and diagnostic criteria for headache disorders, cranial neuralgias and facial pain. *Cephalalgia* 1988;**7**(Suppl.):1–96.

17. Scher AI, Lipton RB, Stewart WF. Demographic factors and migraine prevalence: the influence of ethnicity and geography. *Med Americas* 2000;**1**:65–70.

18. Stovner LJ, Hagen K, Jensen R, et al. The global burden of headache: a documentation of headache prevalence and disability worldwide. *Cephalalgia* 2007;**27**:193–210.

19. Lyngberg AC, Rasmussen BK, Jorgensen T, Jensen R. Incidence of primary headache: a Danish epidemiologic follow-up study. *Am J Epidemiol* 2005;**161**:1066–73.

20. Stewart WF, Wood C, Reed ML, Roy J, Lipton RB, on behalf of the AMPP advisory group. Cumulative lifetime migraine incidence in women and men. *Cephalalgia* 2008;**28**: 1170–8.

21. Stewart WF, Linet MS, Celentano DD, Van Natta M, Ziegler D. Age-and sex-specific

incidence rates of migraine with and without visual aura. *Am J Epidemiol* 1991;**134**:1111–20.

22. Natoli JL, Manack A, Dean B, et al. Global prevalence of chronic migraine: a systematic review. *Cephalalgia* 2010;**30**:599–609.

23. Olesen J, Bousser MG, Diener HC, et al. New appendix criteria open for a broader concept of chronic migraine. *Cephalalgia* 2006;**26**: 742–6.

24. Bigal ME, Serrano D, Buse D, Scher A, Stewart WF, Lipton RB. Acute migraine medications and evolution from episodic to chronic migraine: a longitudinal population-based study. *Headache* 2008;**48**:1157–68.

25. World Health Organization. *The World Health Report 2001. Mental Health: New Understanding, New Hope*. Geneva: WHO; 2001. Available at: www.who.int/whr/2001/en/index.html (accessed September 2012).

26. Buse DC, Bigal MB, Rupnow M, Reed, M, Serrano D, Lipton RB. Development and validation of the Migraine Interictal Burden Scale (MIBS): a self-administered instrument for measuring the burden of migraine between attacks. *Neurology* 2007;**68**(Suppl. 1):A89.

27. Peres MF, Mercante JP, Guendler VZ, et al. Cephalalgiaphobia: a possible specific phobia of illness. *J Headache Pain* 2007;**8**: 56–9.

28. Buse DC, Lipton RB. Facilitating communication with patients for improved migraine outcomes. *Curr Pain Headache Rep* 2008; **12**:230–6.

29. Holmes WF, MacGregor EA, Sawyer JP, Lipton RB. Information about migraine disability influences physicians' perceptions of illness severity and treatment needs. *Headache* 2001;**41**:343–50.

30. Stewart WF, Lipton RB, Kolodner K, Liberman J, Sawyer J. Reliability of the Migraine Disability Assessment (MIDAS) score in a population based sample of headache sufferers. *Cephalalgia* 1999;**19**:107–14.

31. Blumenfeld A, Varon S, Wilcox TK, et al. Disability, HRQoL and resource use among chronic and episodic migraineurs: results from the International Burden of Migraine Study (IBMS). *Cephalalgia* 2011;**31**: 301–15.

32. Buse DC, Manack AN, Serrano D, et al. Headache-impact of chronic and episodic migraine: results from the AMPP Study. *Headache* 2012;**52**:3–17.

33. Hahn SR, Lipton RB, Sheftell FD, et al. Healthcare provider-patient communication and migraine assessment: results of the American Migraine Communication Study (ACMS) Phase II. *Curr Med Res Opin* 2008;**24**:1711–8.

34. Turner-Bowker DM, Bayliss MS, Ware JE, Kosinski M. Usefulness of the SF-8 Health Survey for comparing the impact of migraine and other conditions. *Qual Life Res* 2003; **12**:1002–12.

35. Lipton RB, Liberman JN, Kolodner KB, Bigal ME, Dowson A, Stewart WF. Migraine headache disability and health-related quality-of-life: a population-based case-control study from England. *Cephalalgia* 2003;**23**:441–50.

36. Hawkins K, Wang S, Rupnow MFT. Indirect cost burden of migraine in the United States. *J Occup Environ Med* 2007;**49**:368–74.

37. Stewart WF, Ricci JA, Leotta C, Chee E, Morganstein D, Lipton R. Lost productive time and cost due to common pain conditions in the US workforce. *JAMA* 2003;**290**:2443–54.

38. Bigal ME, Rapoport AM, Lipton RB, Tepper SJ, Sheftell FD. Assessment of migraine disability using the Migraine Disability Assessment (MIDAS) questionnaire: a comparison of chronic migraine with episodic migraine. *Headache* 2003;**3**:336–42.

39. Bigal ME, Serrano D, Reed M, Lipton RB. Chronic migraine in the population: burden, diagnosis, and satisfaction with treatment. *Neurology* 2008;**71**:559–66.

40. Meletiche DM, Lofland JH, Young WB. Quality of life differences between patients with episodic and transformed migraine. *Headache* 2001;**41**:573–8.

41. Chen YC, Tang CH, Ng K, Wang SJ. Comorbidity profiles of chronic migraine sufferers in a national database in Taiwan. *J Headache Pain* 2012;**13**:311–9.

42. Stewart WF, Wood GC, Manack A, Varon SF, Buse DC, Lipton RB. Employment and work impact of chronic migraine and episodic migraine. *J Occup Environ Med* 2010;**52**: 8–14.

43. Scher AI, Bigal ME, Lipton RB. Comorbidity of migraine. *Curr Opin Neurol* 2005;**18**: 305–10.

44. Rhode AM, Hosing VG, Happe S, Biehl K, Young P, Evers S. Comorbidity of migraine and restless legs syndrome-a case-control study. *Cephalalgia* 2007;**27**:1255–60.

45. De Tommaso M, Sardaro M, Serpino C, et al. Fibromyalgia comorbidity in primary headaches. *Cephalalgia* 2008;**29**:453–64.

46. Etminan M, Takkouche B, Isorna FC, Samii A. Risk of ischemic stroke in people with migraine: systemic review and meta-analysis of observational studies. *BMJ* 2005; **330**:63.

47. Stang PE, Carson AP, Rose KM, et al. Headache, cerebrovascular symptoms, and stroke: the Atherosclerosis Risk in Communities Study. *Neurology* 2005;**64**:1573–7.

48. Scher AI, Terwindt GM, Picavet HSJ, Verschuren WMM, Ferrari MD, Launer LJ. Cardiovascular risk factors and migraine: the GEM population-based study. *Neurology* 2005;**64**:614–20.

49. Kurth T, Slomke MA, Kase CS, et al. Migraine, headache, and the risk of stroke in women: a prospective study. *Neurology* 2005;**64**: 1020–6.

50. Kurth T, Gaziano JM, Cook NR, Logroscino G, Diener HC, Buring JE. Migraine and the risk of cardiovascular disease in women. *JAMA* 2006;**296**:283–91.

51. Kurth T, Schurks M, Logroscino G, Gaziano JM, Buring JE. Migraine, vascular risk, and cardiovascular events in women: prospective cohort study. *BMJ* 2008;**337**:a636.

52. Kurth T, Gaziano JM, Cook NR, et al. Migraine and risk of cardiovascular disease in men. *Arch Intern Med* 2007;**167**:795–801.

53. Kruit MC, van Buchem MA, Hofman PAM, et al. Migraine as a risk factor for subclinical brain lesions. *JAMA* 2004;**291**:427–34.

54. Palm-Meinders IH, Koppen H, Terwindt GM, et al. Structural brain changes in migraine. *JAMA* 2012;**308**:1889–97.

55. Schurks M, Rist PM, Bigal ME, Buring JE, Lipton RB, Kurth T. Migraine and cardiovascular disease: systematic review and meta-analysis. *BMJ* 2009;**339**:1–11.

56. Schwedt TJ, Demaerschalk BM, Dodick DW. Patent foramen ovale and migraine: a quantitative systematic review. *Cephalalgia* 2008;**28**:531–40.

57. Dowson A, Wilmshurst P, Muir KW, et al. A prospective, multicenter, randomized, double blind, placebo-controlled trial to evaluate the efficacy of patent foramen ovale closure with the STARFlex septal repair implant to prevent refractory migraine headaches: the MIST trial: S61.002. *Neurology* 2006;**67**:185.

58. Haut SR, Bigal ME, Lipton RB. Chronic disorders with episodic manifestations: focus on epilepsy and migraine. *Lancet Neurol* 2006;**5**:148–57.

59. Ottman R, Lipton RB. Comorbidity of migraine and epilepsy. *Neurology* 1994;**44**: 2105–10.

60. Ottman R, Lipton RB. Is the comorbidity of epilepsy and migraine due to a shared genetic susceptibility? *Neurology* 1996;**47**: 918–24.

61. Patel NV, Bigal ME, Kolodner KB, Leotta C, Lafata JE, Lipton RB. Prevalence and impact of migraine and probable migraine in a health plan. *Neurology* 2004;**63**:1432–8.

62. Zwart JA, Dyb G, Hagen K, et al. Depression and anxiety disorders associated with headache frequency. The Nord-Trondelag Health Study. *Eur J Neurol* 2003;**10**:147–52.

63. Jette N, Patten S, Williams J, Becker W, Wiebe S. Comorbidity of migraine and psychiatric disorders—a national population-based study. *Headache* 2008;**48**:501–16.

64. Peterlin BL, Tietjen G, Meng S, Lidicker J, Bigal M. Post-traumatic stress disorder in episodic and chronic migraine. *Headache* 2008;**48**:517–22.

65. McWilliams LA, Goodwin RD, Cox RJ. Depression and anxiety associated with three pain conditions: results from a nationally representative sample. *Pain* 2004;**111**: 77–83.

66. Spitzer R, Kroenke, K., Williams, J. Validation and utility of a self-report version of PRIME-MD: the PHQ primary care study. *JAMA* 1999;**282**, 1737–44.

67. Stokes MS, Werner JB, Lipton RB, Sullivan SD, Wilcox TK, Wells L. Cost of health care among patients with chronic migraine and episodic migraine in Canada and the USA: results from the International Burden of

Migraine Study (IBMS). *Headache* 2011 **51**:1058–77.

68. Bigal ME, Lipton RB. Clinical course in migraine: conceptualizing migraine transformation. *Neurology* 2008;**71**:848–55.

69. Bigal ME, Lipton RB. The prognosis of migraine. *Curr Opin Neurol* 2008;**21**: 301–8.

70. Boardman HF, Thomas E, Millson DS, Croft PR. The natural history of headache: predictors of onset and recovery. *Cephalalgia* 2006;**26**:1080–8.

71. Manack A, Buse D, Serrano D, Turkel C, Lipton RB. Rates, predictors, and consequences of remission from chronic migraine to episodic migraine. *Neurology* 2011;**76**: 711–8.

72. Visudtibhan A, Thampratankul L, Khongkhatithum C, et al. Migraine in junior high-school students: a prospective 3-academic-year cohort study. *Brain Dev* 2010;**32**:855–62.

73. Wang SJ, Fuh JL, Lu SR. Chronic daily headache in adolescents: an 8-year follow-up study. *Neurology* 2009;**73**:416–22.

74. Lipton RB, Bigal ME. Looking to the future: research designs for study of headache disease progression. *Headache* 2008;**48**: 58–66.

75. Lipton RB, Bigal ME. Migraine: epidemiology, impact, and risk factors for progression. *Headache* 2005;**45**(Suppl. 1):S3–13.

76. Bigal ME, Lipton RB. When migraine progresses: transformed or chronic migraine. *Expert Rev Neurother* 2006;**6**:297–306.

77. Scher AI, Stewart WF, Ricci JA, Lipton RB. Factors associated with the onset and remission of chronic daily headache in a population-based study. *Pain* 2003;**106**: 81–9.

78. Scher AI, Lipton RB, Stewart WF. Habitual snoring as a risk factor for chronic daily headache. *Neurology* 2003;**60**:1366–8.

79. Couch JR, Lipton RB, Stewart WF, Scher AI. Head or neck injury increases the risk of chronic daily headache: a population-based study. *Neurology* 2007;**69**:1169–77.

80. Scher AI, Stewart WF, Lipton RB. The comorbidity of headache with other pain syndromes. *Headache* 2006;**46**:1416–23.

81. Shapiro RE. Caffeine and headaches. *Curr Pain Headache Rep* 2008;**12**:311–5.

82. Scher AI, Stewart WF, Lipton RB. Caffeine as a risk factor for chronic daily headache. *Neurology* 2004;**63**:2022–7.

83. Scher AI, Stewart WF, Buse D, Krantz DS, Lipton RB. Major life changes before and after the onset of chronic daily headache: a population-based study. *Cephalalgia* 2008; **28**:868–76.

84. Welch KM, Nagesh V, Aurora SK, Gelman N. Periaqueductal gray matter dysfunction in migraine: cause or the burden of illness? *Headache* 2001;**41**:629–37.

85. Bahra A, Walsh M, Menon S, Goadsby PJ. Does chronic daily headache arise de novo in association with regular use of analgesics? *Headache* 2003;**43**:179–90.

86. Buse DC, Pearlman SH, Reed ML, Serrano D, Ng-Mak DS, Lipton RB. Opioid use and dependence among persons with migraine: results of the AMPP study. *Headache* 2012;**52**:18–36.

87. Burstein R, Yarnitsky D, Goor-Aryeh I, Ransil BJ, Bajwa ZH. An association between migraine and cutaneous allodynia. *Ann Neurol* 2000;**47**:614–24.

88. Lipton RB, Bigal ME, Ashina S, et al. Cutaneous allodynia in the migraine population. *Ann Neurol* 2008;**63**:148–58.

89. Bigal ME, Ashina S, Burstein R, et al. Prevalence and characteristics of allodynia in headache sufferers: a population study. *Neurology* 2008;**70**:1525–33.

90. Ashina S, Buse, D, Bigal, M, Serrano D, Reed M, Lipton RB. Cutaneous allodynia—a predictor of migraine chronification: a longitudinal population-based study. *Cephalalgia* 2009;**29**:58–9.

91. Burstein R, Jakubowski M. Analgesic triptan action in an animal model of intracranial pain: a race against the development of central sensitization. *Ann Neurol* 2004;**55**: 27–36.

92. Burstein R, Collins B, Jakubowski M. Defeating migraine pain with triptans: a race against the development of cutaneous allodynia. *Ann Neurol* 2004;**55**:19–26.

93. Bigal ME, Liberman JN, Lipton RB. Obesity and migraine: a population study. *Neurology* 2006;**66**:545–50.

94. Bigal ME, Lipton RB. Obesity is a risk factor for transformed migraine but not chronic tension-type headache. *Neurology* 2006;**67**:252–7.

95. Bigal ME, Tsang A, Loder E, Serrano D, Reed ML, Lipton RB. Body mass index and episodic headaches: a population-based study. *Arch Intern Med* 2007;**167**:1964–70.

96. Bigal ME, Lipton RB, Holland PR, Goadsby PJ. Obesity, migraine, and chronic migraine: possible mechanisms of interaction. *Neurology* 2007;**68**:1851–61.

97. Bigal ME, Lipton RB. Putative mechanisms of the relationship between obesity and migraine progression. *Curr Pain Headache Rep* 2008;**12**:207–12.

98. Jennum P, Sjol A. Epidemiology of snoring and obstructive sleep apnea in a Danish population, age 30–60. *J Sleep Res* 1992;**1**:240–4.

99. Dworkin SF, LeResche L. Research diagnostic criteria for temporomandibular disorders: review, criteria, examinations and specifications, critique. *J Craniomandib Disord* 1992;**6**:301–55.

100. Bevilaqua Grossi D, Lipton RB, Bigal ME. Temporomandibular disorders and migraine chronification. *Curr Pain Headache Rep* 2009;**13**:314–8.

101. Bevilaqua-Grossi D, Lipton RB, Napchan U, Grosberg B, Ashina S, Bigal ME. Temporomandibular disorders and cutaneous allodynia are associated in individuals with migraine. *Cephalalgia* 2009;**29**:75–6.

102. Ashina S, Serrano D, Lipton RB, et al. Depression and risk of transformation of episodic to chronic migraine: results of the American Migraine Prevalence and Prevention Study. Enrico Greppi Award 2012. *J Headache Pain* 2012;**13**:615–24.

103. Wang SJ, Fuh JL, Lu SR, Juang KD. Outcomes and predictors of chronic daily headache in adolescents: a 2-year longitudinal study. *Neurology* 2007;**68**:591–6.

104. Smitherman TA, Penzien DB, Maizels M. Anxiety disorders and migraine intractability and progression. *Curr Pain Headache Rep* 2008;**12**:224–9.

105. Ashina S, Buse DC, Maizels M, et al. Self-reported anxiety as a risk factor for migraine chronification. results from the American Migraine Prevalence and Prevention (AMPP) study. *Headache* 2010;**50**(Suppl. 1):S4.

106. Manack AN, Serrano D, Turkel CC, Lipton RB, Buse DC. Rates of stressful life events in chronic and episodic migraine. results from the American Migraine Prevalence and Prevention (AMPP) Study. *Neurology* 2012;**8**(Suppl. 1):P04240.

107. Russell MB, Hilden J, Sorensen SA, Olesen J. Familial occurrence of migraine without aura and migraine with aura. *Neurology* 1993;**43**:1369–73.

108. Russell MB, Olesen J. Migrainous disorder and its relation to migraine without aura and Migraine with aura. A genetic epidemiological study. *Cephalalgia* 1996;**16**:431–5.

109. Ulrich V, Gervil M, Fenger K, Olesen J, Russell MB. The prevalence and characteristics of migraine in twins from the general population. *Headache* 1999;**39**:173–80.

110. Lemos C, Castro MJ, Barros J, et al. Familial clustering of migraine: further evidence from a Portuguese study. *Headache* 2009;**49**:404–11.

111. Stewart WF, Bigal ME, Kolodner K, Dowson A, Liberman JN, Lipton RB. Familial risk of migraine: variation by proband age at onset and headache severity. *Neurology* 2006;**66**:344–8.

112. Stewart WF, Staffa J, Lipton RB, Ottman R. Familial risk of migraine: a population-based study. *Ann Neurol* 1997;**41**:166–72.

113. Arruda MA, Guidetti V, Galli F, Albuquerque RCAP, Bigal ME. Frequency of headaches in children is influenced by parental headache status. *Headache* 2010;**50**:973–80.

114. Nackley AG, Tan KS, Fecho K, Flood P, Diatchenko L, Maixner W. Catechol-O methyltransferase inhibition increases pain sensitivity through activation of both beta2- and beta3-adrenergic receptors. *Pain* 2007;**128**:199–208.

115. Diatchenko L, Nackley AG, Slade GD, et al. Catechol-O methyltransferase gene polymorphisms are associated with multiple pain-evoking stimuli. *Pain* 2006;**125**:216–24.

116. Bond DS, Vithiananthan S, Nash JM, Thomas JG, Wing RR. Improvement of migraine

headaches in severely obese patients after bariatric surgery. *Neurology* 2011;**76**: 1135–8.

117. Calhoun AH, Ford S. Behavioral sleep modification may revert transformed migraine to episodic migraine. *Headache* 2007;**47**: 1178–83.

118. Boudreau GP, Grosberg BM, McAllister PJ, Sheftell FD, Lipton RB, Buse DC. Open-label, multicenter study of the efficacy and outcome of onabotulinumtoxin-A treatment in patients with chronic migraine and comorbid depressive disorders. Presented at the 2nd European Headache and Migraine Trust (EHMTIC) International Congress, Nice, France, October 28–31, 2010.

119. Silberstein SD. Practice parameter: evidence-based guidelines for migraine headache (an evidence-based review): report of the Quality Standards Subcommittee of the American Academy of Neurology. *Neurology* 2000;**55**:754–62.

120. Buse DC, Rupnow MF, Lipton RB. Assessing and managing all aspects of migraine: migraine attacks, migraine-related functional impairment, common comorbidities, and quality of life. *Mayo Clinic Proc* 2009; **84**:422–35.

121. Buse DC, Andrasik F. Behavioral medicine for migraine. *Neurol Clin* 2009;**27**:445–65.

122. Buse DC, Sollars CM, Steiner TJ, Jensen RH, Al Jumah MA, Lipton RB. Why hurt? A review of clinical instruments for headache management. *Curr Pain Headache Rep* 2012;**16**:237–54.

123. Stewart WF, Lipton RB. Work-related disability: results from the American Migraine Study. *Cephalalgia* 1996;**16**:231–8.

124. Lipton RB, Bigal ME, Diamond M, Freitag F, Reed ML, Stewart WF. Migraine prevalence, disease burden and the need for preventive therapy (AMPP). *Neurology* 2007;**68**:343–9.

125. Katsarava Z, Schneeweiss S, Kurth T, et al. Incidence and predictors for chronicity of headache in patients with episodic migraine. *Neurology* 2004;**62**:788–90.

126. Plesh O, Adams SH, Gansky SA. Self-reported comorbid pains in severe headaches or migraines in a US national sample. *Headache* 2012;**52**:946–56.

Pathophysiology and Genetics of Migraine

Peter J. Goadsby

University of California, San Francisco, CA, USA

Introduction

Migraine is likely to be a brain disorder involving a disordered regulation and control of afferents, with a particular focus on the cranium [1]. An understanding of the pathophysiology of migraine should be based upon the anatomy and physiology of the pain-producing structures of the cranium, integrated with a knowledge of their central nervous system modulation. Current views concerning migraine will be reviewed, concluding that the disorder is a disturbance in the brain of the subcortical aminergic sensory modulatory systems, in addition to other brainstem, hypothalamic, and thalamic structures.

Migraine—explaining the clinical phenotype

Migraine is in essence a familial episodic disorder whose key marker is headache with certain associated features (Tables 6.1 and 6.2). It is these features that give crucial clues to its pathophysiology, and ultimately will provide insights leading to new treatments.

The essential elements to be considered are:

- the genetics of migraine;
- the physiologic basis for the aura;
- the anatomy of head pain, particularly that of the trigeminovascular system;
- the physiology and pharmacology of activation of the peripheral branches of ophthalmic branch of the trigeminal nerve;
- the physiology and pharmacology of the trigeminal nucleus, in particular its caudal most part, the trigeminocervical complex;
- brainstem and diencephalic modulatory systems that influence trigeminal pain transmission and processing of other sensory modalities.

Migraine is a form of sensory processing disturbance with wide ramifications for CNS function, and while pain is used as the exemplar symptom, a brain-centered explanation provides a framework to understand all the manifestations of migraine.

Genetics of migraine

One of the most important aspects of the pathophysiology of migraine is the inherited nature of the disorder [3]. It is clear from clinical practice that many patients have first-degree relatives who also suffer from migraine. Transmission of migraine from parents to children has been

Headache, First Edition. Edited by Matthew S. Robbins, Brian M. Grosberg, and Richard B. Lipton.
© 2013 John Wiley & Sons, Ltd. Published 2013 by John Wiley & Sons, Ltd.

reported as early as the 17th century, and numerous published studies have reported a positive family history.

Genetic epidemiology

Studies of twin pairs are the classical method to investigate the relative importance of genetic and environmental factors. A Danish study included 1013 monozygotic and 1667 dizygotic twin pairs of the same gender, obtained from a population-based twin register. The pairwise concordance rate was significantly higher among monozygotic than dizygotic twin pairs ($P < 0.05$).

Several studies have attempted to analyze the possible mode of inheritance in families with migraine, but conflicting results have been obtained. Both twin studies and population-based epidemiologic surveys strongly suggest that migraine without aura is a multifactorial disorder, caused by a combination of genetic and environmental factors. An unexplained but epidemiologically well-established predisposition relates to a methyltetrahydrofolate reductase C677T gene mutation that is certainly over-represented in migraine with aura. The presence of aura seems to be associated, in rarer inherited cases, such as CADASIL (cerebral autosomal dominant arteriopathy with subcortical infarcts and leukoencephalopathy) or autosomal dominant retinal vasculopathy with cerebral leukodystrophy, with structural protein dysfunction [4], and perhaps with an embryonic syndrome that includes patent foramen ovale. Such a view makes the small excess stroke risk for young migraineurs unsurprising [5], and suggests a common genetics as opposed to a pathophysiologic link for migraine pain. Remarkably, and importantly for patients and clinicians, the most recent population-based epidemiologic data suggest that migraine carries no excess risk for cognitive function compared to age- and sex-matched controls. In that French cohort, the

Table 6.1. Features of migraine as included in the second edition of the International Classification of Headache Disorders [2]

Repeated episodic headache (4–72 hours) with the following features:	
Any two of:	*Any one of:*
• Unilateral	• Nausea/vomiting
• Throbbing	• Photophobia and
• Worsened by	phonophobia
movement	
• Moderate or severe	

Table 6.2. Neuroanatomical processing of vascular head pain

	Structure	Comments
Target innervation • Cranial vessels • Dura mater	Ophthalmic branch of the trigeminal nerve	
First-order neuron	Trigeminal ganglion	Middle cranial fossa
Second-order neuron	Trigeminal nucleus (quintothalamic tract)	Trigeminal nucleus caudalis and C1/C2 dorsal horns
Third-order neuron	Thalamus	Ventrobasal complex Medial nucleus of posterior group Intralaminar complex
Modulatory	Midbrain Hypothalamus	PAG Orexinergic mechanisms
Final	Cortex	• Insulae • Frontal cortex • Anterior cingulate cortex • Basal ganglia

presence or absent of changes in brain MRI was also not predictive of cognitive decline.

Familial hemiplegic migraine

In approximately 50% of the reported families, familial hemiplegic migraine (FHM) has been assigned to chromosome 19p13. Few clinical differences have been found between chromosome 19-linked and unlinked FHM families. Indeed, the clinical phenotype does not associate particularly with the known mutations. The most striking exception is cerebellar ataxia, which occurs in approximately 50% of the chromosome 19-linked, but none of the unlinked, families. Another less striking difference includes the fact that patients from chromosome 19-linked families are more likely to have attacks that can be triggered by minor head trauma or are that associated with coma.

The biologic basis for the linkage to chromosome 19 is mutations involving the $Ca_v2.1$ (P/Q) type voltage-gated calcium channel *CACNA1A* gene [6]. Responsible for what is now known as FHM-I, this mutation is accounts for about 50% of identified families. One consequence of this mutation may be enhanced glutamate release. Mutations in the *ATP1A2* gene have been identified to be responsible for about 20% of FHM families [7]. Interestingly, the phenotype of some FHM-II involves epilepsy. The gene codes for an Na^+/K^+ ATPase, and the mutation results in a smaller electrochemical gradient for sodium ions. One effect of this change is to reduce or inactivate astrocytic glutamate transporters, leading to a build-up of synaptic glutamate. A mis-sense mutation (Q1489K) in *SCN1A* has been reported in three German families, thus characterizing the genetic defect of what is now known as FHM-III [8]. This mutation affects a highly conserved amino acid in a part of the channel that contributes to its rapid closure after opening in response to membrane depolarization (fast inactivation). This represents a gain of function: instead of the channel rapidly closing, allowing the membrane to repolarize fully after an action potential, the mutated channel allows a persistent sodium influx.

Taken together, the known mutations suggest that migraine, or at least the neurologic manifestations currently called the aura, are ionopathies. Linking the channel disturbance for the first time to the aura process has demonstrated that human mutations expressed in a knockin mouse produce a reduced threshold for cortical spreading depression (CSD) [9]. Further, studies of trigeminal durally evoked nociceptive activation using Fos protein expression in these knockin mice demonstrate reduced second-order neuronal activation compared to wild-type animals and enhanced Fos protein expression in certain thalamic nuclei. The data suggest the brunt of the pathophysiologic burden in this mutation may fall on thalamocortical mechanisms.

Migraine aura

Migraine aura is defined as a focal neurologic disturbance manifest as visual, sensory, or motor symptoms. It is seen in about 30% of patients, and it is clearly neurally driven. The case for the aura being the human equivalent of the CSD of Leão has been well made [10]. In humans, the visual aura has been described as affecting the visual field, suggesting the visual cortex, and it starts at the centre of the visual field, propagating to the periphery at a speed of 3 mm/min. This is very similar to the spreading depression described in rabbits. Blood flow studies in patients have also shown that a focal hyperemia tends to precede the spreading oligemia, and again this is similar to what would be expected with spreading depression. After this passage of oligemia, the cerebrovascular response to hypercapnia in patients is blunted while autoregulation remains intact [11]. Again, this pattern is repeated with experimental spreading depression. An interesting recent study suggested that female mice are more susceptible generally to CSD than male mice, which would be consistent with the excess risk of migraine in females after menarche that is still with them, on a population basis, into menopause and afterwards.

Human observations, including a recent study showing that ketamine, which is well known to block CSD in animals, can ameliorate prolonged aura in patients, have rendered the arguments reasonably sound that human aura has as its equivalent in animal CSD. An area of controversy surrounds whether aura in fact triggers the rest of the attack, and is indeed painful. The current data in humans, in particular the very well-recognized phenomenon of migraine aura without headache, suggest that it is indeed not painful.

Therapeutic manipulation of aura

Tonabersat (SB-220453) is a CSD inhibitor that has completed clinical trials in migraine. Tonabersat inhibits CSD, CSD-induced nitric oxide release, and cerebral vasodilation. Tonabersat does not constrict isolated human blood vessels, but does inhibit trigeminally induced craniovascular effects. It has been shown to be ineffective in migraine when reduced attacks of pain are taken as the end-point, yet it can reduce frequency of aura [12].

Remarkably, topiramate, a proven preventive agent in migraine, also inhibits CSD in cats and rats, and in the rat with prolonged dosing. Topiramate inhibits trigeminal neurons activated by nociceptive intracranial afferents, but not by a mechanism local to the trigeminocervical complex, and thus CSD inhibition may be a model system to contribute to the development of preventive medicines, particularly agents to prevent aura. The model predicts that agents interacting with Na^+-based mechanisms might be effective, as would glutamate–α-amino-3-hydroxy-5-methylisoxazole-4-propionate (AMPA) receptor mechanisms, but not gamma-aminobutyric acid (GABA)-ergic mechanisms, at least directly. Glutamate N-methyl-D-aspartate (NMDA)-mediated effects have been reported to important in CSD, and in an active-controlled study of migraine with prolonged aura. These may suggest some way forward for the management of at least the most disabled group who have persistent or prolonged aura.

Headache—anatomy

Trigeminal innervation of pain-producing intracranial structures

Surrounding the large cerebral vessels, pial vessels, large venous sinuses, and dura mater is a plexus of largely unmyelinated fibres that arise from the ophthalmic division of the trigeminal ganglion, and in the posterior fossa from the upper cervical dorsal roots. Trigeminal fibers innervating cerebral vessels arise from neurons in the trigeminal ganglion that contain substance P and calcitonin gene-related peptide (CGRP), both of which can be released in either humans or cats when the trigeminal ganglion is stimulated. Stimulation of the cranial vessels, such as the superior sagittal sinus, is certainly painful in humans. Human dural nerves that innervate the cranial vessels largely consist of small-diameter myelinated and unmyelinated fibers that almost certainly subserve a nociceptive function.

Headache physiology—peripheral connections

Plasma protein extravasation

A series of laboratory experiments in the 1990s suggested that migraine pain may be due to a sterile, neurogenically driven inflammation of the dura mater [13]. Neurogenic plasma extravasation can be seen during electrical stimulation of the trigeminal ganglion in the rat. Plasma extravasation can be blocked by ergot alkaloids, indomethacin, acetylsalicylic acid, and the serotonin–$5-HT_{1B/1D}$ agonist sumatriptan. Further, preclinical studies have suggested that CSD may be a sufficient stimulus to activate trigeminal neurons, although this has been controversial. In addition, there are structural changes in the dura mater that are observed after trigeminal ganglion stimulation. These include mast cell degranulation and changes in postcapillary venules including platelet aggregation. While it is generally accepted that such changes, and particularly the initiation of a sterile inflammatory response, would cause pain, it is not clear whether this is sufficient of itself, or requires other stimulators or promoters. Preclinical studies suggest that CSD may be a sufficient stimulus to activate trigeminal neurons, although this has been a controversial area. What neurogenic dural plasma extravasation fails to predict is whether new targets, when engaged, are effective in either the acute or preventive treatment of migraine. Blockade of neurogenic plasma protein extravasation is not predictive of antimigraine efficacy in humans, as evidenced by the failure in clinical trials of substance P, neurokinin-1 receptor antagonists, specific plasma protein extravasation blockers CP122,288 and 4991w93, an endothelin antagonist, a neurosteroid, and an inhibitor of the inducible form of nitric oxide synthase known as GW274150 [14].

Sensitization and migraine

While it is highly doubtful that there is a significant sterile inflammatory response in the dura mater during migraine, it is clear that some form of sensitization takes place during migraine. About two-thirds of patients complain of pain from non-noxious stimuli: allodynia [15]. A particularly interesting aspect is the demonstration of allodynia in the upper limbs ipsilateral and contralateral to the pain. This finding is consistent with at least third-order neuronal involvement, such as a sensitization of thalamic neurons, and firmly places the pathophysiology within the central nervous system. Sensitization in migraine may also have a peripheral component with a local release of inflammatory markers, which would certainly activate trigeminal nociceptors, although a peripheral component is not necessary to explain the symptoms. More likely, in migraine there is a form of central sensitization, which may be classical central sensitization, or a form of disinhibitory sensitization with dysfunction of the descending modulatory pathways. Interestingly, the presence or absence of allodynia does not predict outcome after acute therapy in randomized-controlled trials.

Just as dihydroergotamine (DHE) can block trigeminovascular nociceptive transmission, probably at least by a local effect in the trigeminocervical complex [16], DHE can block central sensitization associated with dural stimulation by an inflammatory soup. Indeed, localization of DHE binding in the midbrain dorsal raphe nucleus and periaqueductal gray (PAG) matter [17], and the antinociceptive effect of naratriptan when injected locally into the PAG or sensory thalamus [18], offer challenges to the orthodoxy that acute antimigraine medicines are simply inhibitors of the trigeminovascular system.

Neuropeptide studies

Electrical stimulation of the trigeminal ganglion in both humans and cats leads to increases in extracerebral blood flow and the local release of both CGRP and substance P. In the cat, trigeminal ganglion stimulation also increases cerebral blood flow by a pathway traversing the greater superficial petrosal branch of the facial nerve, again releasing a powerful vasodilator peptide, vasoactive intestinal polypeptide (VIP). Interestingly, the VIPergic innervation of the cerebral vessels is predominantly anterior rather than posterior, and this may contribute to this region's vulnerability to spreading depression, explaining why the aura is so very often seen to commence posteriorly.

Stimulation of the more specifically pain-producing superior sagittal sinus increases cerebral blood flow and jugular vein CGRP levels. Human evidence that CGRP is elevated in the headache phase of severe migraine [19], although not in less severe attacks, in cluster headache, and in chronic paroxysmal hemicrania supports the view that the trigeminovascular system may be activated in a protective role in these conditions [20]. Moreover, nitric oxide donor-triggered migraine, which is typical migraine in all regards, also results in increases in CGRP that are blocked by sumatriptan, just as in spontaneous migraine [21]. It is of interest in this regard that compounds that have not shown activity in migraine, notably the conformationally restricted analogue of sumatriptan, CP122,288, and the conformationally restricted analogue of zolmitriptan, 4991w93, were both ineffective inhibitors of CGRP release after superior sagittal sinus stimulation in the cat. The development of nonpeptide, highly specific CGRP receptor antagonists, and the successful results of now at least four different CGRP receptor antagonists in acute migraine, firmly establishes this as a novel and important new emerging principle for acute migraine [22]. Interestingly, given the variability, it will probably not provide a biomarker for migraine. At the same time, the lack of any effect of CGRP receptor antagonists on plasma protein extravasation explains in some part why that model has proved inadequate for translation into human therapeutic approaches.

Headache physiology—central connections

The trigeminocervical complex

Fos immunohistochemistry is a method for looking at activated cells by plotting the expression of Fos protein. After meningeal irritation with blood, Fos expression is noted in the trigeminal nucleus caudalis, while after stimulation of the superior sagittal sinus, Fos-like immunoreactivity is seen in the trigeminal nucleus caudalis and in the dorsal horn at the C1 and C2 levels in the cat and monkey [23]. These latter findings are in accord with similar data using 2-deoxyglucose measurements with superior sagittal sinus stimulation [24]. Similarly, stimulation of a branch of C2, the greater occipital nerve, increases metabolic activity in the same regions, i.e. trigeminal nucleus caudalis and the C1/2 dorsal horn. In experimental animals, one can record directly from trigeminal neurons with both supratentorial trigeminal input and input from the greater occipital nerve, a branch of the C2 dorsal root. Stimulation of the greater occipital nerve for 5 minutes results in substantial increases in responses to supratentorial dural stimulation, which can last for over an hour. Conversely, stimulation of the dura mater over the middle meningeal artery with the C-fiber irritant mustard oil sensitizes responses to occipital muscle stimulation. It can be shown, again using the Fos method, that this interaction is likely to involve at least activation of the NMDA-subtype glutamate receptors. Taken together, these data suggest a convergence of cervical and ophthalmic inputs at the level of the second-order neuron [25]. Moreover, stimulation of a lateralized structure, the middle meningeal artery, produces Fos expression bilaterally in both cat and monkey brain. This group of neurons from the superficial laminae of the trigeminal nucleus caudalis and C1/2 dorsal horns should be regarded functionally as the *trigeminocervical* complex.

These data demonstrate that trigeminovascular nociceptive information comes by way of the most caudal cells. This concept provides an anatomic explanation for the referral of pain to the back of the head in migraine. Moreover, experimental pharmacologic evidence suggests that drugs that act to abort migraines, such as ergot derivatives, acetylsalicylic acid, sumatriptan, eletriptan, naratriptan, rizatriptan, and zolmitriptan, and the novel approach of CGRP receptor antagonists can have actions at these second-order neurons that reduce cell activity, and suggests a further possible site for therapeutic intervention in migraine [26]. The triptan action can be dissected out to involve each of the 5-HT_{1B}, 5-HT_{1D}, and 5-HT_{1F} receptor subtypes, consistent with the localization of these receptors on peptidergic nociceptors. Interestingly, triptans also influence the CGRP promoter, regulate CGRP secretion from neurons in culture, and may not access their receptors until the trigeminovascular system is activated. Further, the demonstration that some part of this action is postsynaptic with either 5-HT_{1B} or 5-HT_{1D} receptors located *non*-presynatically offers the prospect of highly anatomically localized targets for treatment. Certainly, the triptan, $5\text{-HT}_{1B/1D/1F}$ receptors are not localized peripherally since they can be identified at every level of sensory input from the trigeminal ganglion through the cervical, thoracic, lumbar, and sacral dorsal root ganglia [27].

Serotonin—5-HT_{1F} receptor agonists and migraine

Some, but not all, of the triptans are not only 5-HT1B/1D receptor agonists, but also potent 5-HT1F receptor agonists. $5\text{-HT}_{1B/1D}$ receptor agonists are also potent 5-HT1F receptor agonists. A notably example is naratriptan, which is highly potent by the injectable route. With the same second messenger activity as the $5HT_{1B}$ and 5-HT_{1D} receptors, adenylate cyclase inhibition, and no contractile effects on blood vessels so far identified, it is a good novel neural target for migraine treatment. It can be shown that 5-HT_{1F} activation inhibits trigeminal nucleus Fos activation and neuronal firing in response to dural stimulation, the latter without cranial vascular effects. One early compound was found to be effective in clinical situations but had toxicologic problems unrelated to the mechanism, and another, lasmiditan (COL-144), has now been shown in a randomized-controlled trial to be an effective acute antimigraine treatment [28]. These data further the concept that vascular mechanisms are not necessary for acute migraine treatments.

Glutamatergic transmission in the trigeminocervical complex

A potential target for antimigraine drugs is the family of glutamate receptors (GluRs), which consist of the ionotropic (iGluRs) NMDA, AMPA, and kainate, and the metabotropic glutamate receptors (mGluRs) 1–8 [29]. NMDA receptor channel blockers have been shown reduce nociceptive trigeminovascular transmission *in vivo*. The AMPA/kainate receptor antagonists 6-cyano-7-nitroquinoxaline-2,3-dione (CNQX) and

2,3-dioxo-6-nitro-1,2,3,4-tetrahydrobenzoqui-noxaline-7-sulfonamide reduced Fos protein expression after activation of the structures involved in nociceptive pathways, and direct application of CNQX to the trigeminocervical complex attenuated neurons with nociceptive trigeminovascular inputs. Regarding the group III mGluR receptor, the agonist L-(+)-2-amino-4-phosphonobutyric acid decreased Fos protein expression in an animal model of trigeminovascular nociceptive processing. It is also notable that the group I mGluR5 modulator ADX10059 has been reported to be effective in the acute treatment of migraine.

Kainate receptors are constituted by the "low-affinity" iGluR5, iGluR6, and iGluR7, and the "high-affinity" KA1 and KA2 subunits, which form different homo- or heteromeric assemblies, giving rise to functional receptors. The presence of iGluR5 subunits in the trigeminal ganglion neurons and at the presynaptic sites of primary afferents indicates a possible role of kainate receptors in trigeminovascular physiology. Most recently, it has been shown that activation of the iGluR5 kainate receptors with the selective agonist iodowillardiine is able to inhibit neurogenic dural vasodilation, probably by inhibiting the prejunctional release of CGRP from the trigeminal afferents. Further, in a double-blinded, randomized, placebo-controlled study in acute migraine, LY466195, an iGluR5 kainate receptor antagonist, was effective at the 2-hour pain-free end-point. In a separate small study of acute migraine, intravenous application of the decahydroisoquinoline AMPA/iGluR5 antagonist LY293558 improved headache pain in two-thirds of migraineurs and relieved the associated symptoms of the attack. Taken together, these studies suggest a strong basis for pursuing glutamate targets, with some care for considering how to do this without attracting unwanted side effects.

Higher order processing

Following transmission in the caudal brainstem and high cervical spinal cord, information is relayed rostrally.

Thalamus

Processing of vascular nociceptive signals in the thalamus occurs in the ventroposteromedial (VPM) thalamus, the medial nucleus of the posterior complex, and the intralaminar thalamus [30]. Application of capsaicin to the superior sagittal sinus activates trigeminal projections with a high degree of nociceptive input that are processed in neurons particularly in the VPM thalamus and in its ventral periphery. These neurons in the VPM can be modulated by activation of $GABA_A$ inhibitory receptors, and perhaps of more direct clinical relevance by propranolol though a beta-1-adrenoceptor mechanism [31]. Remarkably, triptans can, through $5-HT_{1B/1D}$ mechanisms, also inhibit VPM neurons locally, as demonstrated by microiontophoretic application, suggesting a hitherto unconsidered locus of action for triptans in acute migraine. Importantly, human imaging studies have confirmed activation of the thalamus contralateral to the pain in acute migraine, cluster headache, short-lasting unilateral neuralgiform headache with conjunctival injection and tearing (SUNCT), and hemicrania continua.

Activation of modulatory regions

Stimulation of nociceptive afferents in the superior sagittal sinus in the cat activates neurons in the ventrolateral PAG. PAG activation in turn feeds back to the trigeminocervical complex with an inhibitory influence [32]. PAG is clearly included in the area of activation seen in positron-emission tomography (PET) studies in migraineurs, and may have a more generic antinociceptive role. This typical negative feedback system will be further considered later as a possible mechanism for the symptomatic manifestations of migraine.

Another potential modulatory region activated by stimulation of nociceptive trigeminovascular input is the posterior hypothalamic gray. This area is crucially involved in several primary headaches, notably cluster headache, SUNCT, paroxysmal hemicrania, and hemicrania continua [33]. Moreover, the clinical features of the premonitory phase, and other features of the disorder, suggest dopamine neuron involvement in some part. It can be shown in the experimental animal that D_2 family receptors are more often seen in rat trigeminocervical neurons than D_1 family receptors, and that dopamine locally iontophoresed into the trigeminocervical complex, but not administered intravenously, inhibits trigeminovascular nociceptive transmission. Moreover, it seems plausible that this effect, at least in part, emanates from the dopamine-containing A11 neurons, which inhibit trigeminovascular nociceptive transmission through a D_2 receptor-mediated mechanism, and after lesioning of this region trigeminal nociceptive transmission is facilitated [34]. Orexinergic neurons in the posterior hypothalamus can have both pro- and antinociceptive downstream effects and are activated when trigeminovascular nociceptive afferents are stimulated. Orexin A activation of the OX_1 receptor can both modulate dural–vascular responses to trigeminal afferent activation and inhibit second-order trigeminovascular neurons in the trigeminocervical complex. Orexinergic mechanisms may be an attractive component of the central matrix of neuronal systems that are dysfunctional in migraine [35].

The "vascular hypothesis"—a good story ruined by the facts

For much of the later part of the 20th century, a rather straightforward concept dominated thinking about migraine. First proposed in some part by Willis and best articulated by Wolff, the theory explained the pain of migraine to be due to dilation of the cranial vessels. By the later part of the 19th century, neuronal theories had been well articulated, and indeed Gowers seemed happy with that concept. It is now clear that the vascular hypothesis is untenable as an explanation for migraine pathophysiology, and some of the data behind this view are covered here.

It has been shown that infusion of pituitary adenylate cyclase activating peptide (PACAP)-38 can produce cranial vasodilation and trigger a delayed migraine in sufferers but not in controls, and not in migraineurs when infused with placebo. The same group using the same methods has shown that VIP, another member, with PACAP, of the secretin/glucagon peptide superfamily, can induce an equal craniovascular vasodilation but does not trigger migraine at all. So it is not the dilation but the receptor site activation—put simply, the vasodilation is an epiphenomenon that is neither sufficient nor necessary [36]. Another lynchpin of the vascular argument came

from the behavior of cranial vessels in migraine sufferers. It had been shown that ergotamine could produce vasoconstriction in line with its efficacy in migraine. When this was more closely examined, it was shown that the vascular changes were unrelated to the phase of the attack, and indeed blood flow could be reduced or normal during the pain phase. Most recently, using high-resolution 3T magnetic resonance angiography, it has been reported that migraine triggered by nitroglycerin occurs without any continuing change in intracranial or extracranial vessels.

An important result for all of us, but more particularly for patients, is that the neuronal–vascular acute treatment debate has now come full circle in favor of a neuronal approach. Triptans, serotonin 5-$HT_{1B/1D}$ receptor agonists, which are extremely effective treatments and were developed initially as cranial vasoconstrictors, have been for some time described to have effects on neuronal transmission in the brain. The most recent studies demonstrate that CGRP receptor antagonists such as olcegepant and telcagepant, developed based on the elevation of CGRP in acute, severe migraine and its normalization with treatment, are both effective and without vascular effects. Similarly, a purely neurally acting 5-HT_{1F} receptor agonist, lasmiditan, is effective and devoid of vasoconstrictor actions. Taken together, be it triggering, measuring, or inducing vascular change with therapies, vascular change is neither necessary, sufficient, nor needed in migraine—in short, it is an epiphenomenon of the neural substrates that are activated by the underlying pathophysiology of the disorder.

Central modulation of trigeminal pain

Brain imaging in humans

Functional brain imaging with PET has demonstrated activation of the dorsal midbrain, including the PAG, and the dorsal pons, near the locus coeruleus, in studies during migraine without aura [37]. Dorsolateral pontine activation is shown by PET in spontaneous episodic and chronic migraine, and with nitroglycerin-triggered attacks. These areas are active immediately after successful treatment of the headache, but are not active interictally. The activation corresponds with the brain regions reported to cause migraine-like headache when stimulated in patients with electrodes implanted for pain control. Similarly, excess iron has been noted in the PAG of patients with episodic and chronic migraine, and chronic migraine can develop after a bleed into a cavernoma in the region of the PAG, or with a lesion of the pons. What could dysfunction of these brain areas lead to?

Animal experimental studies of sensory modulation

It has been shown in the experimental animal that stimulation of the nucleus locus coeruleus, the main central noradrenergic nucleus, reduces cerebral blood flow in a frequency-dependent manner through an alpha-2-adrenoceptor-linked mechanism [38]. This reduction is maximal in the occipital cortex. While a 25% overall reduction in cerebral blood flow is seen, extracerebral vasodilatation occurs in parallel. In addition, the main serotonin-containing nucleus in the brainstem, the midbrain dorsal raphe nucleus, can increase cerebral blood flow when activated [39]. Further, stimulation of the PAG will inhibit sagittal sinus-evoked trigeminal neuronal activity in the cat, while blockade of P/Q-type voltage-gated calcium channels in the PAG facilitates trigeminovascular nociceptive processing with the local GABAergic system of the PAG still intact.

Electrophysiology of migraine in humans

Studies of evoked potentials and event-related potentials provide some link between animal studies and human functional imaging. Authors have shown changes in neurophysiologic measures of brain activation, but there is much discussion of how to interpret such changes. Perhaps the most reliable theme is that the migrainous brain does not habituate to signals in a normal way, nor indeed does that of patients who have first-degree relatives with migraine. Similarly, contingent negative variation, an event-related potential, is abnormal in migraineurs compared to controls. Changes in contingent negative variation predict attacks, and preventive therapies alter or normalize such changes; recent evidence suggests the involvement of thalamocortical relays in these habituation deficits [40]. Attempts to correlate clinical phenotypes with electro-

physiologic changes may enhance further studies in this area.

Conclusion: what is migraine?

Migraine is an inherited, episodic disorder involving sensory sensitivity (Figure 6.1). Patients complain of pain in the head that is throbbing, but there is no reliable relationship between the vessel diameter and the pain, or its treatment. They complain of discomfort caused by normal lights and the unpleasantness of routine sounds. Some mention that otherwise pleasant odours are unpleasant. Normal movement of the head causes pain, and many mention a sense of unsteadiness as if they have just stepped off a boat, having been nowhere near the water. The anatomic connections of, for example, the pain pathways are clear; the ophthalmic division of the trigeminal nerve subserves sensation within the cranium and perhaps underpins why the top of the head equates to headache, while the maxillary division relates to *facial pain*. The convergence of cervical and trigeminal afferents explains why neck stiffness or pain is so common in primary headache. The genetics of channelopathies is opening up a plausible way to think about the episodic nature of migraine. However, where is the lesion, and what is actually the pathology?

Migraine aura cannot be the trigger—there is no evidence at all after 4000 years that it occurs in aura more than 30% of migraine patients. Aura can be experienced without pain at all, and is seen in the other primary headaches. There is not a photon of extra light that migraine patients receive over others, so for that symptom, and phonophobia and osmophobia, the basis of the problem must be abnormal central processing of a normal signal. Perhaps electrophysiologic changes in the brain have been mislabelled as *hyperexcitability* whereas dyshabituation might be a simpler explanation. If migraine were basically a sensory attentional problem with changes in cortical synchronization—*hypersynchronization*—all its manifestations could be accounted for in a single overarching pathophysiologic hypothesis of a disturbance of subcortical sensory modulation systems. While it seems likely that the trigeminovascular system, and its cranial autonomic reflex connections, the trigeminal–autonomic reflex, act as a feedforward system to

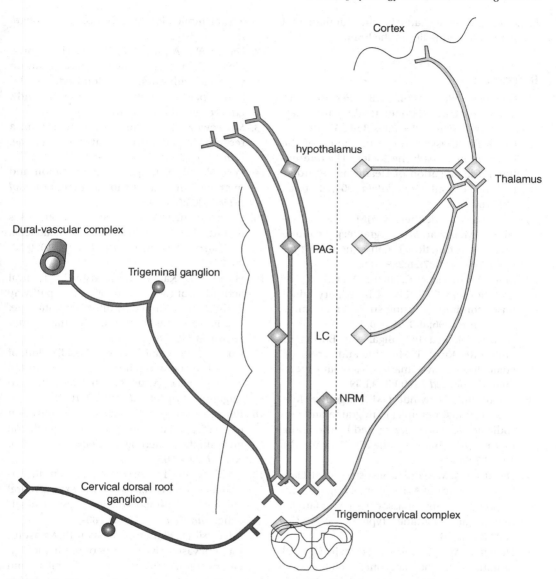

Figure 6.1. Pathophysiology of migraine. Diagram of some of the structures involved in the transmission of trigeminovascular nociceptive input and the modulation of that input that form the basis of a model of the pathophysiology of migraine. Afferents from the dural–vascular complex innervated predominantly by branches of the first (ophthalmic) division of the trigeminal nerve, whose cell bodies are found in the trigeminal ganglion, project to second-order neurons in the trigeminocervical complex (TCC). The TCC extends from the trigeminal nucleus caudalis to the caudal portion of the dorsal horn of the C2 spinal cord. Input from cervical structures, such as joints or muscles, projects through cell bodies in the upper cervical dorsal root ganglia to the TCC. TCC neurons project to the ventrobasal thalamus (thalamus) and thence to the cortex. Sensory modulation can occur by descending influences onto the TCC that largely respect the midline (dashed line), such as those from the hypothalamus, midbrain PAG, pontine locus coeruleus (LC), and nucleus raphe magnus (NRM). These influences are represented in the figure as being direct, but both direct and indirect projections are recognized. In addition sensory modulation can occur from at least the LC, PAG, and hypothalamic projections to the thalamic nuclei as ascending systems again that largely respect the midline.

facilitate the acute attack, the fundamental problem in migraine lies in the brain.

References

1. Goadsby PJ, Lipton RB, Ferrari MD. Migraine—current understanding and treatment. *New Engl J Med* 2002;**346**:257–70.

2. Headache Classification Committee of the International Headache Society. The International Classification of Headache Disorders (second edition). *Cephalalgia* 2004;**24**(Suppl. 1):1–160.

3. van den Maagdenberg AMJM, Haan J, Terwindt GM, Ferrari MD. Migraine: gene mutations and functional consequences. *Curr Opin Neurol* 2007;**20**:299–305.

4. Joutel A, Corpechot C, Ducros A, et al. Notch3 mutations in CADASIL, a hereditary adult-onset condition causing stroke and dementia. *Nature* 1996;**383**:707–10.

5. Schurks M, Rist PM, Bigal ME, Buring JE, Lipton RB, Kurth T. Migraine and cardiovascular disease: systematic review and meta-analysis. *Br Med J* 2009;**339**:b3914.

6. Ophoff RA, Terwindt GM, Vergouwe MN, et al. Familial hemiplegic migraine and episodic ataxia type-2 are caused by mutations in the Ca^{2+} channel gene CACNL1A4. *Cell* 1996;**87**:543–52.

7. De Fusco M, Marconi R, Silvestri L, et al. Haploinsufficiency of ATP1A2 encoding the Na^+/K^+ pump α2 subunit associated with familial hemiplegic migraine type 2. *Nat Gen* 2003;**33**:192–6.

8. Dichgans M, Freilinger T, Eckstein G, et al. Mutation in the neuronal voltage-gated sodium channel *SCN1A* causes familial hemiplegic migraine. *Lancet* 2005;**366**: 371–7.

9. van den Maagdenberg AMJM, Pietrobon D, Pizzorusso T, et al. A Cacna1a knock-in migraine mouse model with increased susceptibility to cortical spreading depression. *Neuron* 2004;**41**:701–10.

10. Lauritzen M. Pathophysiology of the migraine aura. The spreading depression theory. *Brain* 1994;**117**:199–210.

11. Olesen J. Cerebral and extracranial circulatory disturbances in migraine: pathophysiological implications. *Cerebrovasc Brain Metab Rev* 1991;**3**:1–28.

12. Hauge AW, Asghar MS, Schytz HW, Christensen K, Olesen J. Effects of tonabersat on migraine with aura: a randomised, double-blind, placebo-controlled crossover study. *Lancet Neurol* 2009;**8**:718–23.

13. Moskowitz MA, Cutrer FM. Sumatriptan: a receptor-targeted treatment for migraine. *Annu Rev Med* 1993;**44**:145–54.

14. Peroutka SJ. Neurogenic inflammation and migraine: implications for therapeutics. *Mol Interv* 2005;**5**:306–13.

15. Selby G, Lance JW. Observations on 500 cases of migraine and allied vascular headache. *J Neurol Neurosurg Psychiatry* 1960;**23**: 23–32.

16. Hoskin KL, Kaube H, Goadsby PJ. Central activation of the trigeminovascular pathway in the cat is inhibited by dihydroergotamine. A c-Fos and electrophysiology study. *Brain* 1996;**119**:249–56.

17. Goadsby PJ, Gundlach AL. Localization of [³H]-dihydroergotamine binding sites in the cat central nervous system: relevance to migraine. *Ann Neurol* 1991;**29**:91–4.

18. Bartsch T, Knight YE, Goadsby PJ. Activation of 5-HT$_{1B/1D}$ receptors in the periaqueductal grey inhibits meningeal nociception. *Ann Neurol* 2004;**56**:371–81.

19. Goadsby PJ, Edvinsson L, Ekman R. Vasoactive peptide release in the extracerebral circulation of humans during migraine headache. *Ann Neurol* 1990;**28**:183–7.

20. Edvinsson L, Ekman R, Goadsby PJ. Measurement of vasoactive neuropeptides in biological materials: problems and pitfalls from 30 years of experience and novel future approaches. *Cephalalgia* 2010;**30**:761–6.

21. Goadsby PJ, Edvinsson L. The trigeminovascular system and migraine: studies characterizing cerebrovascular and neuropeptide changes seen in humans and cats. *Ann Neurol* 1993;**33**:48–56.

22. Ho TW, Edvinsson L, Goadsby PJ. CGRP and its receptors provide new insights into migraine pathophysiology. *Nat Rev Neurol* 2010;**6**:761–6.

23. Goadsby PJ, Hoskin KL. The distribution of trigeminovascular afferents in the nonhu-

man primate brain *Macaca nemestrina*: a c-fos immunocytochemical study. *J Anat* 1997;**190**:367–75.

24. Goadsby PJ, Zagami AS. Stimulation of the superior sagittal sinus increases metabolic activity and blood flow in certain regions of the brainstem and upper cervical spinal cord of the cat. *Brain* 1991;**114**:1001–11.

25. Bartsch T, Goadsby PJ. Anatomy and physiology of pain referral in primary and cervicogenic headache disorders. *Headache Curr* 2005;**2**:42–8.

26. Andreou AP, Summ O, Charbit AR, Romero Reyes M, Goadsby PJ. Animal models of headache—from bedside to bench and back to beside. *Expert Rev Neurother* 2010;**10**:389–411.

27. Classey JD, Bartsch T, Goadsby PJ. Distribution of 5-HT$_{1B}$, 5-HT$_{1D}$ and 5-HT$_{1F}$ receptor expression in rat trigeminal and dorsal root ganglia neurons: relevance to the selective anti-migraine effect of triptans. *Brain Res* 2010;**1361**:76–85.

28. Ferrari MD, Farkkila M, Reuter U, et al. Acute treatment of migraine with the selective 5-HT1F receptor agonist lasmiditan – a randomised proof-of-concept trial. *Cephalalgia* 2010;**30**:1170–8.

29. Andreou AP, Goadsby PJ. Therapeutic potential of novel glutamate receptor antagonists in migraine. *Expert Opin Investig Drugs* 2009;**18**:789–803.

30. Zagami AS, Lambert GA. Stimulation of cranial vessels excites nociceptive neurones in several thalamic nuclei of the cat. *Exp Brain Res* 1990;**81**:552–66.

31. Shields KG, Goadsby PJ. Propranolol modulates trigeminovascular responses in thalamic ventroposteromedial nucleus: a role in migraine? *Brain* 2005;**128**:86–97.

32. Knight YE, Bartsch T, Kaube H, Goadsby PJ. P/Q-type calcium channel blockade in the PAG facilitates trigeminal nociception: a functional genetic link for migraine? *J Neurosci* 2002;**22**(RC213):1–6.

33. Goadsby PJ, Cittadini E, Cohen AS. Trigeminal autonomic cephalalgias: paroxysmal hemicrania, SUNCT/SUNA and hemicrania continua. *Semin Neurol* 2010;**30**:186–91.

34. Charbit AR, Akerman S, Holland PR, Goadsby PJ. Neurons of the dopaminergic/CGRP A11 cell group modulate neuronal firing in the trigeminocervical complex: an electrophysiological and immunohistochemical study. *J Neurosci* 2009;**29**:12532–41.

35. Holland PR, Goadsby PJ. The hypothalamic orexinergic system: pain and primary headaches. *Headache* 2007;**47**:951–62.

36. Goadsby PJ. The vascular theory of migraine—a great story wrecked by the facts. *Brain* 2009;**132**:6–7.

37. Sprenger T, Goadsby PJ. What has functional neuroimaging done for primary headache . . . and for the clinical neurologist? *J Clin Neurosci* 2010;**17**:547–53.

38. Goadsby PJ, Lambert GA, Lance JW. Differential effects on the internal and external carotid circulation of the monkey evoked by locus coeruleus stimulation. *Brain Res* 1982;**249**:247–54.

39. Goadsby PJ, Piper RD, Lambert GA, Lance JW. The effect of activation of the nucleus raphe dorsalis (DRN) on carotid blood flow. I. The Monkey. *Am J Physiol* 1985;**248**:R257–62.

40. Schoenen J, Ambrosini A, Sandor PS, Maertens de Noordhout A. Evoked potentials and transcranial magnetic stimulation in migraine: published data and viewpoint on their pathophysiologic significance. *Clin Neurophysiol* 2003;**114**:955–72.

Multidisciplinary Approach to Patients with Migraine

Lucille A. Rathier[1], Dawn C. Buse[2], Robert A. Nicholson[3], and Frank Andrasik[4]

[1]The Miriam Hospital, Providence, RI, USA
[2]Albert Einstein College of Medicine, Ferkauf Graduate School of Psychology and Montefiore Headache Center, Bronx, NY, USA
[3]Saint Louis University School of Medicine, Mercy Health Research and Ryan Headache Center, St. Louis, MO, USA
[4]University of Memphis, Memphis, TN, USA

Introduction

The effective long-term management of patients with migraine can be challenging because migraine is a complex, not yet fully understood disease with heterogeneous triggers, expression, and impact [1, 2]. Although the biomedical model has led to important insights into the pathophysiologic mechanisms of migraine, there are limitations to this model, including the marked varied individual responses to identical treatments [1]. As with any other pain condition, migraine involves both sensory (e.g., pain location, intensity, and quality) and affective (e.g., depression, anxiety, and distress) components [3]. At its core, the pain experience involves the interconnectivity of physical vulnerabilities (e.g., genetics), psychological predispositions (e.g., prior learning history), biologic changes, psychological issues, and biopsychosocial contexts that influence an individual's appraisal of and response to migraine [1]. As a result, the effective treatment of migraine cannot rely solely on regulating the chemical and electrical signals within the pain pathways associated with migraine, but must also address the cognitive, affective, and behavioral components of migraine.

For most of the history of headache medicine, nonpharmacologic treatment for migraine was considered an option only when the patient's presentation fell outside the normative patient experience. As migraine has begun to be conceptualized as a chronic disease [4], treatment also needs to reflect this conceptualization. This means that relying on pharmacologic prophylaxis alone is suboptimal care [5, 6]. Rather, a comprehensive, multidisciplinary treatment program to prevent migraine is appropriate.

> ★ TIPS AND TRICKS
>
> Educating patients about why migraine is a chronic disease and how diaries can help to identify trigger and treatment patterns, and

teaching the patient strategies for managing triggers and stress are all parts of an optimal migraine prevention plan. When a provider takes the time either to directly discuss these techniques or provide the patient with access to educational materials (along with an endorsement and rationale for why this will be useful for the patient), the patient is far more likely to engage in these activities. Moreover, in the follow-up visits with the patient, the patient will be more likely to continue utilizing self-management strategies if the provider reviews the patient's diary and checks in with the patient about what they have learned from the diary.

The overwhelming majority of persons with headache can benefit from patient education, identifying triggers through diaries, managing triggers, and stress management [7]. However, some patients require a more formal multidisciplinary treatment plan in order to achieve optimal outcomes. Although numerous nonpharmacologic interventions can be utilized in a multidisciplinary program, biobehavioral approaches (e.g., cognitive-behavioral therapy [CBT], relaxation training, biofeedback, and stress management) and acupuncture have the strongest efficacy. Other nonpharmacologic interventions (e.g., physical medicine approaches including physical therapy, chiropractic medicine, massage, and yoga) do not, to date, have the evidence to support using them as a first-line intervention; however, individual patients may benefit based on their presentation.

Evidence supports the benefits of utilizing nonpharmacologic approaches alone or in combination with pharmacologic intervention (Table 7.1). Using educational and office-based management strategies improves various migraine-related outcomes [8, 9, 10, 11], as do multidisciplinary treatments [12, 13, 14, 15, 16]. A full review of each of these studies is beyond the scope of the current chapter, the goal of which is to provide an overview of the treatment modalities that are commonly included in a multidisciplinary treatment program for migraine

management. We begin with the group of treatments with the greatest evidence for efficacy: biobehavioral interventions.

> ### ⚖ SCIENCE REVISITED
>
> Evidence supports using nonpharmacologic approaches alone or in combination with pharmacologic intervention to prevent migraine. Simply providing tools for migraine self-management in the office (often by the nursing staff) or via educational media (group classes, printed materials, and tailored education) can improve patient outcomes when used with pharmacologic intervention. When higher level interventions aimed at lowering physiologic arousal (e.g., biofeedback, relaxation, and CBT) are employed in conjunction with pharmacologic intervention and self-management training, many patients see an increased improvement in migraine-related outcomes.

Biobehavioral treatments for migraine

Biobehavioral techniques focus on managing the physiologic and cognitive/affective components of stress. Biofeedback and relaxation focus mainly on the individual recognizing and managing the physiologic consequences of the stress, whereas CBT focuses on the patient modifying what they consider "stressful" and how they respond to such stressors. Moreover, biobehavioral techniques facilitate skill development aimed toward increasing the patient's ability to cope with pain and reduce migraine-related distress [17].

> ### ⚖ SCIENCE REVISITED
>
> Reviews of biobehavioral treatments consistently show that biofeedback, relaxation, and CBT (including stress management) produce a 30%–60% reduction in migraine activity. The US Headache Consortium [18] assigned the

Table 7.1. Recommendations for multidisciplinary treatments for migraine based on level of evidence

Intervention type	Specific procedure	Level of evidence for prevention/ modification of headache/migraine[a]	Author recommendations
Biobehavioral	Psychoeducation, trigger management, diary-keeping	I	First-line intervention
Biobehavioral	Relaxation training	I	First-line intervention if patient is considered appropriate, and based on patient preference
Biobehavioral	Biofeedback	I	First-line intervention if patient is considered appropriate, and based on patient preference
Biobehavioral	Cognitive-behavioral therapy	I	First-line intervention if patient is considered appropriate, and based on patient preference
Physical medicine	Acupuncture	II	Secondary intervention if patient is considered appropriate, and based on patient preference
Physical medicine	Spinal manipulation therapy	III	Secondary intervention if deemed medically appropriate
Physical medicine	Physical therapy	III	Secondary intervention if deemed medically appropriate
Physical medicine	Occupational therapy	II	Secondary intervention if deemed medically appropriate
Physical medicine	Exercise	III	First-line intervention if patient is considered appropriate, and based on patient preference
Physical medicine	Massage	IV	Secondary intervention if deemed medically appropriate, and based on patient preference
Physical medicine	Yoga	II	First-line intervention if patient is considered appropriate, and based on patient preference
Physical medicine	Reflexology	IV	Tertiary intervention/based on patient preference

[a]Level of evidence from I (highest level of evidence) to IV (lowest level of evidence).

following treatments "Grade A" evidence (multiple well-designed, randomized clinical trials that yielded a consistent pattern of findings): relaxation training, thermal biofeedback combined with relaxation training, electromyographic biofeedback, and CBT (for prevention of migraine). "Grade B" evidence (some evidence from randomized clinical trials, but the scientific support was not optimal) was given for CBT combined with preventive drug therapy to achieve added clinical improvement for migraine. Figure 7.1 displays the reported efficacy of biobehavioral treatments across multiple meta-analyses.

There are various aspects of the patient's presentation that suggest biobehavioral treatment would be an appropriate option within a multidisciplinary treatment for migraine. Individuals with clinical depression or anxiety, those with moderate to severe migraine-related disability or difficulty managing triggers (including stress), patients with other significant psychological issues (e.g., a history of abuse/maltreatment), and those with a preference for biobehavioral approaches are all ideal candidates for biobehavioral intervention [18]. Two of these issues, stress and comorbid depression/anxiety, are typically a focus of biobehavioral interventions.

♻ SCIENCE REVISITED

STRESS AND MIGRAINE
All individuals are vulnerable to the effects of stress. Stress involves the situation as well as the physiologic, cognitive, and affective responses to the situation. When an individual experiences a situation they perceive to be "stressful" (i.e., the individual perceives the event as threatening to their well-being), the individual's physiologic,

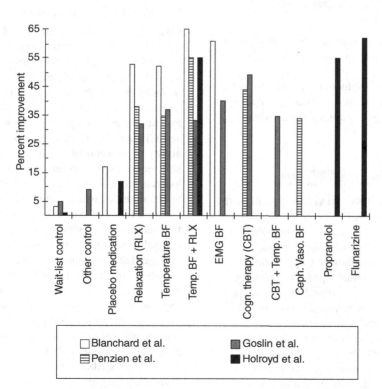

Figure 7.1. Meta-analyses of behavioral and pharmacologic treatments for migraine. Percent improvement scores are reported by treatment condition [7, 25, 69, 70, 71, 72, 73, 74]. Data from [25] and [69].

cognitive, and affective response elicits various physiologic changes including cerebral vasoconstriction and neurogenic inflammation. Stress increases sympathetic arousal and may increase neuronal hyperexcitability.

There are five ways that stress can potentially contribute to the expression and maintenance of individual episodes of migraine:

1. *Predisposer.* Stress contributes to the onset or expression of migraine in a person with a pre-existing vulnerability.
2. *Precipitant.* Stress precipitates individual migraine episodes.
3. *Exacerbator.* Stress exacerbates the progression of migraine, including transformation from an episodic to a chronic condition.
4. *Perpetuator.* Stress worsens migraine-related disability and quality of life.
5. *Consequence.* Migraines can serve as a stressor [19].

Also, after a stressful period, there may be a letdown phase that can, in itself, trigger a migraine.

Relaxation, biofeedback, and CBT are all potential methods to produce efficacious stress management within individuals.

⬡ SCIENCE REVISITED

COMORBID PSYCHIATRIC DISORDERS AND MIGRAINE

Depression and anxiety are more common among patients with migraine relative to the general population. Depression and anxiety are especially prevalent among those with chronic migraine, with more than half experiencing depression and nearly one-third experiencing anxiety. Experiencing depression or anxiety is associated with more severe migraines, increased disability, reduced adherence, increased medication use, and lower efficacy for actively managing migraine. In

fact, psychological distress may play a greater role in the progression of migraine from episodic to chronic than medication overuse.

The prevalence and impact of abuse and maltreatment is beginning to receive greater attention within the migraine community. As many as one-third of individuals with chronic migraine may have a childhood history of abuse or maltreatment. For a portion of these individuals, this trauma impairs their ability to cope with various aspects of life, including how to manage migraine. As a result, when there is a history of trauma, the individual would be well served by including psychotherapy into the multidisciplinary treatment program.

Cognitive-behavioral therapy

CBT, a Grade A treatment for migraine prevention [18], employs both cognitive and behavioral migraine management strategies. Cognitive strategies focus on identifying and challenging maladaptive or dysfunctional thoughts, beliefs, and responses to stress [20]. Cognitive foci of CBT for migraine management include enhancing self-efficacy (i.e., the patient's belief in his or her ability to succeed or accomplish a certain task) [21], encouraging patients to adopt an internal locus of control (i.e., a belief that the mechanism for change lies within oneself as opposed to an external locus of control, or the belief that only the healthcare provider, medication, or medical procedures have the power to bring about change) [22], and eliminating catastrophizing (a hopeless and overwhelming way of thinking). Research has demonstrated that among persons with migraine, low self-efficacy, having an external locus of control, and catastrophizing predict poor treatment outcomes [23]. Behavioral strategies include replacing behaviors that may maintain or exacerbate migraines with healthier behaviors. CBT may also provide the patient with tools to avoid triggering a migraine, improve overall coping, and help the migraine sufferer manage comorbid symptoms of depression and anxiety.

Biofeedback

Biofeedback has received Grade A evidence for its use [24, 25, 26, 27]. It involves monitoring physiologic processes that the patient may not be consciously aware and/or does not believe that he or she voluntarily controls. Digital processes take the patient's physiologic information and convert it into a signal that the patient receives in either visual or auditory form. Through biofeedback training, patients develop increased awareness of physiologic functions associated with migraine and stress, and learn to control their physiologic states [28, 29, 30]. Various relaxation skills, such as diaphragmatic breathing or visualization to induce the "relaxation response" [31], are often incorporated into biofeedback training [32].

During or preceding a migraine, the body may enter the "fight or flight" state (activation of the sympathetic nervous system). As sympathetic activity increases, circulation to the extremities and finger temperature both decrease. Conversely, as parasympathetic activity increases and the relaxation response is activated, circulation and extremity temperature increase. Biofeedback procedures are designed to help reduce sympathetic nervous system activity while increasing parasympathetic nervous system activity [26, 29]. Many modalities may be monitored through biofeedback, including peripheral skin temperature, blood-volume–pulse, and electromyographic, electroencephalographic, and galvanic skin response feedback. The strongest evidence for migraine management is for thermal, electromyographic, and blood-volume–pulse biofeedback and relaxation training [18]. Thermal biofeedback, also known as "hand-warming biofeedback" or "autogenic feedback," involves monitoring finger temperature (a measure of circulation) with a sensitive thermometer. Patients are taught that a higher finger temperature corresponds to a more relaxed state, with the goal being to raise their finger temperature.

Recently published meta-analyses have revealed medium to large mean effect sizes for biofeedback for the treatment of migraine, and found that treatment effects were maintained over an average follow-up period of 14 months, both in completer and intention-to-treat analyses [33, 34]. In addition to reduced attack frequency, significant effects were also found for improved self-efficacy, symptoms of depression and anxiety, and medication use.

Relaxation training

Relaxation techniques possess Grade A evidence for their use [18]. The focus is on helping patients to minimize physiologic responses to stress and decrease sympathetic arousal. The classic procedure, progressive muscle relaxation training, first published in 1938, involves tensing and relaxing various muscle groups while attending to the resulting contrasting sensations [35]. Other relaxation techniques include visual or guided imagery, cue-controlled relaxation, diaphragmatic breathing, hypnosis, and self-hypnosis [32, 36]. To achieve the benefits from relaxation, patients may use any techniques or tools that help them quiet the mind and calm the body (e.g., meditation, prayer, yoga, pleasant music, or guided relaxation). To achieve maximum benefit from these techniques, the patient must be motivated to regular practice in order to utilize these skills during migraine attacks or stressful situations.

Patient education

Patients often benefit from detailed education that highlights the complex nature of migraine difficulties [37, 38]. Indeed, 46% of patients want an explanation for their pain during a consultation, while 31% want pain relief [39, 40]. Explanations of the pathophysiology of migraine can improve patients' understanding of the rationale for both pharmacologic and biobehavioral treatment. Information shared may include the role of genetic predispositions, hormonal factors, the stress response, and relevant cognitive, emotional, and behavioral issues. Keeping a patient headache diary and having it reviewed at medical visits helps both the patient and the provider to understand the various factors involved in migraines and direct treatment. Helping patients to understand that they can learn self-management skills for coping with many of the factors involved in migraine can lead to greater self-efficacy and acceptance of a referral for biobehavioral treatment.

MIGRAINE PROGRESSION
Modifiable risk factors for migraine chronification include medication overuse, obesity, caffeine overuse, snoring, depression, and stressful life events. This emphasizes the importance of self-management as part of the multidisciplinary program. This puts the onus on the healthcare provider to provide the patient with proper medication, education, and skills. It also puts the onus on the patient to actively utilize the education and tools provided in order to optimally manage their migraine. For example, patients can benefit from making lifestyle behavior changes designed to help them maintain a healthy weight and achieve a state of physical well-being (i.e., proper nutrition and eating habits, reduced consumption of caffeine, and regular physical activity). Interventions that encourage patients to improve sleep hygiene, quit smoking (as smoking worsens snoring), reduce alcohol intake, reduce the use of sedative medications, and adhere to the use of continuous positive airway pressure (if diagnosed with sleep apnea) may also be provided by a psychologist.

Food triggers

Many foods have been reported idiosyncratically to trigger migraine [41]. In general, patients are encouraged to stay hydrated and eat at regular intervals in order to maintain the body's homeostasis. Failure to do so likely increases the patient's susceptibility to experiencing a migraine attack. Martin and Behbehani [42] wrote a comprehensive review of the evidence for and against certain foods, food additives, and beverages as potential triggers of migraine. Another review of foods often said to trigger migraine attacks (e.g., cheese, chocolate, alcohol, and citrus fruit) has not shown that they do so in clinical trials [43]. A specific concern in migraine management has been the role played by caffeine. This substance is frequently avoided by migraine sufferers, and some have suggested that overusing caffeine

alone can account for migraine development [44]. Moreover, some have suggested that a popular no-calorie sweetener, Sucralose, can be responsible for triggering migraine [45]. A complete review of the data on the role of food and food additives in migraine is beyond the scope of the current chapter; however, the interested reader is encouraged to read the excellent reviews on this topic [42, 43].

Physical treatments: acupuncture, chiropractic, physical and occupational therapies, and massage

Primary headache disorders, especially migraine, are often accompanied by neck pain or other symptoms [46]. Significant levels of muscle tenderness along with postural and mechanical abnormalities have been reported in migraines [47, 48]. Head pain can be referred from the cervical spine or soft tissues of the neck [46]. Physical treatments such as physical therapy, massage, chiropractic therapy, and osteopathic manipulation that focus on the cervical spine may benefit certain patients for whom various soft tissue, neurogenic, or osseous structures of the head, neck, and upper body actively contribute to triggering a migraine [49, 50]. However, the efficacy data for most physical treatments is lacking [46], and thus caution needs to be taken when considering their use.

Data on the efficacy of physical treatments for migraine are limited by small sample size, poor study design, and weak results. Healthcare providers and patients are advised to make cautious and individualized judgments about the utility of physical treatments for migraine. In some cases, these modalities may provide valuable addition to first-line pharmacologic and biobehavioral treatments; however, cost, time, and potential adverse effects should be weighed carefully. It is also important to note that patients who believe that a physical treatment will work are excellent candidates for their use given their beliefs (this may result in placebo-induced positive outcomes).However, providers need to ensure that patients understand that these are not first-line interventions with a strong evidence base. This will help to guard against patients believing that the provider failed to inform them about the realistic potential benefit of physical treatment for migraine.

Acupuncture

Data on the efficacy of acupuncture for migraine treatment and management are mixed. In 1998, the National Institutes of Health Consensus Development Program expressed concerns about the methodology used in acupuncture studies [51]. However, recent randomized-controlled trials have increased the confidence in acupuncture as a potential component of multidisciplinary treatment [52, 53, 54, 55]. For example, a Cochrane Review of acupuncture initially concluded that the evidence was "promising but not sufficient" for preventing migraine. However, an updated review included 12 additional migraine trials and concluded that acupuncture was a valuable non-pharmacologic tool in migraine management [55]. It is important, however, to keep in mind that the mechanisms whereby acupuncture work for migraine are unknown. Some have theorized that placebo effects play a significant role in the benefits of acupuncture due to needles being used (regardless of whether they are used following classical acupuncture techniques) [51].

Spinal manipulative therapies

Spinal manipulative therapies (SMTs) include such treatments as chiropractic, osteopathy, and physiotherapy. The contribution of cervicogenic dysfunction to migraine has been debated for many years. To patients, who often suffer neck pain or tender muscle-point activation in the neck with different types of migraine, it can frequently seem obvious that some sort of physical treatment needs to be given to help their pain. This is the case despite evidence that the presence of cervicogenic pain and stiffness may well be a consequence, rather than a cause, of migraine [56].

The chiropractic literature is replete with single cases, case series, and uncontrolled studies that suggest the beneficial effects of cervical spine manipulation for migraine. However, the methodology of these trials is weak [57]. There have been at least two reviews of SMT [57] and physical treatments for migraine [46]. Both reported a lack of evidence in controlled trials to firmly establish SMT as a first-line treatment option in any kind of primary headache. In the presence of cervical signs and symptoms combined with a normal neurologic examination, SMT might benefit the patient [58, 59, 60]; however, it cannot be considered a first-line multidisciplinary option at this time.

> ### ✋ CAUTION!
>
> SMT has been implicated as causing some forms of stroke. This is taken very seriously among the chiropractic community, even if the risk is probably not high, especially in those without pre-existing risk factors. One review identified 136 references to complications of cervical spine manipulation from 1966 to 1996. Twenty-three of these occurred when headache was the presenting complaint, but the authors concluded that serious complications of cervical spine manipulation have a very low incidence of 10–20 per 10 million manipulations. Even so, patients undergoing SMT should be aware of the potential risk of stroke or vascular injury from the procedure.

Physical therapy, occupational therapy, and exercise

Exercise improves physical functioning, may reduce BMI, and may reduce the somatic and cognitive experience of pain [61]. Exercise can also improve depression, anxiety, and quality of life, and help regulate basic needs (sleep–wake cycles and appetite). Occupational therapists help patients to incorporate effective pain-management strategies (e.g., goal-setting, group programs, pacing techniques, assertive communication, using appropriate body mechanics, and suggesting environmental modifications) into their everyday life. A structured review of data on physical treatments for migraine reported that physical therapy is potentially effective as a secondary intervention when combined with other first-line pharmacologic and non-pharmacologic treatments [46]. However, there is no evidence that exercise, physical therapy, or occupational therapy is an effective first-line option for migraine prevention.

Massage

Few data exist on the efficacy of massage as a treatment for migraine. However, two studies found that massage led to a reduction in migraine frequency and an improvement in sleep quality when compared to control participants [62]. Massage cannot be considered a first-line migraine prevention option; however, massage may benefit a patient who expresses interest in its use.

Yoga and meditation

Yoga is an ancient Indian practice that includes breathing techniques, mindfulness, meditation, and building strength, flexibility, and stamina through physical postures and routines. Meditation and yoga have been demonstrated to produce positive physiologic effects (e.g., in terms of heart rate, blood pressure, galvanic skin response, and respiratory rate) [63, 64]. Benefit has been demonstrated with a combined pharmacologic and yoga approach in one randomized trial among migraine sufferers [64]. However, yoga must be considered to be a secondary intervention because there is not enough evidence to recommend it for first-line migraine prevention.

Reflexology

This therapy relies on the theoretical notion that all parts of the body and any dysfunction in them, including the head, are in some way reflected in "reflex zones" in the feet. Although one uncontrolled study using reflexology for migraine exists [65], there is no evidence that reflexology has any use as a treatment for migraine.

Referrals to multidisciplinary providers

Discussing the referral with patients

Establishing a collaborative provider–patient interaction facilitates treatment adherence and

acceptance of a multidisciplinary referral. Collaboration involves the provider listening to and reflecting back the patient's thoughts, feelings, and behaviors about their migraines, how they manage and cope with migraine, and the impact of migraine on their lives. Doing so exudes empathy so that the patient will believe that the provider understands and values the patient and their situation. In turn, when patients believe that their provider is empathetic, they will be more likely to follow treatment recommendations. In addition, shared decision-making about treatment will promote collaboration.

★ TIPS AND TRICKS

FINDING PSYCHOLOGISTS WHO TREAT PATIENTS WITH MIGRAINE
Psychologists who treat migraines can be found using a variety of locator services. These include the American Headache Society (http://www.americanheadachesociety.org), the American Psychological Association (http://locator.apa.org), the Association for Behavioral and Cognitive Therapies (http://www.abct.org), the Association for Applied Psychophysiology and Biofeedback (http://www.resourcenter.net/scripts/4disapi9.dll/4dcgi/resctr/search.html), the Biofeedback Certification International Alliance (http://www.resourcenter.net/Scripts/4Disapi6.dll/4DCGI/resctr/search.html), and health insurers' provider panels.

Anticipate barriers to a referral and educating patients

Patients with migraine often interpret referrals to multidisciplinary treatment as a suggestion that the pain is not "real," not important, that the migraine is "all in their head," that the patient does not need medication, or that the provider is simply trying to terminate the relationship [66]. It is important to emphasize that nonpharmacologic is not antipharmacologic [38], and that multidisciplinary does not mean the provider no longer wants to see the patient.

Patients often benefit from detailed education that highlights the complex nature of migraine difficulties [37, 38]. Explaining the pathophysiology of migraine, and learning about the role of genetic predisposition and how trigger factors (e.g., hormones, stress, and sleep) are important in migraine can all benefit the patient. Helping patients to understand that they can learn migraine self-management skills can lead to greater self-efficacy and acceptance of a referral. However, it is also crucial to assess the patient's level of "readiness" to actively engage in self-management and multidisciplinary migraine treatment. The transtheoretical model [67] posits that patients have different levels of readiness or motivation to change, which warrant tailored responses. The interested reader can see Nicholson [68] for a review of the model and strategies for addressing each stage of the model as it applies to migraine management. In essence, the physician can help "prime the pump" for success when they listen to the patient, acknowledge the patient's situation, questions, and concerns, educate the patient about various aspects of the development and management of migraine, and engage in collaborative decision-making about the benefits of multidisciplinary treatment.

★ TIPS AND TRICKS

EFFECTIVE COMMUNICATION INCREASES THE ACCEPTANCE OF REFERRALS

Exuding empathy toward patients about how migraine impacts their life is a tenet of effective treatment. Even so, making a referral for multidisciplinary treatment is a challenge no matter the level of collaboration between the provider and patient. The following are ways to discuss the referral using a psychologist as an example.

- Present the psychologist as a consultant: "I know you are still having quite a bit of disability from your migraines. Dr. X is a psychologist whose specialty is helping me better understand how to best treat you. Would you be willing to meet with her to talk about how the migraines are impacting your life?

- Put "behavioral issues" in context as part of the development and management of migraine:
"Looking at what migraines are doing to your life, your migraine pain is obviously real. I think the stress you've told me about may play a role in why the migraines are so severe. Stress can cause changes in your body that can make it more likely you will get a migraine or make it more severe. I think talking with Dr. Y, one of our psychologists who specialize in stress management, may help make the medications work even better. Dr. Y and I will work together with you."

Conclusion

Migraine is more than just a series of changes in neurophysiology and neurochemistry. It involves individuals experiencing pain and attempting to manage the impact of that pain on their lives. As a result, migraine is best conceptualized in a biopsychosocial framework, as involving physiologic, cognitive/affective, and behavioral phenomena. Although pharmacologic treatment is considered a basis of involvement in migraine management and prevention, many individuals with migraine will benefit from other multidisciplinary treatments in conjunction with or in lieu of pharmacologic therapies. In the current chapter, the theoretical assumptions and evidence base for various multidisciplinary treatments were reviewed. Strategies for improving patient participation, motivation, adherence, and communication were also reviewed. As with any chronic disease, it is vital that patients take an active role in self-managing their migraines. In order to maximize the likelihood of this happening, it is vital that the provider and patient together establish a collaborative relationship whereby the patient perceives that the provider is empathetic. This will, in turn, make it more likely that the patient will trust that the provider has his or her best interests at heart. This will optimize patient adherence and improve multidisciplinary treatment outcomes.

Acknowledgments

The authors would like to thank C. Mark Sollars, MS, and Michael T. Lynch, BA, for editorial assistance.

References

1. Andrasik F, Flor H, Turk DC. An expanded view of psychological aspects in head pain: the biopsychosocial model. *Neurol Sci* 2005;**26**:S87–91.
2. Ramadan NM, Silberstein FD, Freitag FG, et al. Evidence-based guidelines for migraine headache in the primary care setting: pharmacological management for prevention of migraine. *US Headache Consortium* 2000;**1**: 1–56.
3. Beecher HK. *Measurement of Subjective Responses*. New York: Oxford University Press; 1959.
4. Lipton RB, Pan J. Is migraine a progressive brain disease? *JAMA* 2004;**291**:493–4.
5. Bodenheimer T, Wagner EH, Grumbach K. Improving primary care for patients with chronic illness. *JAMA* 2002;**288**:1775–9.
6. Lorig KR, Solomon H. Self-management education: history, definition, outcomes, and mechanisms. *Ann Behav Med* 2003; **26**:1–7.
7. Buse DC, Andrasik F. Behavioral medicine for migraine. *Neurol Clin* 2009;**27**(2):445–65.
8. Blumenfeld A, Tischio M. Center of Excellence for Headache Care: Group model at Kaiser Permanente. *Headache* 2003;**43**: 431–40.
9. Cady R, Farmer K, Beach M, Tarrasch, J. Nurse-based education: an office-based comparative model for education of migraine patients. *Headache* 2008;**48**:564–9.
10. Rothrock JF, Parada VA, Sims C, Key K, Walters NS, Zweifler RM. The impact of intensive patient education on clinical outcome in a clinic-based migraine population. *Headache* 2006;**46**:726–31.
11. Smith TR, Nicholson RA, Banks JW. Migraine education improves quality of life in a primary care setting. *Headache* 2010; **50**(4):600–12.
12. Gunreben-Stempfle B, Grießinger N, Lang E, Muehlhans B, Sittl R, Ulrich K. Effectiveness of an intensive multidisciplinary headache treatment program. *Headache* 2009;**49**:990–1000.
13. Lemstra M, Stewart B, Olszynski WP. Effectiveness of multidisciplinary intervention in the treatment of migraine: a randomized clinical trial. *Headache* 2002;**42**:845–54.
14. Magnusson JE, Riess CE, Becker WJ. Effectiveness of a multidisciplinary treatment program for chronic daily headache. *Can J Neurol Sci* 2004;**31**:72–9.
15. Marcus DA, Scharff L, Mercer S, Turk DC. Musculoskeletal abnormalities in chronic headache: a controlled comparison of headache diagnostic groups. *Headache* 1999; **39**(1):21–7.
16. Zeeburg P, Olesen J, Jensen, R. Efficacy of multidisciplinary treatment in a tertiary referral headache centre. *Cephalalgia* 2005; **25**:1159–167.
17. Lipchik GL, Smitherman TA, Penzien DB, Holroyd KA. Basic principles and techniques of cognitive-behavioral therapies for co-morbid psychiatric symptoms among headache patients. *Headache* 2006;**S3**: S119–32.
18. Campbell JK, Penzien DB, Wall EM. Evidence-based guidelines for migraine headaches: behavioral and physical treatments. 25 Apr 2000. Available at: http://www.aan.com/professionals/practice/pdfs/gl0089.pdf (accessed March 2011).
19. Nash J, Thebarge R. Understanding psychological stress, its biological processes, and impact on primary headache. *Headache* 2006;**46**:1377–86.
20. Beck AT, Rus AJ, Shaw BF, Emery G. *Cognitive Therapy of Depression*. New York: Guilford Press; 1979.
21. Bandura A. Self-efficacy: toward a unifying theory of behavior change. *Psychol Rev* 1977;**84**:191–215.
22. Heath RL, Saliba M, Mahmassini O, Major SC, Khoury BA. Locus of control moderates the relationship between headache pain and depression. *J Headache Pain* 2008;**9**:301–8.
23. Nicholson RA, Houle TT, Rhudy JL, Norton PJ. Psychological risk factors in headache. *Headache* 2007;**47**:413–26.
24. Andrasik F. Biofeedback in headache: an overview of approaches and evidence. *Cleve Clin J Med* 2010;**77**(Suppl. 3):S72–6.

25. Andrasik F. What does the evidence show? Efficacy of behavioural treatments for recurrent headaches in adults. *Neurol Sci* 2007;**26**:S70--7.

26. Andrasik F, Flor H. Biofeedback. In Breivik H, Campbell WI, Nicholas MK (eds.), *Clinical Pain Management: Practice and Procedures* (2nd edn.). London: Hodder & Stoughton; 2008: pp. 153–66.

27. Eccleston C, Morley S, Williams A, *et al*. Systematic review of randomised controlled trials of psychological therapy for chronic pain in children and adolescents, with a subset meta-analysis of pain relief. *Pain* 2002;**99**:157–65.

28. Penzien DB, Holroyd KA. Psychosocial interventions in the management of recurrent headache disorders. II. Description of treatment techniques. *Behav Med* 1994;**20**:64–73.

29. Schwartz MS, Andrasik F. *Biofeedback: A Practitioner's Guide* (3rd edn.). New York: Guilford Press; 2003.

30. Sovak M, Kunzel M, Sternbach RA, Dalessio DJ. Mechanism of the biofeedback therapy of migraine: volitional manipulation of the psychophysiological background. *Headache* 1981;**21**:89–92.

31. Benson H. *The Relaxation Response*. New York: William Morrow; 1975.

32. Rime C, Andrasik F. Relaxation techniques and guided imagery. In Waldman SD (ed.), *Pain Management* (Vol. 2, 2nd edn.). Philadelphia, PA: Saunders/Elsevier; 2011: pp. 967–77.

33. Nestroriuc Y, Martin A. Efficacy of biofeedback for migraine: a meta-analysis. *Pain* 2007;**128**:111–27.

34. Nestroriuc Y, Martin A, Rief W, Andrasik F. Biofeedback treatment for headache disorders: a comprehensive efficacy review. *Appl Psychophysiol Biofeedback* 2008;**33**:125–40.

35. Jacobsen E. *Progressive Relaxation*. Chicago: University of Chicago Press; 1938.

36. Bernstein DA, Borkovec TD, Hazlett-Stevens H. *New Directions in Progressive Relaxation Training: A Guidebook for Helping Professions*. Westport, CT: Praeger; 2000.

37. Holroyd KA, Andrasik F. A cognitive-behavioral approach to recurrent tension and migraine headache. In Kendall PC (ed.), *Advances in Cognitive-behavioral Research and Therapy* (Vol. 1). New York: Academic Press; 1982: pp. 275–320.

38. Weeks RE. Integration of behavioural techniques into clinical practice. *Neurol Sci* 2007;**28**:S84–8.

39. Packard RC. What does the headache patient want? *Headache* 1979;**19**:370–4.

40. Lipton RB, Stewart WF. Acute migraine therapy: do doctors understand what patients with migraine want from therapy? *Headache* 1999;**28**:S20–6.

41. Peatfield RC, Glover V, Littlewood JT, Sandler M, Clifford-Rose F. The prevalence of diet-induced migraine. *Cephalalgia* 1984;**4**:179–83.

42. Martin VT, Behbehani MM. Toward a rational understanding of migraine triggers. *Med Clin N Am* 2001;**85**(4):911–41.

43. Crawford P, Simmons M. What dietary modifications are indicated for migraines? *J Fam Pract* 2006;**55**:62–6.

44. Hering-Hanit R, Gadoth N. Caffeine-induced headache in children and adolescents *Cephalalgia* 2003;**23**:332–5.

45. Patel RM, Sarma R, Grimsley E. Popular sweetener sucralose as a migraine trigger. *Headache* 2006;**46**:1303–4.

46. Biondi D. Physical treatments for headache: a structured review. *Headache* 2005;**45**:738–46.

47. Blau JN, MacGregor EA. Migraine and the neck. *Headache* 1994;**34**:88–90.

48. Tfelt-Hansen P, Lous I, Olesen J. Prevalence and significance of muscle tenderness during common migraine attacks. *Headache* 1981;**21**:49–54.

49. Bartsch T, Goadsby PJ. Increased response in trigeminocervical nociceptive neurons to cervical input after stimulation of the dura mater. *Brain* 2003;**126**:1801–13.

50. Jansen J, Bardosi A, Hildebrant J, Lucke A. Cervicogenic, hemicranial attacks associated with vascular irritation or compression of the cervical nerve root C2: clinical manifestations and morphological findings. *Pain* 1989;**39**:203–12.

51. NIH Consensus Conference. Acupuncture. *JAMA* 1998;**280**:1518–24.

52. Linde K, Streng A, Jurgens S, et al. Acupuncture for patients with migraine: a randomized controlled trial. *JAMA* 2005;**293**:2118–25.

53. Vickers AJ, Rees RW, Zollman CE, et al. Acupuncture for chronic headache in primary care: large, pragmatic, randomised trial. *BMJ* **328**;2004:744.

54. Linde, K., Allais G, Brinkhaus B, Manheimer E, Vickers A, White AR. Acupuncture for migraine prophylaxis. *Cochrane Database Syst Rev* 2009;(1):CD001218.

55. Linde K, Allais G, Brinkhaus B, Manheimer E, Vickers A, White AR. Acupuncture for tension-type headache. *Cochrane Database Syst Rev* 2009(1):CD007587.

56. Vernon H, Jansz G, Goldsmith CH, McDermai C. A randomized, placebo-controlled clinical trial of chiropractic and medical prophylactic treatment of adults with tension-type headache: results from a stopped trial. *J Manipulative Physiol Ther* 2009;**32**:344–51.

57. Bronfort G, Assendelft WJ, Evans R, Haas M, Bouter L. Efficacy of spinal manipulation for chronic headache: a systematic review. *J Manipulative Physiol Ther* 2001;**24**:457–66.

58. Hurwitz EL, Aker PD, Adams AH, Meeker WD, Shekelle PG. Manipulation and mobilization of the cervical spine: a systematic review of the literature. *Spine* 1996;**21**:1746–60.

59. Shekelle PG, Coulter I. Cervical spine manipulation: summary report of a systematic review of the literature and a multidisciplinary expert panel. *J Spinal Disord* 1997; **10**:223–8.

60. Whitmarsh T, Buse, D. Biobehavioral, complementary, and alternative treatments for headache. In Martelletti P, Steiner T (eds.), *Handbook of Headache*. New York: Springer, 2011: pp. 667–86.

61. Darabaneanu S, Overath CH, Rubin D, et al. Aerobic exercise as a therapy option for migraine: a pilot study. *Int J Sports Med.* 2011;**32**(6):455–60.

62. Lawler SP, Cameron LD. A randomized controlled trial of massage therapy as a treatment for migraine. *Ann Behav Med* 2006; **32**(1):50–9.

63. Ospina MB, Bond K, Karkhaneh M, et al. Meditation practices for health: state of the research (AHRQ). *Evidence Report/ Technology Assessment* 2007;(155):1–263.

64. John PJ, Sharma N, Sharma CM, Kankane A. Effectiveness of yoga therapy in the treatment of migraine without aura: a randomized controlled trial. *Headache* 2007;**47**:654–61.

65. Launso L, Brendstrup E, Arnberg S. An exploratory study of reflexological treatment for headache. *Altern Ther Health Med* 1999;**5**:57–65.

66. Lipsitt DR. Helping primary care physicians make psychiatric referrals: some practical considerations *UBM Medical Psychiatric Times* 2010. Available at: http://www.psychiatrictimes.com/display/article/10168/1759296 (accessed March 2011).

67. Prochaska JO, Redding A, Evers KE. The transtheoretical model and stages of change. In Glanz K, Lewis FM, Rimer BK (eds.), *Health Behavior and Health Education*. San Francisco, CA: Jossey-Bass; 1997: pp. 60–84.

68. Nicholson RA. The role of the psychologist in chronic headache. *Curr Pain Head Rep* 2010;**14**(1):47–54.

69. Penzien DB, Rain JC, Andrasik F. Behavioral management of recurrent headache: three decades of experience and empiricism. *Appl Psychophysiol Biofeedback* 2002;**27**:163–81.

70. Blanchard EB, Andrasik F, Ahles TA, et al. Migraine and tension headache: a meta-analytic review. *Behav Ther* 1980;**14**:613–31.

71. Goslin RE, Gray RN, McCrory DC, et al. Behavioral and physical treatments for migraine headache. Technical review 2.2 February 1999. Prepared for the Agency for Health Care Policy and Research under Contract No. 290-94-2025. Available at http://www.clinpol.mc.due.edu (accessed May 2011).

72. Holroyd KA, Penzien DB, Cordingley GE. Propranolol in the management of recurrent migraine: a meta-analytic review. *Headache* 1991;**3**:333–40.

73. Holroyd KA, Penzien DB, Rokicki LA, Cordingley GF. Flunarizine vs. propranolol: a meta-analysis of clinical trials. *Headache* 1992;**32**:256.

74. Penzien DB, Holroyd KA, Holm JE, Hursey KG. Behavioral management of migraine: results from five-dozen group outcome studies. *Headache* 1985;**25**:162.

Acute Treatments for Migraine

Dagny Holle and Hans-Christoph Diener

University of Duisburg-Essen, Essen, Germany

Introduction

Various treatment options are available for the acute treatment of migraine. Successful therapy essentially depends on an individual treatment concept for each patient, considering specific clinical features (e.g., severity, degree of temporary disability, and accompanying symptoms such as nausea and vomiting) and a distinct personal medical history that takes into account cardiovascular risk and age. Additionally, prior response rates to and tolerance for specific medications must be considered. A thorough screening of a patient's medical history and clinical examination are important for choosing the best acute treatment strategy.

The US Headache Consortium has identified several goals for successful treatment of acute migraine attacks [1]:

- Treat attacks rapidly and consistently without recurrence.
- Restore the patient's ability to function.
- Minimize the use of back-up and rescue medications.
- Optimize self-care and reduce the subsequent use of resources.
- Provide the best cost-effectiveness for overall management.
- Ensure there are minimal or no adverse events.

As well as setting treatment goals, establishing realistic expectations concerning the response rates and efficacy of pain-relieving medication is important. In most cases, patients will find that the recommended medication is not 100% effective. Patients will sometimes experience little change in their headache intensity or no effect at all. Therefore, acute treatment is considered to be effective only if the headache disappears completely within 2 hours after drug intake or if the headache intensity is reduced from severe to mild within 2 hours. Response rates usually range between 50% and 80%. To avoid patient disappointment, therapeutic goals should be discussed and expectations should be put into proper perspective.

Acute migraine attack medication can be divided into nonspecific and specific compounds. Nonspecific treatment approaches include analgesics (e.g., nonsteroidal anti-inflammatory drugs [NSAIDs], nonopioids and

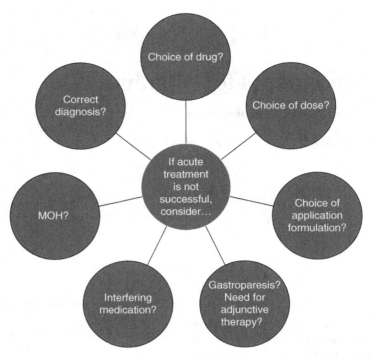

Figure 8.1. What to consider if administered acute treatment is not working.

combination analgesics), opioid analgesics, and corticosteroids, combined with support therapy that includes antiemetics and neuroleptics. These drugs can be used for migraine treatment, but they are also effective in other pain conditions. Specific migraine medications include selective 5-hydroxytryptamine $_{1B/1D}$ (5-HT $_{1B/1D}$) receptor agonists, also known as triptans, ergot alkaloids, and ergot derivates, which can selectively control migraine headaches but are not effective in other pain disorders.

As a basic principle, all medication for acute migraine treatment should be taken early after the onset of headache and at a sufficient dosage to achieve the best efficacy. To evaluate the efficacy of acute treatment (Figure 8.1), patients should be asked to keep a headache diary.

General pain management: nonpharmacologic strategies

Nonpharmacologic strategies should be tried first in acute migraine treatment before considering drug therapy as they increase the efficacy of drug therapy and have a positive impact on treatment outcome. Migraine trigger factors should be minimized by resting in a cool, dark, quiet room. Some patients report an improvement in their migraine pain by applying a cold compress or ice pack to the area that hurts. It might be also helpful to use relaxation techniques to ease stress and calm the pain.

Pain-relieving medication and adjunctive therapy

NSAIDs, nonopioids, and combination analgesics

NSAIDs such as acetylsalicylic acid (ASA), ibuprofen, diclofenac, and naproxen are the most commonly used drugs in acute migraine therapy and first-choice treatment for mild or moderate migraine attacks (Table 8.1). Although acetaminophen is also often used, it seems to have a

Table 8.1. NSAIDs, non-opioid, and combined analgesics for treatment of acute migraine attacks

Drug	Available forms	Single dosage (maximum dosage per day)	Side effects	Contraindications
ASA	Oral, i.v.	1000 mg	Gastrointestinal, nausea, inhibition of platelet aggregation	Gastrointestinal ulcers, hemorrhagic diathesis, last trimester of pregnancy
Ibuprofen	Oral	200–600 mg	As for ASA, edema	As for ASA, less hemorrhagic diathesis; renal insufficiency, lupus erythematosus
Naproxen	Oral	500–1000 mg	As for ibuprofen	As for ibuprofen
Diclofenac	Oral	50–100 mg	As for ibuprofen	As for ibuprofen
Metamizol	Oral, suppository, i.v., i.m.	500–1000 mg	Anaphylactic reactions, Stevens–Johnson syndrome, Lyell's syndrome, agranulocytosis, inhibition of platelet aggregation	
Acetaminophen	Oral, suppository, i.v., i.m.	500–1000 mg	Liver damage, renal failure, asthmatic symptoms, eczema	Hepatic or renal insufficiency, alcoholism, dehydration, glucose-6-phosphate dehydrogenase deficiency
ASA + acetaminophen + caffeine	Oral	2 × 250 mg + 200 mg + 50 mg	See ASA and acetaminophen	See ASA and acetaminophen

i.m., intramuscular; i.v., intravenous.

lower response rate than NSAIDs. Combinations of ASA, acetaminophen, and caffeine are more effective than one single substance or a dual combination of these compounds [2]. Combined analgesics, however, show a higher risk of rebound headache and MOH, and should be administered infrequently. Single substances should be not taken for more than 15 days per month, and combined substances only on 10 days or fewer per month. Special forms of appli-

cation, such as effervescent tablets, are preferable as they produce faster absorption and higher serum levels within the first 30 minutes of administration.

Most common side effects from NSAID treatment, mainly due to prostaglandin synthesis inhibition, are gastrointestinal symptoms such as nausea, vomiting, diarrhea, gastric pain, gastric ulcers, and occult bleeding. Allergic reactions and impairment of renal or liver function occur

Table 8.2. Antiemetics and neuroleptics for supportive treatment of acute migraine attack

Drug	Dosage	Side effects	Contraindications	Comments
Metoclopramide	10 mg i.m. 10 mg oral 20 mg per rectum 0.1 mg/kg i.v. for 1–3 doses to 10 mg	Extrapyramidal symptoms, sedation, drowsiness, postural hypotension	Children below the age of 12	
Chlorpromazine	0.1 mg/kg i.m. for 1–3 doses to 1 mg/kg 12.5–37.5 mg i.v.			
Prochlorperazine	25 mg per rectum 5–15 mg oral 10 mg i.m. 10 mg i.v.			
Domperidone	30–120 mg per rectum 10 mg oral			No extrapyramidal effects, can be given to children

i.m., intramuscular; i.v., intravenous.

infrequently. In patients with such pre-existing conditions, the use of NSAIDs should be restrained and cautiously monitored.

Acetaminophen rarely causes side effects, although infrequently it induces liver dysfunction or allergic reactions. In case of a severe renal insufficiency, an 8-hour interval should be recommended between two intakes. Patients must adhere to a maximal acetaminophen dosage of 4 g per day to avoid life-threatening liver failure.

Antiemetics: adjunctive therapy

Migraine attacks are often associated with nausea and vomiting. Antiemetics (metoclopramide and domperidone) and neuroleptics (chlorpromazine and prochlorperazine) improve accompanying vegetative symptoms (Table 8.2). Additionally, these compounds are gastroprokinetic agents and facilitate gastric emptying, which increases the absorption rates of pain-relieving drugs and improves therapy outcome. Metoclopramide also displays intrinsic pain-relieving effects [3, 4].

Most antiemetics and neuroleptics are available as oral, intravenous, intramuscular, and rectal suppository applications, but in most cases intravenous application shows the best efficacy. All drugs share common side effects including, pre-dominantly, drowsiness and sedation. Aside from akathisia, extrapyramidal adverse effects such as acute dystonic reactions are only rarely reported and do not occur after intake of domperidone as this drug does not cross the blood–brain barrier. In children or very old patients, metoclopramide and neuroleptics should be avoided for this reason.

In summary, antiemetic medications are appropriate for acute migraine treatment and should usually be combined with pain-relieving medication. Importantly, antiemetics should not be restricted to patients who vomit or are very likely to vomit as nausea itself might be the disabling symptom.

> ✋ CAUTION!
>
> Metoclopramide as an antiemetic drug can induce extrapyramidal side effects, especially in children and elderly patients. Therefore, when available, domperidone should be rather chosen in these patient groups.

5-HT$_{1B/D}$ receptor agonists (triptans)

Sumatriptan, zolmitriptan, naratriptan, rizatriptan, almotriptan, eletriptan, and frovatriptan are agonists at the 5-HT $_{1B/D}$ receptor [5]. 5-HT $_{1B}$ receptors are found in the meningeal arteries, and their activation causes vasoconstriction of the dural blood vessels. 5-HT$_{1D}$ receptors are primarily located in the trigeminal nuclei and nerve, and in vascular smooth muscle. Receptor activation downregulates the release of inflammatory neuropeptides that are involved in the pathophysiology of migraine, and inhibits the propagation of trigeminal pain signals.

Triptans are specific migraine medications and are not effective in patients with pure tension-type headaches or other pain conditions. Triptans are termed abortive migraine medications. They cannot prevent migraine attacks.

All triptans have shown their efficacy in large placebo-controlled trials (Table 8.3) [6, 7]. Triptans are effective at every point within the attack, although their efficacy increases when they are taken early within the attack or when the headache is still mild [8, 9]. Migraneurs should be encouraged to take triptans as quickly as possible. Despite their pain-relieving properties, triptans also have a positive impact on typical

Table 8.3. 5HT$_{1B/D}$- agonists for treatment of acute migraine attacks

Drug	Dosage	Side effects	Contraindications	Comments
Sumatriptan	25, 50–100 mg oral 10–20 mg nasal spray 6 mg subcutaneous	Chest tightness, paresthesia of the extremities, sensation of cold, nausea, dizziness, muscle weakness Local reaction at site of injection	Arterial hypertension, coronary heart disease, angina pectoris, myocardial infarction in history, Raynaud's disease, transient ischemic attack, stroke, multiple cardiovascular risk factors, liver and renal failure	Subcutaneous formulation shows the fastest therapeutic effect (10 min)
Zolmitriptan	2.5 or 5 mg oral, 2.5 mg disintegrating tablet 5 or 10 mg nasal spray	Equal to sumatriptan	See sumatriptan	
Naratriptan	1, 2.5 mg Oral	Less than sumatriptan	See sumatriptan	Better tolerability than sumatriptan
Rizatriptan	5 or 10 mg oral or disintegrating tablet	Equal to sumatriptan	See sumatriptan	Better efficacy than sumatriptan
Almotriptan	6.25 or 12.5 mg oral	Less than sumatriptan	See sumatriptan	Better tolerability than sumatriptan
Frovatriptan	2.5 mg oral	Equal to sumatriptan	See sumatriptan	Better tolerability than sumatriptan
Eletriptan	20 mg or 40 mg oral	Equal to sumatriptan	See sumatriptan	80 mg Better efficacy than sumatriptan (but not universally available)

migraine-associated features such as nausea, vomiting, and phono- and photophobia. In addition, triptans improve disability and help to reduce the need for other pain-relieving medications.

There are only minor differences between the specific triptans. Subcutaneous sumatriptan shows the fastest onset of action, within about 10 minutes. Oral rizatriptan and eletriptan need about 30 minutes to abort pain, whereas oral sumatriptan, almotriptan, and zolmitriptan take about 45–60 minutes. Naratriptan and frovatriptan are rather slow-onset triptans and take up to 4 hours to work after application, but they are long-acting and cause rather rarely recurrent headache. In general, nasal application forms are faster in onset than oral formulations. Subcutaneous sumatriptan shows the best results in regard to 2-hour efficacy (with a response rate of up to 80%) compared with other results, but patients often experience a rebound headache. Trials suggest that naratriptan and frovatriptan are substantially less effective than other triptans, but side effects and recurrent headache are only rarely reported.

Patients should treat three consecutive migraine attacks with the same triptan before judging its efficacy as up to 40% of patients fail to respond to a particular medication in that class. Triptans have a response rate of between 60% and 80%. If one triptan does not work adequately, it is well worthwhile trying other triptans. Finally, if treatment is still insufficient, subcutaneous sumatriptan should be administered in another migraine attack before considering a patient to be a real triptan nonresponder.

★ TIPS AND TRICKS

Before you consider a patient to be a triptan nonresponder:

- Try the same triptan in three different headache attacks
- Try another triptan
- Try subcutaneous application of a triptan (sumatriptan) to rule out a lack of resorption

It is important to inform patients in detail about possible side effects in order to increase their compliance. Common side effects are chest tightness and parasthesias of the extremities. Uninformed patients sometimes misinterpret these side effects as symptoms of angina pectoris or myocardial infarction, and in turn refuse another application. Contraindications due to the vasoconstrictive characteristics of triptans include coronary heart disease, prior cerebrovascular events, arterial occlusive disease, uncontrolled arterial hypertension, multiple vascular risk factors, and Raynaud's syndrome. In patients with cardiovascular risk factors, a distinct evaluation of a clinical history and an examination should be performed before considering triptan therapy. Taking these contraindications into account, triptan therapy is safe, and an increased risk of stroke or myocardial infarction has not been observed. Severe side effects occur in fewer than 1 in 1,000,000 applications.

A well-known phenomenon in triptan treatment is headache recurrence after the initially successful treatment of the migraine attack. Recurrence is defined as an increase in headache intensity from no or mild headache to moderate or severe headache in a time period of between 2 and 24 hours after the first successful triptan treatment [10]. This therapeutic problem also occurs with ergotamine and NSAIDs but is more frequently encountered in patients who use triptans. Up to 40% of patients describe a recurrence of their headache within a few hours after oral or subcutaneous triptan application. In such cases, a second intake of the same triptan is successful in most patients [11]. Triptans with longer half-lives are less often associated with a recurrent headache. The combined intake of a triptan and an NSAID initially might help to avoid recurrence of the headache [12]. One combination pill containing sumatriptan and naproxen has been recently approved by the US Food and Drug Administration for the treatment of migraine.

★ TIPS AND TRICKS

If patients have headache recurrence after triptan use, consider the following options:

- Give a second intake of the same triptan
- Switch to a long-duration triptan such as frovatriptan or naratriptan
- Adding a NSAID to acute triptan therapy

Table 8.4. Ergot alkaloids and derivatives for treatment of acute migraine attacks

Drug	Dosage	Side effects	Contraindications	Comments
DHE	1 mg subcutaneous 1 mg i.m. 1–2 mg i.v.	Nausea, vomiting, dysphoria, flushing, restlessness, anxiety, diarrhea, muscle cramps, paresthesia, tachy- and bradycardia	Risk for ischemic heart disease, uncontrolled arterial hypertension coronary heart disease, Raynaud's disease, arterial occlusion disease, stroke, acute porphyria	Useful in long-standing headache
DHE	Nasal spray	Nasal congestion, nausea, vomiting		Treatment option for patients with nausea and vomiting
Ergotamine (without caffeine)	1–2 mg per rectum	See DHE	See DHE	
Ergotamine plus caffeine	Per rectum 2 mg plus 200 mg caffeine		See DHE	

DHE, dihydroergotamine; i.m., intramuscular; i.v., intravenous.

All triptans can ultimately lead to an increase in headache frequency and MOH. Intake of triptans should be restricted to fewer than 10 treatment days per month.

For safety reasons, triptans should not be taken during an aura, or by patients with basilar-type or hemiplegic migraine. Triptans should not be combined with other triptans, or taken together with ergots.

Ergot alkaloids and derivates

Ergotamines are also migraine-specific drugs (Table 8.4). They inhibit neurogenic inflammation and the secretion of vasoactive neuropeptides. Several receptors are activated by ergots—serotonin receptors, alpha-adrenergic receptors, dopamine receptors, and histamine receptors.

⚓ CAUTION!

Simultaneous administration of triptans and ergotamines should be strictly avoided as the vasoconstrictive side effects of both drugs might be additive. After ergotamine application, triptans should not be taken for the next 24 hours. Ergots should not be administered until 12 hours or more following triptan application. Multiple triptans should not be mixed. It is recommended that these substances should be combined with NSAIDs or antiemetics.

There are only a few prospective studies that have evaluated the efficacy of ergots in the acute treatment of migraine [13]. Ergots have been less effective in head-to-head trials than triptans, but they show a longer duration of action [14]. In contrast to triptans ergotamines are thought to be primarily effective at the beginning of a migraine attack and for this reason should be taken as early as possible after onset of headache.

Ergot alkaloids as well as ergotamine combinations (plus caffeine, plus caffeine and pentobarbital, or plus metoclopramide) are often associated with side effects such as nausea and vomiting. These symptoms should not be mistaken as associated symptoms of the migraine attack and should not lead to reapplication of an ergot. Additional side effects include diarrhea, muscle cramps, paresthesia of the legs and arms, thoracic pain, and tachy- or bradycardia. As with triptans, ergots are contraindicated in patients with uncontrolled arterial hypertension, coronary heart disease, Raynaud's disease, arterial occlusion disease, prior myocardial infarction, stroke, and acute porphyria. Vasoconstrictive properties are more pronounced in ergots than triptans [15]. In a few cases, the regular intake of ergots can lead to ergotism with life-threatening vascular complications. Also as with triptans, ergots carry a high risk for inducing MOH. Patients should receive a restricted number of ergot applications as rescue medication (<10 intake days per month).

Ergots and triptans *must not* be combined. After an intake of ergots, triptan application must be postponed for at least 24 hours. After triptan application, ergots should not be taken within the following 12 hours.

Opioids and barbiturates

Medications containing narcotics are sometimes used in migraineurs with intractable pain in the emergency room when triptans or ergots are contraindicated. Additionally, opioids might be used for the therapy of severe migraine attacks during pregnancy. Common side effects of opioids include nausea and vomiting. Frequent intake causes MOH and dependency. Opioids should only be used as last resort in acute migraine therapy as they are habit-forming.

Barbiturates are *no longer recommended* in acute migraine therapy as they increase the risk of dependency, withdrawal symptoms, and MOH.

Steroids

Evidence concerning steroid therapy in migraine is insufficient, and study results are inconsistent. Steroids may be considered for rescue therapy in patients with status migrainosus when the headache lasts for over 72 hours and triptans or ergots are no longer effective.

Acute treatment strategies in specific clinical conditions

Self-administered drug treatment in acute migraine

Early drug intake is critical in acute migraine treatment. Medication should be taken when the headache is still mild to moderate in intensity as early intake improves the therapeutic outcome. Prior treatment approaches implied a stepped care therapy, but new data support the concept of stratified care [16]. Stratified care means that the initial treatment is based on patients' perception of the severity of headache and other factors. If the patient considers the headache to be mild, NSAIDs, nonopioid analgesics, and combined analgesics with additional antiemetics are recommended. If the headache is considered to be moderate to severe, the first-choice treatment is a triptan or ergot. The initial dosage should be sufficient to avoid redosing with the drugs. In case of headache recurrence, a second application of medication is recommended when the initial intake has aborted pain. Triptans and ergots *must not be taken together*. Similarly, different triptans *must not be mixed*.

> ★ TIPS AND TRICKS
>
> Do not restrict antiemetics to patients who are vomiting or are very likely to vomit, as nausea itself can be one of the most disabling symptoms of migraine attacks and should be treated appropriately. Antiemetics facilitate gastric empting and support resorption of the pain-relieving drugs. Further, metoclopramide has intrinsic analgesic properties.

Emergency room

Patients that come to the emergency room because of an acute migraine attack usually have already tried several oral medications without success. It is mandatory to make sure that the ongoing headache is a migraine attack and not a secondary headache (e.g., subarachnoidal bleeding, meningitis, or tumor). At this stage, the medication of first choice is a drug to be administered intravenously, such as ketorolac or, where available, ASA. Antiemetics such as metoclopramide may be administered in combination with an NSAID or as monotherapy. If there are no contraindications, subcutaneous sumatriptan or intravenous dihydroergotamine can be tried.

Status migrainosus

Expert consensus recommends the application of 50–100 mg of prednisone or 10 mg of dexamethasone, but placebo-controlled trials have not shown consistent results concerning this treatment. Usually, parenteral medication should be administered, but evidence-based data on appropriate therapy are still lacking. It is important to consider comorbidities that might evolve during this condition, such as dehydration and electrolyte abnormalities.

Migraine with pronounced nausea and vomiting

Nausea with or without vomiting is a common accompanying clinical feature in migraine and is closely associated with decreased absorption rates of pain-relieving medication. In this subgroup of patients, a nonoral administration route, such as a nasal spray, subcutaneous application, or suppository, should be selected. In some patients, a combined therapy of oral migraine medication and antiemetics might be also effective.

★ TIPS AND TRICKS

Select a nonoral administration form (nasal spray, suppository, or injection) of acute medication in migraineurs who present with distinct nausea or vomiting.

Menstrual migraine

In general, therapy of perimenstrual migraine attacks does not differ from that of nonmenstruation-associated migraine attacks. However, it is reasonable to apply long-acting triptans such as frovatriptan or ergots in combination with slow-release NSAIDs for therapy.

Migraine with aura, and aura without headache

Up to now, there has been no aura-specific treatment or strong evidence to suggest medications that successfully abort aura. Analgesics and migraine-specific drugs, if taken during the aura, do not reliably treat or prevent the following migraine pain. Previous data suggested that triptans and ergots should not be given because they are not effective and might even be harmful due to their vasoconstrictive effects. In contrast, a more recent study has shown the efficacy of pre-emptive triptan therapy during the aura phase of migraine attacks [6].

Basilar-type migraine and hemiplegic migraine

In basilar-type migraine and hemiplegic migraine, triptans and ergot alkaloids are not yet recommended based on a lack of safety data in migraine patients with these aura symptoms. Treatment options include antiemetics, NSAIDs, and non-narcotic pain relievers.

Chronic migraine

Acute treatment in chronic migraine is challenging as not all headache episodes can be treated early and efficiently with pain-relieving medications to avoid MOH. Almost all acute medications have the ability to cause MOH, especially triptans, ergots, caffeine-containing drugs, and in particular opioids and barbiturates. The last two drugs are therefore not used in Europe, but unfortunately they remain widely prescribed in North America. Migraine-specific drugs should be limited to 10 intake days per month, and nonmigraine-specific drugs can be used on up to 15 days a month. It is crucial that application days are counted rather than single dosages. If, for instance, triptans and NSAIDs are taken on one day, one intake day would be measured. In contrast, when triptan application is on one day and NSAIDs application on the following day, two application days would be counted.

The therapeutic aim in chronic migraine has to be to reduce the frequency of migraine attacks by initiating preventive therapy to a number below 10 days requiring acute medications so that an adequate acute treatment becomes possible.

Migraine in pregnancy

The main available data concerning the safety of migraine treatment in pregnancy are derived from pregnancy registers and a few prospective studies. Acetaminophen is a safe drug during all trimesters of pregnancy but is often not effective.

NSAIDs can be given in the second trimester and probably also in the first. In the third trimester, NSAIDs (especially ASA) are known to increase the risks of premature closure of the ductus arteriosus and the development of fetal pulmonary hypertension, inhibition of uterine contraction, and increase of maternal and newborn bleeding. Some data suggest that NSAIDs might inhibit embryo implantation and should be therefore avoided during attempted conception.

So far, no association has been observed between exposure to triptans during pregnancy and increased risk for major malformation. Triptan therapy during the second or third trimester is associated with a slightly increased risk of atonic uterus and blood loss during labour. However, no risk of adverse fetal outcomes have been observed. Opioids are considered to be relatively safe in pregnancy, but should only be considered as second choice because of their side effects. Regular use of opioids should be avoided as they cause an increased risk for fetal mortality during delivery and premature labor associated with fetal opioid withdrawal. In cases of intractable migraine attacks, a single dose of corticosteroids can be given.

Dihydroergotamine and ergotamine are contraindicated in pregnancy as the risks outweigh any possible treatment effect. They are known to cause impaired placental blood flow and may lead to spontaneous abortion and fetal distress, intestinal atresia, poor cerebral development, and Möbius syndrome.

Antiemetics might be also necessary to treat nausea and vomiting and improve the absorption of pain-relieving medication. Metoclopramide, chlorpromazine, and promethazine are compatible with pregnancy. Phenothiazines are used in hyperemesis gravidarum on a regular basis, and no teratogenic or embryotoxic effects have been observed.

Migraine and breastfeeding

Information on treatment options during breast-feeding period is scarce. Medications with a relative infant dose less than 10% of the maternal dose are considered to be compatible with breastfeeding. Acetaminophen and ibuprofen are drugs of first choice during lactation. Occasional intake of ASA is also safe. To what extent triptans can be used is controversial. Sumatriptan is considered to be compatible with breastfeeding, although small amounts have been measured in breast milk after maternal intake. To avoid any influence of sumatriptan on the child, the breast milk should be discarded over the 12 hours following triptan intake. Ergots are generally contraindicated as they inhibit prolactin secretion and induce diarrhea, vomiting, and convulsions in infants. Metoclopramide also passes into breast milk. Although no effects on infants have been observed up to now, indications for intake should be discussed thoroughly for each individual case.

Migraine in children

Migraine attacks in children should be treated with acetaminophen 15 mg/kg body weight or ibuprofen 10 mg/kg body weight. Ibuprofen has been shown to be superior to acetaminophen with regard to 2-hour efficacy. Both drugs can be given as tablets, liquids, or suppositories. When available, domperidone should be chosen rather than metoclopramide as an antiemetic to avoid extrapyramidal side effects.

Data on the efficacy of triptans in children below the age of 12 years are less promising than those for adults or teenagers. The younger the child, the less likely triptans are to be effective. There are two explanations for this. First, migraine attacks in children are clearly shorter than those in adults. Second, the placebo effect is much higher in children, which makes it difficult to show an efficacy of triptans in traditional parallel group studies. For intractable migraine attacks, nasal sumatriptan might be used for adolescents between the ages of 12 and 17 years. In younger children, the benefit of a triptan therapy should be considered and discussed with a headache specialist.

Migraine precursor syndromes such as periodic vomiting syndrome, periodic vertigo, and abdominal migraine are quite common during childhood. In these conditions, priority should be given to symptomatic therapy. In periodic vomiting syndrome, intravenous fluids containing adequate glucose should be given to avoid dehydration. Analgesics seem to be useful, and some patients also respond to triptans and ergot-amine compounds; however, these drugs are not approved in children. The application should be therefore only considered in severe cases.

Ondansetron might be effective for treating nausea and vomiting in these patients. Abdominal migraine responds very well to rest and sleep. In severe cases, triptan or ergots in combination with antiemetics are reported to be helpful.

Migraine in elderly patients

If triptans are being considered for migraine management in elderly patients, the increased numbers of comorbidities in this age group has to be taken into account. In particular, cardiovascular risk factors, prior myocardial infarction, and prior ischemic stroke have to be considered as migraine-specific drugs such as triptans or ergots would then be contraindicated. Additionally, blood tests should be performed to rule out renal or liver insufficiency. NSAIDs and non-opioid pain-relieving medication are contraindicated in such cases. Elderly patients are more prone to develop extrapyramidal side effects under metoclopramide therapy.

Conclusion

Acute migraine treatment should be adapted to the needs of individual patients with regard to headache characteristics, accompanying symptoms, and prior diseases. Treatment should always include nonpharmacologic treatment and, when needed, pharmacologic treatment. Pain-relieving drugs should be taken as early as possible after the beginning of the migraine attack to reach best efficacy. A stratified therapy should be favored: mild attacks can be treated with nonmigraine-specific drugs combined with antiemetics, and severe attacks should be treated from the beginning with migraine-specific drugs. For successful treatment, it is important to apply a sufficient dosage of the drug initially as redosing jeopardizes successful therapy. The formulation of the application has to be adapted to the accompanying symptoms, such as in cases of vomiting, where a suppository or nasal spray would be preferable. Frequent intake of specific and unspecific migraine medication can cause MOH and should be therefore avoided.

References

1. Ramadan NM, Silberstein SD, Freitag FG, Gilbert TT, Frishberg BM. Evidence-based guidelines for migraine headache in the primary care setting: pharmacological management for prevention of migraine. 2000. Available at http://www.aan.com/professionals/practice/pdfs/gl0087.pdf (accessed April 2013).
2. Lipton RB, Stewart WF, Ryan RE Jr, Saper J, Silberstein S, Sheftell F. Efficacy and safety of acetaminophen, aspirin, and caffeine in alleviating migraine headache pain: three double-blind, randomized, placebo-controlled trials. *Arch Neurol* 1998;**55**(2): 210–7.
3. Ellis GL, Delaney J, DeHart DA, Owens A. The efficacy of metoclopramide in the treatment of migraine headache. *Ann Emerg Med* 1993;**22**(2):191–5.
4. Friedman BW, Corbo J, Lipton RB, et al. A trial of metoclopramide vs sumatriptan for the emergency department treatment of migraines. *Neurology* 2005;**64**(3):463–8.
5. Goadsby PJ. The pharmacology of headache. *Prog Neurobiol* 2000;**62**(5):509–25.
6. Aurora SK, Barrodale PM, McDonald SA, Jakubowski M, Burstein R. Revisiting the efficacy of sumatriptan therapy during the aura phase of migraine. *Headache* 2009;**49**(7): 1001–4.
7. Ferrari MD, Roon KI, Lipton RB, Goadsby PJ. Oral triptans (serotonin 5-HT(1B/1D) agonists) in acute migraine treatment: a meta-analysis of 53 trials. *Lancet* 2001;**358**: 1668–75.
8. Burstein R, Collins B, Jakubowski M. Defeating migraine pain with triptans: a race against the development of cutaneous allodynia. *Ann Neurol* 2004;**55**(1):19–26.
9. Dowson AJ, Massiou H, Lainez JM, Cabarrocas X. Almotriptan improves response rates when treatment is within 1 hour of migraine onset. *Headache* 2004;**44**(4):318–22.
10. Ferrari M. How to assess and compare drugs in the management of migraine: success rates in terms of response and recurrence. *Cephalalgia* 1999;**19**(Suppl. 23):2–4; discussion 4–8.
11. Ferrari MD, James MH, Bates D, et al. Oral sumatriptan: effect of a second dose, and incidence and treatment of headache recurrences. *Cephalalgia* 1994;**14**(5):330–8.
12. Brandes JL, Kudrow D, Stark SR, et al. Sumatriptan-naproxen for acute treatment

of migraine: a randomized trial. *JAMA* 2007;**297**(13):1443–54.

13. Goadsby PJ, Lipton RB, Ferrari MD. Migraine—current understanding and treatment. *N Engl J Med* 2002;**346**(4):257–70.

14. A randomized, double-blind comparison of sumatriptan and Cafergot in the acute treatment of migraine. The Multinational Oral Sumatriptan and Cafergot Comparative Study Group. *Eur Neurol* 1991;**31**(5):314–22.

15. Wammes-van der Heijden EA, Rahimtoola H, Leufkens HGM, Tijssen CC, Egberts ACG. Risk of ischemic complications related to the intensity of triptan and ergotamine use. *Neurology* 2006;**67**(7):1128–34.

16. Lipton RB, Stewart WF, Stone AM, Láinez MJ, Sawyer JP. Stratified care vs step care strategies for migraine. The Disability in Strategies of Care (DISC) Study: a randomized trial. *JAMA* 2000;**284**(20):2599–605.

Preventive Treatments for Migraine

William B. Young

Thomas Jefferson University, Philadelphia, PA, USA

Introduction

Pharmaceutical management for migraine typically consists of treating symptomatic migraine attacks at the time of their occurrence, sometimes combined with daily preventive treatment intended to modify or decrease the probability of future migraine attacks. A third type of treatment that is sometimes used is "bridge," or short-term preventive/abortive, treatment given for 3–21 days to temporarily decrease headache intensity during an ongoing or anticipated exacerbation (e.g., during menses or drug withdrawal). Successful control of migraine often requires a comprehensive therapeutic program, of which medications are one component and behavioral treatments another.

Migraine ranks as approximately the 20th most frequent cause of disability in Westernized societies [1]. It affects the patient not only during, but also between attacks, and may affect not only the patient, but family members, friends, and coworkers as well. Migraines are often triggered by everyday occurrences and exposures, requiring patients to limit their activities and forego career pursuits or social events [2].

Abortive treatments do not always work; in addition, they may cause their own side effects,

require more adjunctive medications, and be very expensive, with visits to the emergency department for intensive evaluation and treatment.

This chapter will focus on the medications that effectively prevent recurrent migraine attacks and how to use them. The goals of migraine prevention are described in Table 9.1.

When to treat migraines preventively

Preventive treatment is necessary when migraine causes undue distress, dysfunction, and spending of healthcare dollars, or the patient is at risk for clinical deterioration. Frequent headaches at baseline predict progression to chronic daily headache at 1 year. The 4-days-per-month threshold for prevention is supported by epidemiologic data. It is based not only on the patient's pain and disability, but also on the risk of the headaches evolving into chronic migraine. The inflection point for progression occurs a little beyond 52 headache days per year (or an average of once weekly) (Figure 9.1). Other factors to consider in deciding who should be taking preventive medications are outlined in Table 9.2 [3].

Treating attacks can be costly, necessitating expensive acute medications, frequent office or

Headache, First Edition. Edited by Matthew S. Robbins, Brian M. Grosberg, and Richard B. Lipton.
© 2013 John Wiley & Sons, Ltd. Published 2013 by John Wiley & Sons, Ltd.

emergency room visits, and diagnostic testing when an attack mimics a secondary headache disorder (e.g., hemiplegic migraine). Prevention can reduce overall costs.

Migraine prevention: general principles

Physicians have many preventive medications from which to choose. The ideal preventive medication is effective across a broad population, has few side effects (or has advantageous ones), and does not interfere with, and may enhance, the treatment of coexistent conditions. Once the treatment has been selected, realistic expectations should be set. A 50% reduction in headache frequency might be a reasonable expectation. Inform the patient of common and serious uncommon side effects and how to manage

Table 9.1. Goals of preventive treatment

- Reduce the frequency, intensity, and duration of attacks
- Improve responsiveness to acute medication
- Improve function and reduce disability
- Reduce costs
- Prevent disease progression

them. Preventive treatment takes several weeks or months to work; it is unlikely to eliminate attacks entirely, but it will make them far more manageable in terms of reduced frequency, intensity, and duration, and may improve their responsiveness to acute treatment.

★ TIPS AND TRICKS

It is widely accepted that medication overuse may interfere with the effectiveness of preventive medications, and steps must be taken to reduce acute medication use. Although several studies have shown that preventive agents can work in the presence of medication overuse, most headache experts continue to hold that discontinuing or limiting overused abortive medications below recognized thresholds is always desirable, and is mandatory when the overused medications are barbiturates, opioids, or mixed analgesics [4]. Many maintain that overusing nonsteroidal anti-inflammatory drugs (NSAIDs) and simple analgesics may also interfere with the effectiveness of preventive medications.

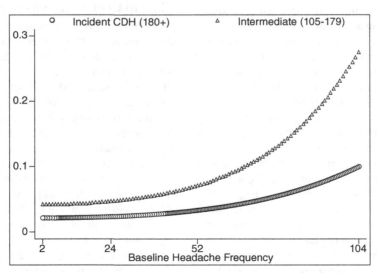

Figure 9.1. Risk of worsening of headache as a function of baseline headache frequency. The estimated 1-year incidence of chronic daily headache (CDH; >180 headaches per year) or very frequent headache (105–179 headaches per year) among patients with 2–104 headaches per year. (Reproduced from Scher AI, Stewart WF, Ricci JA, Lipton RB. Factors associated with the onset and remission of chronic daily headache in a population-based study. *Pain* 2003;106:81–89.)

Table 9.2. Criteria for initiating migraine prevention

- Migraine significantly interferes with the patient's daily routine, despite acute treatment
- Frequent headaches (>4 attacks/month)
- Acute medications are:
  - Ineffective
  - Contraindicated
  - Overused
  - Associated with troublesome adverse events
- Presence of uncommon migraine conditions with potentially disastrous consequences:
  - Hemiplegic migraine
  - Basilar-type migraine
  - Migraine with prolonged aura
  - Migrainous infarction
- Patient preference

discontinuation, an ineffective drug, a need for combination therapy, adverse effects, and poor adherence. Excessive initial doses of a preventive medication may lead to treatment-limiting side effects; inadequate final doses may result in limited or no efficacy. Generally, all preventive agents take weeks to months before benefit is noted. Premature discontinuation may occur if a patient takes a preventive medication on an irregular basis or for an inadequate duration of treatment. Variable responses can be seen among patients who are treated with the same preventive agent. Sometimes, a preventive agent may not be effective even if taken at the appropriate dose for the appropriate duration. Finally, in some patients rational polytherapy is necessary.

Preventive medications should be given at an adequate dose for an adequate length of time. It is best to start preventive medications at a low dose and then gradually increase the dose, as tolerated and if necessary. Start with 10%–30% of the target dose of preventive medication and increase this incrementally and gradually, allocating 3–14 days between dose escalations. A typical preventive trial lasts 2–3 months. Waiting longer delays finding an effective preventive agent, and waiting for a shorter time may cause one to discard a perfectly good medication. If the first preventive trial fails, revisit any issue of medication overuse. Consider a preventive medication with a different mechanism. If multiple single trials fail, consider using a combination of two or more preventive medications [5, 6].

Preventive medications for migraine are generally *not* chosen based on the demonstrated superior *efficacy* of some medications relative to others, since there is no evidence of such therapeutic superiority. Therefore, preventive medications are often selected to take advantage of the opportunity to treat migraine and comorbid conditions with a single medication, thereby possibly reducing costs, drug interactions, and side effects. Likewise, choices of preventive medication may hinge on avoiding potential side effects or drug interactions. Other considerations include costs, convenience or frequency of dosing, and previous response to medications.

Sometimes changes in headache characteristics are not obvious and require a headache calendar to document them. Patients are often mistaken about their baseline headache frequency and patterns. Patients should keep track of their headaches to monitor for changes in frequency, intensity, responsiveness to acute medications, and temporal pattern. Daily calendars are useful in establishing whether any type of gains are being made (frequency, intensity, or responsiveness to acute treatment) and can also reveal unrecognized medication overuse. Ongoing assessment of the success and appropriateness of preventive treatment is essential.

✋ CAUTION!

Most patients respond well to prophylactic treatment, but some patients do not. It is important to identify the reason or reasons why these patients have not responded appropriately. Common reasons for preventive treatment "failure" include improper dosing strategies, premature

Table 9.3. Principles of preventive treatment

- Communicate realistic expectations
- Choose treatment based on:
  - Efficacy
  - Adverse event profile
  - Coexistent medical and psychiatric conditions
- Assure adequate contraception
- Start at a predetermined low dose and gradually increase until efficacy is achieved, side effects develop, or the dose is reached
- Explain that benefits develop slowly (over months)
- Treatment is often not fully effective until overuse has been addressed; eliminate it either during treatment or before
- If the first-choice agent fails, choose a second from another therapeutic class
- Monotherapy is preferred, but combination therapy is often necessary
- Evaluate therapy:
  - Use a calendar
  - If side effects are present at the target dose, taper down to the lowest effective dose

Once adequate control has been attained and maintained for 6 months, consider tapering the preventive medication. Evidence suggests that some people can sustain an improvement in headache frequency for at least 6 months after discontinuing the preventive, while others will have a recurrence. Patients can often taper medication without worsening their condition, and can maintain control with lifestyle changes and nonprescription supplements (Tables 9.3, 9.4, 9.5, and 9.6) [7].

How preventive agents work

Preventive medications may work by reducing neuronal hyperexcitability. Evidence from an animal model of migraine supports this: in the animal model, preventives operating with a wide variety of mechanisms decreased the number of cortical spreading depressions induced by a stimulus (Figure 9.2) [8].

The mechanisms by which this may occur are diverse, as similarly effective treatments have completely different mechanisms of action (Table 9.7). Recent evidence suggests that the anticonvulsants valproic acid and topiramate may have an inhibitory effect on histone deacetylation, suggesting epigenetic effects that might explain the lag between achieving adequate blood levels and reducing headache frequency. At least one preventive treatment, OnabotulinumtoxinA, appears to be *ineffective* for most cases of episodic migraine, while it is proven to be effective for chronic migraine. As more treatments are discovered to be helpful in migraine prevention (indeed, almost all discoveries have been serendipitous—none but methysergide was engineered for migraine treatment), more light will be shed on the pathophysiologic underpinnings of migraine.

Migraine preventives

Preventive medications generally come from four categories: anticonvulsants, antidepressants, antihypertensives, and others. Tables 9.3–9.6 have detailed examples from each category, putative relative efficacies, starting and target doses, and considerations for coexistent/comorbid conditions [6]. It is also important to remember, especially in patients with comorbidities, to avoid unnecessary polypharmacy and drug–drug interactions.

Anticonvulsants

Among the anticonvulsants, the strongest evidence for efficacy exists for valproic acid and topiramate. Several studies have demonstrated the efficacy of sodium valproate, divalproex sodium, or extended-release divalproex sodium. In general, the goal dose is 1000 mg daily (500 mg twice daily or 1000 mg nightly if an extended-release formulation is used). It is not useful to assess drug levels, except when one suspects toxicity or nonadherence. Common adverse events include nausea and gastrointestinal distress, which decrease over time. Tremor, alopecia, and weight increase tend to occur later.

Table 9.4. Practical categories of migraine preventives based (in part) upon US Consortium recommendations

Most effective	Weaker evidence	Less effective	Unproven, often used	Ineffective for routine use
Anticonvulsants	**Anticonvulsants**	**Anticonvulsants**	**Antidepressants**	**Anticonvulsants**
Topiramate	Gabapentin	Carbamazepine	Nortriptyline	Lamotrigine
Divalproex sodium			Protriptyline	Oxcarbazepine
Antidepressants	**Antidepressants**	**Calcium channel blockers**	Imipramine	Clonazepam
Amitriptyline	Fluoxetine	Verapamil	Doxepin	
	Venlafaxine	Diltiazem	Fluvoxamine	**Others**
Beta-blockers	**Beta-blockers**	Nimodipine	Paroxetine	Acetazolamide
Timolol	Atenolol	Nifedipine	Sertraline	Lanepitant
Propranolol	Nadolol	Nicardipine	Phenelzine	Montelukast
Metoprolol				Omega-3
Serotonin antagonist	**Angiotensin system**	**Alpha-agonists**	**Serotonin antagonist**	Vitamin E
Methysergide	Lisinopril	Clonidine[b]	Methylergonovine	Onabotulinumtoxin A[c]
	Candesartan			
Other	**Other**			
Petasites (butterbur)	Coenzyme Q10			
Neurotoxin	Riboflavin			
Onabotulinumtoxin A[a]	Feverfew			
Triptan	**Serotonin agonist**			
Frovatriptan	Naratriptan[b]			
	Zolmitriptan[b]			
	NSAIDs			

Groups of medications used for migraine prevention based on levels of evidence for efficacy according the Quality Standards Subcommittee of the American Academy of Neurology. [a]For chronic migraine. [b]For short-term prophylaxis of menstrually related migraine. [c]For episodic migraine.

Table 9.5. Using various preventive medications

Drug	Starting dose	Target dose
Anticonvulsants (Although used as mood stabilizers, be vigilant for destabilization of mood with any of these)		
Topiramate	25 mg	100–200 mg/day
Divalproex sodium	250 mg	1500–2000 mg/day
Gabapentin	300 mg	1800–4800 mg/day
Zonisamide	25 mg	150–300 mg/day
Lamotrigine	25 mg	100–200 mg/day
Antidepressants (All below can cause sexual dysfunction; caution with bipolar patients, adolescents, and the elderly due to potential for mood destabilization and suicidality)		
Tricyclics		
Amitriptyline	10 mg	50–75 mg
Nortriptyline	10 mg	30–50 mg
Protriptyline	5 mg tid	10–20 mg tid
Imipramine	10 mg	30–50 mg
Doxepin	10 mg	30–100 mg
Tetracyclic		
Mirtazapine	7.5 mg	15–30 mg
Serotonin–norepinephrine reuptake inhibitors		
Venlafaxine	25–37.5 mg	150–300 mg/day
Duloxetine	20–30 mg	60–120 mg/day
Fluoxetine	10 mg	40 mg/day
Sertraline	25–50 mg	100–200 mg/day
MAOIs (Many dangerous drug–drug interactions, low-tyramine diet required, not good for unreliable/noncompliant patients)		
Phenelzine	15 mg bid/tid	90 mg/day
Antihypertensives (All below can cause hypotension and fatigue; can be used in patients with normal or low blood pressure, just "start low and go slow")		
Beta-blockers		
Propranolol	10–60 mg	120 mg
Timolol	2.5–10 mg/day	20 mg/day
Metoprolol	25 mg	50–100 mg/day
Atenolol	25 mg	50–100 mg/day
Nadolol	10 mg	20–120 mg/day
Calcium channel blockers		
Verapamil	40–120 mg/day	240–480 mg/day
Diltiazem	30–120 mg/day	180–360 mg/day
Flunarizine	5 mg	10 mg
Angiotensin system		
Lisinopril	2.5–5 mg	10–20 mg
Candesartan	4–8 mg	16 mg
Telmisartan	80 mg	80 mg
Olmesartan	5 mg	10–40 mg

Table 9.5. (*Continued*)

Drug	Starting dose	Target dose
Others		
Methysergide	2 mg bid	2 mg tid/qid
Methergine	0.2 mg bid/tid	0.4 mg tid
Onabotulinum neurotoxin	100 U	300 U
Cyproheptadine	2–4 mg	4–12 mg
Memantine	5 mg	20 mg/day
Minocycline	50–100 mg	100 mg/bid
"Natural" remedies		
Feverfew	6.25 mg tid	6.25 mg tid
Petasites	75 mg bid	50–75 mg bid
Riboflavin	400 mg/day	400 mg/day
Magnesium	200 mg/day	1200 mg/day divided
Coenzyme Q10	150–300 mg/day	300 mg/day
Thioctic (alpha-liproic) acid	600 mg/day	600 mg/day

bid, twice a day; qid, four times a day; tid, three times a day.

⚓ CAUTION!

Very rarely, valproic acid can cause severe hepatotoxicity or pancreatitis. The frequency of fulminant liver failure is greatest in very young children, in persons on multiple anticonvulsants, and in the presence of genetic or metabolic abnormalities. Two approaches to monitoring are commonly used. One approach checks liver function tests prior to initiating treatment and does not check them again unless symptoms develop, because fulminant liver failure develops so rapidly that even frequent testing is unlikely to capture the start to the process; the other checks liver function tests and a complete blood count at intervals after starting therapy—perhaps at 3, 6, and 12 months and yearly thereafter. Because of the teratogenic risk and the possibility of inducing polycystic ovarian syndrome, valproic acid should be used with extra caution in teenage girls and women with reproductive potential.

The effectiveness of topiramate has been shown in several high-quality placebo-controlled or active treatment comparator trials. The doses studied have varied from 50 to 200 mg, with 100 mg emerging as the optimal dose for episodic migraine. In one study, topiramate was as effective as propranolol for migraine prevention. The most common adverse events are paresthesias, fatigue, nausea, anorexia, and abnormal taste. Patients should be prepared for the paresthesias that occur in about half of those initiating therapy; the symptoms only rarely lead to discontinuation unless they are unexpected or particularly severe. The paresthesias are usually mild to moderate and might be controlled with potassium supplementation. Weight loss may also occur. The average patient loses approximately 8 lb [3.6 kg] on topiramate [9]. CNS side effects, including concentration and memory disturbances and word-finding difficulties, occur with some regularity. If these side effects occur, many patients can lower the dose and still find effective relief.

Table 9.6. Considering comorbidities in selecting a preventive agent

Drug	Efficacy	Side effects	Relative indications	Relative contraindications
Anticonvulsants				
Topiramate	4+	2+	Epilepsy, obesity, medication overuse headache?	Calcium phosphate kidney stones
Divalproex	4+	2+	Epilepsy, bipolar disorder	Obesity, hepatic dysfunction, bleeding disorder, fertile woman
Gabapentin	2+	2+	Epilepsy, neuropathic pain	Obesity
Antidepressants				
TCAs	4+	2+	Depression, anxiety, insomnia, other pain disorder	Bipolar disorder, heart block, urinary retention, obesity
SSRIs	2+	1+	Depression, anxiety, obsessive-compulsive disorder	Bipolar disorder
SNRIs	3+	2+	Depression, anxiety, fibromyalgia	Bipolar disorder, hypertension
Antihypertensives				
Beta-blockers	4+	2+	Hypertension, angina	Asthma, depression, congestive heart failure, diabetes, Raynaud's disease
Calcium channel blockers	2+	1+	Raynaud's disease, migraine with unusual aura	Heart block, chronic constipation
ACEs	3+	1+	Hypertension	Chronic cough
ARBs	3+	1+	Hypertension	Chronic cough
Others				
Riboflavin	2+	1+	Preference for nutraceutical	None
Coenzyme Q10	2+	1+	Fatigue	None
Magnesium	1+	1+	Constipation	Diarrhea, renal impairment
Petasites	3+	1+	Preference for nutraceutical	None
Onabotulinum neurotoxin	1+ for episodic 4+ for chronic	1+	Chronic migraine	Local infection, neuromuscular disorder

ACE, angiotensin-converting enzyme; ARB, angiotensin receptor blocker; SNRI, serotonin–norepinephrine reuptake inhibitor; SSRI, selective serotonin reuptake inhibitor; TCA, tricyclic antidepressant.

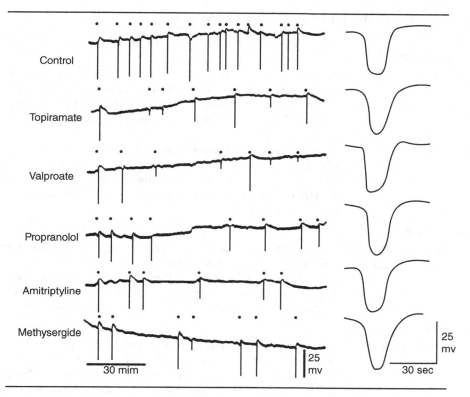

Figure 9.2. Inhibition of cortical spreading depression after chronic treatment with migraine prophylactic drugs. Representative electrophysiologic tracings from cortex after saline control or drug treatment. After chronic treatment, significantly fewer cortical spreading depressions (CSDs) were observed in response to topical KCl application. There was no significant difference in waveform amplitude or morphology. Individual CSDs from representative experiments are shown on the right on an expanded time scale. (Reproduced with permission from Wiley. Dodick DW, Silberstein SD. Migration prevention. *Practical Neurology* 2007;7:383–93.)

✋ CAUTION!

A rare and potentially serious adverse event of topiramate is the development of acute angle-closure glaucoma, the symptoms of which are eye pain and decreased vision. For nonspecific visual symptoms, check the intraocular pressure before discontinuing the medication and potentially depriving a patient of an effective preventive drug. Decreased sweating may occur in association with hyperthermia; most such cases are reported in children. Rarely, patients may also develop nephrolithiasis. Therefore, it is important to advise patients on topiramate to maintain adequate fluid hydration.

Gabapentin may be effective for migraine control, but the data are less convincing based on a single placebo-controlled trial with a high drop-out rate. The effective dose appears to be high, 1800–2400 mg daily. At these doses, weight gain is a particularly onerous problem. Side effects include sedation, dizziness, fatigue, ataxia, nausea, dry mouth, blurred vision, and peripheral edema.

Lamotrigine and oxcarbazepine appear to be *ineffective* for prevention of migraine. On the other hand, based on case series, lamotrigine may be effective at preventing migraine auras. One drug, tonabersat, which is not being taken to market, has been proven to be effective at controlling auras but not migraine without aura [5].

Table 9.7. Possible mechanism of action of some preventive agents

Class/drug	Suspected mechanism of action
Anticonvulsants	
Valproic acid	Enhances postsynaptic responses to GABA. Increases GABA in synaptosomes. Increases potassium (K^+) conductance of GABA receptors. Turns off firing of serotonin (5-HT) neurons in the dorsal raphi nucleus. Inhibits histone deacetylase, producing diverse epigenetic effects
Topiramate	Binds to membrane channel complexes, preventing protein kinase A phosphorylation of AMPA/kainate receptor, $GABA_A$ receptor, and some sodium and calcium ion channels. Carbonic anhydrase IV and II inhibitor. Inhibits histone deacetylase, producing diverse epigenetic effects
Antidepressants	
Amitriptyline (and other tricyclics and venlafaxine)	Increases synaptic norepinephrine and serotonin. Decreases beta-adrenergic receptor density and response. Increases sensitivity of postsynaptic $5\text{-}HT_{1A}$ receptors. Upregulates GABA-β receptor. Augments adenosine actions that contribute to antinociception. Increases BDNF mRNA via $5\text{-}HT_{2A}$ and beta-adrenoreceptors
Antihypertensives	
Propranolol (and other beta-blockers)	Inhibits central beta-receptors, interfering with vigilance. Enhances adrenergic pathway. Interacts with 5-HT receptors. Cross-modulation of serotonin system. Inhibits nitrous oxide reduction by blocking inducible nitrous oxide synthase. Inhibits kainate-induced currents
Lisinopril	Blocks degradation of calcitonin gene-related peptide
Other	
Magnesium	Blocks NMDA activity
Riboflavin	Promotes mitochondrial function
Coenzyme Q	Promotes mitochondrial function

AMPA, α-amino-3-hydroxy-5-methyl-4-isoxazolepropionic acid; BDNF, brain-derived neurotrophic factor; GABA, gamma-aminobutyric acid; NMDA, N-methyl-D-aspartic acid.

Antidepressants

Amitriptyline is one of the most widely used preventive medications for migraine. Several placebo-controlled studies with high drop-out rates have been published demonstrating efficacy in studies that would now be considered to be Class II. The side effects of the tricyclic antidepressants include anticholinergic effects (increased appetite and weight gain, urinary retention, sexual dysfunction, sedation, and restlessness). QTc prolongation may occur, but less than with venlafaxine. Mania and suicidal ideation may rarely occur. If tricyclics are used for a suicide attempt, they are particularly dangerous. Many practices use nortriptyline in preference to amitriptyline in the hope of minimizing sedation, weight gain, and anticholinergic side effects. Other tricyclics that are frequently used include doxepin and desipramine. Protriptyline may be used because of its absence of sedation and tendency *not* to cause weight gain, but it produces more dry mouth and constipation.

Venlafaxine has been shown to be an effective preventive agent. A 150 mg dose of venlafaxine has been shown to be more effective than a 75 mg dose, which in turn was more effective than placebo. In another study, the efficacy of venlafaxine was similar to that of amitriptyline. Comparative studies with venlafaxine and propranolol also suggest efficacy. Side effects include insomnia, nervousness, mydriasis, and, very rarely, seizures. Weight gain is common. Venlafaxine may raise the blood pressure slightly, so this parameter must be tracked. We sometimes use duloxetine, which may have side effect advantages, although only case series supports its use.

Fluoxetine has been effective in migraine prevention in some studies but not others. Some evidence suggests that treatment results may improve from month 3 to month 6, in contrast to other preventive treatments that work more quickly. In practice, many clinicians use other selective serotonin reuptake inhibitors that have fewer side effects or potential drug interactions. Sexual dysfunction, sweating, insomnia, and nausea may occur.

Monoamine oxidase inhibitors (MAOIs) are still used for some patients with refractory migraine based upon anecdotal evidence. Phenelzine is the most commonly used MAOI, with the dose ranging from 30 to 90 mg a day in divided doses. All patients must be on a tyramine-restricted diet, and sympathomimetic drugs must be assiduously avoided. Adverse events, such as sedation and orthostatic hypotension, are common, and weight gain can be a severe problem [9].

Antihypertensives

A number of beta-blockers have been shown to be effective migraine preventives. Propranolol, timolol, and metoprolol have the strongest evidence of efficacy. Nebivolol, atenolol, and nadolol have some evidence supporting their efficacy. Beta-blockers that are partial agonists with intrinsic sympathomimetic activity are not effective. Metoprolol may be an option for patients with mild asthma, for whom less selective beta-blockers are contraindicated. Adverse events include hypotension, bradycardia, bronchospasm, dizziness, sexual dysfunction, and bizarre dreams. Beta-blockers may further reduce cardiac contractility in patients with acute congestive heart failure. Beta-blockers may rarely produce depression, but they may be useful for anxiety.

Verapamil and nimodipine are considered to be weak migraine prophylactic agents. Studies are less conclusive than for beta-blockers, and the magnitude of the response to treatment is generally less than with other preventive agents.

Unlike the doses used for cluster headache, migraine doses in excess of 480 mg per day are generally not used. Adverse effects include bradycardia, first-degree atrioventricular block, hypotension, constipation, gingival hyperplasia, and ankle edema. Rare adverse events include higher order atrioventricular block and pulmonary edema. Outside the USA, flunarizine is widely used in migraine prophylaxis. It is probably a much more effective preventive than the other calcium channel blockers. Adverse events are troublesome, with sedation, weight gain, and depression being most problematic.

Lisinopril, candesartan, and telmisartan have been studied in placebo-controlled trials. Results were positive for lisinopril and candesartan, but positive for telmisartan only after adjustment for baseline characteristics. Based on anecdotal evidence, we sometimes use olmesartan. The target dose for lisinopril is 20 mg daily, although one case series suggests that 5 mg may be effective. For candesartan, the target dose is 16 mg daily. Common adverse events of lisinopril include hypotension, rash, and cough. The cough caused by lisinopril usually does not improve with continued use and is a common cause of discontinuation. Rare angioedema of the face, lips, and throat can occur. Hyperkalemia and renal impairment may occur. Adverse effects of candesartan and telmisartan are similar to those of lisinopril, except that cough does not occur.

Clonidine has been extensively studied, but evidence suggests that it is only minimally and not conclusively effective. Dry mouth, hypotension, impotence, vivid dreams, rash, nausea, and depression are notable adverse events. Bradycardia, QTc prolongation, and atrioventricular block may occur at higher dose. Rapid withdrawal can cause rebound hypertension. Weight gain is unusual [9].

Other migraine preventives

NSAIDs

Studies of daily aspirin in the 325–650 mg range have found reductions in migraine frequency of around 20%–30%. Studies of several other NSAIDs have shown them also to be effective. Because of the association of higher dose aspirin with medication overuse headache, and the possibility that NSAIDs may cause medication overuse headache, some caution is necessary. Daily NSAIDs may cause gastrointestinal bleeding and kidney injury.

Botulinum toxin A

The results for episodic migraine have been mixed, in contrast to the results for chronic migraine. The US Academy of Neurology's practice parameter has determined that botulinum toxin is "probably not effective" for episodic migraine, in contrast to chronic migraine, for which there is strong evidence of efficacy.

Histamine

N-Methylhistamine was positive in a double-blind, placebo-controlled trial for migraine prevention, but it is not commercially available. Histamine injections were given twice weekly. Typically, other histamine formulations are given as a single intramuscular or subcutaneous injection.

Cyproheptadine

Cyproheptadine is widely used in the preventive treatment of pediatric migraine, but controlled trials show limited evidence to uphold this. The total daily doses range from 12 to 36 mg in divided doses, two or three times a day. Common adverse events are sedation and weight gain.

Methysergide

Methysergide is an ergot-derived Food and Drug Administration (FDA)-approved medication for migraine prevention, although there are no placebo-controlled trials to support its efficacy. It is no longer sold in the USA but is available in Canada. It is a vasoconstrictor and thus must be used with care in patients who have potential cardiovascular disease or are users of triptans and other ergots. It commonly causes weight gain. Retroperitoneal fibrosis may occur after 6 months of use. Patients on methysergide should be given a month-long holiday every 6 months or have a chest X-ray, erythrocyte sedimentation rate, and CT scan of the abdomen and pelvis. Some also recommend yearly echocardiography.

Methylergonovine

Methylergonovine is sometimes used in preference to methysergide. It is better tolerated and the risk of retroperitoneal fibrosis is believed to be much less, as is the weight gain and risk of interactions with triptans and other ergots. Nonetheless, as with methysergide, we give holidays or test after 6 months.

Pizotifen

Pizotifen is used in most of the world, but it is not FDA approved or sold in the USA. The dose is 0.5 mg three times daily, which is increased as needed to a maximum of 1.5 mg three times a day. Weight gain and sedation are common. Nausea, dry mouth, depression, sexual dysfunction, and urinary retention may occur.

Memantine

Based on several case series, memantine may be an effective migraine preventive medication, although no placebo-controlled trial for headache disorder has been carried out. Doses range from 5 mg daily to 10 mg twice a day. Adverse events are minimized by slow titration. Hypertension, dizziness, constipation, coughing, ataxia, and vertigo may occur.

"Natural" preventives

Petasites

The purified extract of the butterbur plant, at a dose of 75 mg twice daily, has been shown to be effective in two high-quality placebo-controlled trials. A lower dose of 50 mg twice daily may be less effective. The only common side effect is eructation (burping). Herbal preparations such as Petasites may contain pyrrolizidine derivatives, which are hepatotoxic and teratogenic. It is important to verify that the brand of Petasites used is certified as pyrrolizidine-free.

Riboflavin

Riboflavin may be effective for migraine prevention based on one Class I study and several anecdotal reports. Stomach irritation occasionally occurs, and urine inevitably turns dark yellow or orange. Efficacy may increase for 3–6 months; thus, a trial of only a few months may be inadequate.

Magnesium

Several studies suggest that magnesium is effective for migraine prevention. Doses vary from

200 mg daily to 1200 mg in divided doses. Magnesium is generally extremely safe except in persons with significant renal insufficiency. One strategy is to titrate to the maximal "subdiarrheal" dose, as diarrhea is an inevitable consequence of higher doses.

Coenzyme Q

One double-blind controlled test suggests that coenzyme Q may be an effective preventive for migraine headache. Side effects are few, and safety is believed to be excellent. The best-studied dose is 150 mg three times a day.

Thioctic acid (alpha-lipoic acid)

One small and underpowered controlled trial has suggested that this putative mitochondrial enhancer, at a dose of 600 mg daily, might be effective for migraine prevention. Adverse events are rare. At higher doses, iron levels may drop (as thioctic acid may be a chelating agent).

Feverfew

Feverfew has been found to be effective in some studies. One formulation, MIG-99, has been found to be effective in a well-designed, placebo-controlled trial. The dose is 6.25 mg three times daily.

Bridge therapy

Bridges are treatments given for 3–21 days for short-term prevention, status migrainosus, or exacerbations of chronic migraine (Table 9.8). Bridge therapy is often useful when the goal is stopping overused medications (triptans, combination drugs, or opioids) before preventive treatments become effective. Steroids are often effective for this, as are combinations of an NSAID and an antiemetic. The goal is to keep the patient functional and avoid intravenous treatments or hospitalization. The risk is in increasing the amount of medicine used and possibly contributing to medication overuse headache. The best studied bridge is frovatriptan for menstrual migraine prophylaxis.

Prevention in pregnancy and lactation

The use of preventive medications during pregnancy is problematic, as accurate information to assess the risk to the fetus or baby is lacking.

Table 9.8. Examples of bridge therapy

Steroids	Dose
Methylprednisolone[a] Prednisone[a]	One-dose pack Start at 60–80 mg, decrease over 3–6 days
Dexamethasone[a]	Start at 12 mg, decrease over 3–6 days
NSAIDs	
Naproxen sodium	550 mg tid × 5 days
Naproxen + metoclopramide	550 mg + 10 mg tid over 3–7 days
Naproxen + prochlorperazine	550 mg + 10 mg over 3–7 days
Ergot/triptan	
DHE	DHE nasal spray: 2 mg bid over 3 days DHE i.m.: 1 mg i.m. bid over 3 days
Frovatriptan	2.5 mg bid—bid day 1, then daily for 6 days
Other	
Tizanidine	2–4 mg tid
Olanzapine	2.5–10 mg bid
Methylergonovine	0.2 mg tid × 2 weeks

[a]Some recommend a limit of a maximum of 3 days per month averaged over several months. bid, twice a day; DHE, dihydroergotamine; i.m., intramuscular; tid, three times a day.

Fortunately, migraine activity tends to lessen in the second and third trimesters. In general, we discontinue all preventive medications, including "naturals," prior to attempting pregnancy, except for magnesium, which we often start prior to a patient's pregnancy and maintain through the pregnancy. Oral magnesium supplementation does not cause magnesium levels to rise above normal values.

In special circumstances, preventives need to be given during pregnancy. The FDA system for describing fetal risk from a drug places medication into categories A, B, C, D, and X based on human or animal studies (Table 9.9). Lactating women should be given preventive medications cautiously.

Table 9.9. Preventive treatments

	FDA fetal risk	Breastfeeding
Beta-blockers		
Atenolol	D	Caution
Metoprolol	C[a]	Compatible
Propranolol	C[a]	Compatible
Timolol	C[a]	Compatible
Neuromodulators		
Gabapentin	C	Probably compatible
Topiramate	D	Caution
Valproate (divalproex)	D	Compatible
Tricylics		
Amitriptyline	C	Concern
Imipramine	C	Concern
Nortriptyline	C	Concern
Other		
Fluoxetine	C/D[b]	May be of concern
Venlafaxine	C/D[b]	Potential toxicity

Please note that FDA ratings may change periodically.
[a]D if used when pregnancy is prolonged or at term.
[b]D is for second half of pregnancy.

The future of migraine prevention

Presently, only five medications are FDA-approved for migraine prevention. These are topiramate (its use limited mainly by cognitive and psychiatric adverse events), divalproex sodium (poorly tolerated and inadvisable for women of childbearing potential, a substantial subset of the migraine population), two nearly identical beta-blockers (propranolol and timolol), and methysergide, which is no longer sold in the USA. Several other medications have proven efficacy, but these are largely variations on the same theme. Some unique drugs and approaches have been helpful, but many have unfavorable adverse event profiles, are costly, or are considered experimental [5]. Because of these limitations, the pursuit of new treatments is ongoing.

Medications targeting unique neurotransmitter and receptor systems are being investigated. As new medications are developed for epilepsy, hypertension, and depression, their potential for benefit in headache must be considered. Finally, the nonmedication approaches of various forms of stimulation (transcranial magnetic, peripheral neural, and deep brain) have shown initial promise, and we eagerly await the optimization and more widespread use of these modalities.

References

1. World Health Organization. Headache disorders. Fact sheet No 277. Available at: http://www.who.int/mediacentre/factsheets/fs277/en/print.html. 2007.
2. Munakata J, Hazard E, Serrano D, et al. Economic burden of transformed migraine: results from the American Migraine Prevalence and Prevention (AMPP) Study. *Headache* 2009;**49**:498–508.
3. Scher AI, Stewart WF, Ricci JA, Lipton RB. Factors associated with the onset and remission of chronic daily headache in a population-based study. *Pain* 2003;**106**: 81–9.
4. Bigal ME, Serrano D, Buse D, Scher A, Stewart WF, Lipton RB. Acute migraine medications and evolution from epoisodic to chronic

migraine: a longitudinal population-based study. *Headache* 2008;**48**:1157–68.

5. Silberstein SD, Freitag FG, Bigal ME. Migraine treatment. In Silberstein SD, Lipton RB, Dodick DW (eds.), *Wolff's Headache and Other Head Pain* (8th edn.). New York: Oxford University Press, 2008: pp. 177–292.

6. Dodick DW, Silberstein SD. Migraine prevention. *Practical Neurol* 2007;**7**:383–93.

7. Diener HC, Agosti R, Allais G, et al. Cessation versus continuation of 6-month migraine pre-ventive therapy with topiramate (PROMPT): a randomised, double-blind, placebo-controlled trial. *Lancet Neurol* 2007;**6**: 1054–62.

8. Ayata C, Jin H, Kudo C, Dalkara T, Moskowitz MA. Suppression of cortical spreading depression in migraine prophylaxis. *Ann Neurol* 2006;**59**:652–61.

9. Silberstein SD, Marmura MJ. *Essential Neuropharmacology: The Prescriber's Guide.* New York: Cambridge University Press, 2010.

Managing the Special Problem of Chronic Migraine

Marcelo E. Bigal

Albert Einstein College of Medicine, Bronx, NY, USA

Introduction

Seen as a purely episodic disorder for a large part of the 20th century [1], more recent evidence supports the concept that migraine is a chronic disorder with episodic attacks [2]. Additionally, evidence shows that migraine has a variable clinical course [3]. Some migraine sufferers enjoy remission, becoming free of migraine. Others have a stable clinical course. Finally, a subset develops chronic migraine (CM), a condition characterized by headaches on 15 or more days per month [4, 5]. CM is one subtype of chronic daily headaches and is the scope of this chapter. We start by briefly presenting the phenotype of CM. We then discuss the differential diagnosis and present strategies for treatment. Risk factors for the onset of CM have been discussed in Chapter 5. Since acute medication overuse is a risk factor for increased headache frequency, we will discuss the management of CM with medication overuse, although, from a classification perspective, this subtype of CM is referred to as medication overuse headache [6, 7]. We close by discussing reasons for the failure of CM treatment.

Classification and phenotype of chronic migraine

CM, the clinical consequence of migraine transformation, evolves from episodic migraine, with an escalating attack frequency over a period of time. CM is more frequent in women with a past history of migraine without aura, although it can affect both genders. Subjects usually report a process of transformation over months or years, and as headache increases in frequency, associated symptoms become less severe and frequent. The process of transformation frequently ends in a pattern of daily or nearly daily headache that resembles chronic tension-type headache, with some or many attacks of full-migraine superimposed [5, 8, 9].

CM is sometimes referred to as transformed migraine. The original criteria for transformed migraine required the following:

- The headache did not develop abruptly in a previously headache-free subject.
- The headache has one of the three following links with migraine present: (1) a prior history of migraine; (2) a period of escalating head-

Headache, First Edition. Edited by Matthew S. Robbins, Brian M. Grosberg, and Richard B. Lipton.
© 2013 John Wiley & Sons, Ltd. Published 2013 by John Wiley & Sons, Ltd.

Table 10.1. Revised ICHD classification criteria for CM

A. Headache on ≥15 days/month for >3 months
B. Occurring in a patient with at least 5 prior migraine attacks
C. On ≥8 days per month, for at least 3 months, headache fills the criteria for migraine (C1 and/or C2)
  1. H Has at least two of a–d:
    a. Unilateral location
    b. Pulsating quality
    c. Moderate or severe pain intensity
    d. Aggravation by physical activity
    And at least one of a or b:
    a. Nausea and/or vomiting
    b. Photophobia and phonophobia
  2. Treated and relieved by triptans or ergotamine compounds
D. No medication overuse and not attributable to another causative disorder

Adapted from [11].

ache frequency; and (3) concurrent superimposed attacks of full-blown migraine [5].

The first edition of the International Classification of Headache Disorders (ICHD-1) [6] did not mention CM or chronic daily headaches. The ICHD-2 included criteria for CM that required 15 or more days of full migraine per month [7], but this criterion was too restrictive in clinical practice and research [10, 11]. As a consequence, revised criteria have been endorsed by the International Headache Society (Table 10.1) [12]. Basically, CM is classified in individuals with 15 days or more of headache per month and 8 or more days of migraine or use of acute migraine medications. If subjects are overusing acute medication, they should be classified as having medication overuse headache.

★ TIPS AND TRICKS

The phenotype of CM is variable with age. The progression of migraine into CM has different characteristics when it occurs in adolescents or in adults. The frequency of full-blown migraine attacks is higher in adolescents relative to adults. Most adults with CM have fewer than 15 days of full-blown migraine per month and more days of headache resembling tension-type headache than of migraine. In contrast, CM in adolescents is replete with migraine attacks. Also, most adults with "CM" (84.0%) overuse acute medication, while most adolescents (58.9%) do not [13].

★ TIPS AND TRICKS

The phenotype of CM changes over time. Evidence suggests that the proportion of migraine attacks decreases with age (with a proportional increase in tension-type headache attacks), from 71% below the age of 30 years to 22% at age 60 or above. In the initial phases of migraine progression, when patients are younger, or when the interval between migraine and the onset of CM is relatively short, CM is characterized by migraine days on almost every day. Subsequently, the frequency of clear-cut migraine attacks diminishes [9, 14].

Diagnosing chronic migraine

An individual with CM presents to the office complaining of headaches on more days than not. Some of the headaches are more disabling than others and can be clearly characterized as being migraine attacks. Other headaches are more diffuse and difficult to characterize. When seeing these patients, basically a three-step approach should be used, as outlined below (modified from Bigal and Lipton [15]). If the response to therapy is less than adequate, a fourth step is required (see the section "When chronic migraine becomes refractory").

Step 1: Distinguishing primary from secondary chronic daily headaches

Although important for headaches overall, distinguishing primary from secondary headaches is of particular importance in individuals with frequent headaches. The strategies to identify or

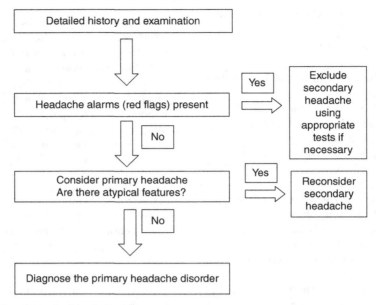

Figure 10.1. Algorithm for headache diagnosis.

exclude secondary headaches are beyond the scope of this chapter. But in brief, the approach is to spot "red flags" that suggest the possibility of secondary headaches (Figure 10.1). Once these features are identified, the physician must conduct the workup indicated by the red flag (Table 10.2) and thereby diagnose any secondary headache disorder that is present.

> ✋ **CAUTION!**
>
> The clear presence of well-established CM does not mutually exclude an incident or coexisting secondary headache disorder. In fact, migraine itself may be a risk factor for certain secondary headaches (e.g., cervical artery dissection) as well as being comorbid with others (idiopathic intracranial hypertension). Extra vigilance must be applied even when a patient with CM possesses new red flags.

Step 2: Approach the primary headaches based on duration and frequency

In a patient with headaches on more days than not but without red flags, the second step is to divide them as a function of duration of attacks into short-duration (<4 hours a day) and long-duration (≥4 hours) headaches (Figure 10.2). CM is a subtype of the high-frequency and long-duration headaches. In a patient with short-duration chronic daily headaches, the differential diagnosis include the trigeminal autonomic cephalalgias (episodic and chronic cluster headache, episodic and chronic paroxysmal hemicrania, and short unilateral neuralgiform headache with conjunctival injection and tearing [SUNCT]), and hypnic headache.

High-frequency headaches of long duration include CM, chronic tension-type headache, new daily persistent headache, and hemicrania continua. The differential diagnosis between CM and chronic tension-type headache is normally not difficult. New daily persistent headache is a primary headache disorder characterized by a new onset of a CDH [13]. In patients with acute headache first seeking care with this syndrome, investigation is necessary to exclude secondary disorders.

Hemicrania continua is probably the most frequently unrecognized primary headache [16, 17]. Hemicrania continua is a chronic, unilateral pain, commonly mistaken for CM. Both disorders are characterized by chronic unilateral pain with superimposed painful exacerbations. In

Table 10.2. Red flags in the diagnosis of headache

Red flag	Consider	Possible investigation(s)
Sudden-onset headache	Subarachnoid hemorrhage, bleed into a mass or AVM, mass lesion (especially in the posterior fossa)	Neuroimaging Lumbar puncture (after neuroimaging)
Worsening-pattern headache	Mass lesion, subdural hematoma, medication overuse	Neuroimaging
Headache with cancer, HIV, or other systemic illness (fever, neck stiffness, cutaneous rash)	Meningitis, encephalitis, Lyme disease, systemic infection, collagen vascular disease, arteritis	Neuroimaging Lumbar puncture Biopsy Blood tests
Focal neurologic signs, or symptoms other than typical visual or sensory aura	Mass lesion, AVM, collagen vascular disease	Neuroimaging Collagen vascular disease evaluation
Papilledema	Mass lesion, pseudotumor, encephalitis, meningitis	Neuroimaging Lumbar puncture (after neuroimaging)
Triggered by cough, exertion, or Valsalva maneuver	Subarachnoid hemorrhage, mass lesion	Neuroimaging Consider lumbar puncture
Headache during pregnancy or postpartum	Cortical vein/cranial sinus thrombosis, carotid dissection, pituitary apoplexy, posterior reversible encephalopathy syndrome, reversible cerebral vasoconstriction syndrome	Neuroimaging

AVM, arteriovenous malformation.

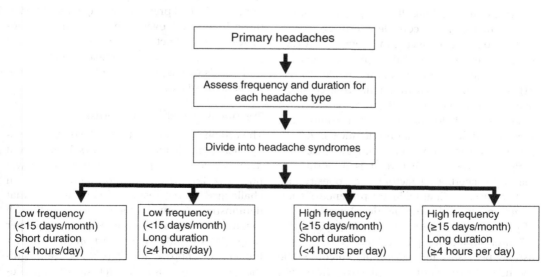

Figure 10.2. Classification of the primary headaches based on frequency and duration.

hemicrania continua, the painful exacerbations are often associated with ipsilateral autonomic features such as conjunctival injection, lacrimation, and ptosis. In CM, exacerbations are more typically accompanied by nausea, photophobia, and phonophobia. In addition, patients with hemicrania continua usually do not have an antecedent history of escalating episodic migraine. In CM, attacks increase in frequency over time. If the headaches are long-standing, the patient may not remember how they began. Although pain fluctuates in hemicrania continua, it does not usually have the morning and end-of-dosing-interval pattern of exacerbations typical of CM.

★ TIPS AND TRICKS

It is advisable to offer patients with unilateral chronic daily headache a therapeutic trial with indomethacin prior to other interventions (doses of indomethacin may need to be increased to up to 225 mg per day for 3–4 days), even if the disorder otherwise resembles CM, as hemicrania continua may be so definitively treated by this specific agent.

Treating chronic migraine

Principles of treatment

As with other life-long illnesses, several fundamental management considerations are important for treatment success in patients with CM. First, CM is comorbid with depression, anxiety, chronic pain, and other conditions [18, 19, 20, 21]. Second, patients with CM may be excessively using acute medications [22]. Third, patents have often sought help (often multiple times) and present with low frustration tolerance, and both physical and emotional dependence [23]. Accordingly, in patients with CM, it is important to identify exacerbating factors (e.g., obesity and caffeine use; see Chapter 5), the presence of analgesic overuse, and comorbidities. A combination of pharmacologic, nonpharmacologic, behavioral, and sometimes physical interventions are usually necessary for a favorable outcome. The essential features of an effective treatment regimen include a combination of the following steps [24, 25, 26, 27]:

1. Educating the patient, and establishing expectations and a follow-up plan.
2. The use of nonpharmacologic therapies when appropriate, such as biofeedback and relaxation therapy, cognitive-behavioral therapy, dietary instructions, chronobiologic therapy, proper sleep hygiene, and a daily exercise program.
3. Identifying, addressing, and treating psychiatric and somatic comorbidities.
4. Discontinuing all potentially offending medications and caffeine by outpatient or inpatient detoxification procedures.
5. Instituting a program of acute care and preventive pharmacologic therapy.

The nonpharmacologic treatment of headache disorders is detailed in Chapter 7.

As already mentioned, risk factors for the development of CM have been identified [28, 29]. Some of the risk factors (obesity, other pain syndromes, depression, caffeine and medication overuse, and snoring) can be addressed by health interventions. Although it is not yet known whether this will translate into better outcomes once CM is already established, it is reasonable to propose their treatment [30]. One such factor, excessive use of acute medications, deserves special comment. We emphasize that, by definition, the ICHD-2 precludes a diagnosis of CM in those individuals overusing medication. Nonetheless, the distinction is not made in clinical practice, and here we will make comments on individuals with a phenotype of CM and overusing acute medication.

Treatment of medication overuse

The established paradigm in individuals overusing acute medication has always been that if detoxification is not performed, prophylaxis will not work [27, 31]. This information has been challenged by the results of clinical trials that demonstrate an improvement of individuals with medication overuse when they are given proper prophylaxis [32, 33]. It is questionable whether the level of improvement is of the same magnitude as if patients are also detoxified. Nonetheless, the take-home message is that *prophylaxis should be started immediately and not only after successful detoxification.*

This said, most studies do and strongly suggest the benefit and necessity of detoxifying the patient from the overused medication (when present), followed by an intensive, long-term treatment plan. If patients discontinue their overused medications, they frequently improve considerably, and if they do not, they are usually difficult to treat effectively [22, 34, 35, 36].

Three outpatient approaches have been used for detoxification. One approach is to taper the overused medication gradually while an effective preventive therapy is established. The second strategy is to abruptly discontinue the overused drug, institute a transitional medication (bridge therapy) to break the cycle of headache, and subsequently taper the transitional medication. The third approach is to combine the two strategies by eliminating the rebound medication rapidly, adding a preventive medication rapidly, but also supplying a temporary bridge, to give the patient the maximum chance to improve without drastically worsening first [37, 38].

No matter what medication is being tapered, it is very useful to use a 3- to 7-day taper of oral corticosteroids, either prednisone starting at 60 mg per day or dexamethasone starting at 4–12 mg per day. Alternatively, triptans or dihydroergotamines are frequently used as bridge therapies [37, 38].

Special comments are required in relation to detoxifying patients who are overusing compounds with butalbital or opioids. Butalbital is a short-acting barbiturate often associated with medication overuse in the USA [39, 40, 41]. For patients suspected of overusing butalbital compounds, it is important to calculate the average daily dose of medication they are using in order to slowly taper the dose over time. One approach is to reduce the dose by one to two tablets every 3–5 days. A more controlled approach is to change the overused butalbital to longer acting phenobarbital, which is easier to withdraw. For each 100 mg of butalbital, give 30 mg of phenobarbital daily. Once this switch has been made, phenobarbital can be tapered by 15–30 mg per day, which will usually avoid withdrawal symptoms and the possibility of seizures

if patients had been using more than 800 mg of butalbital per day (16 tablets, since each mixed butalbital capsule or tablet contains 50 mg of butalbital) [42].

As for opioids, one approach is to taper the opiate by 10%–15% every day over 7–10 days. Adding clonidine 0.05 mg or 0.1 mg two or three times a day during withdrawal of an opiate usually helps [42].

Establishing an effective preventive treatment

With the exception of botulinum toxin [43], most of the commonly used preventive agents for CM have not been evaluated in well-designed, double-blind studies. They are usually the same medications that are tried for migraine prevention. Table 10.3 summarizes the medications commonly used in CM, and we emphasize that their use is off label.

The choice of a preventive drug is based on its proven efficacy, the patient's preferences and headache profile, the drug's side effects, and the presence or absence of coexisting or comorbid disease. The clinician should select the drug with the best risk:benefit ratio for the individual patient and minimize the side effects that are most concerning.

When chronic migraine becomes refractory

When a patient fails to respond as expected to appropriate therapy, or announces at the first consultation that he or she has already tried everything and nothing will work, it is important to identify the reason or reasons that treatment has failed. Lipton et al. [44] provide a detailed discussion on this topic. Nonetheless, when treatment fails, the following steps should be followed (Table 10.4).

1. Reassess the diagnosis

Perhaps the most common reason for treatment failure is that the *diagnosis is inaccurate or incomplete.* This issue takes three major forms: a secondary headache disorder goes undiagnosed (e.g., a brain tumor is a cause of the daily headaches), a primary headache disorder is misdiagnosed (e.g., hemicrania continua is misdiagnosed as CM), or two or more headache disorders are present and at least one goes unrecognized (e.g.,

Table 10.3. Selected preventive therapies for migraine that may be used in the treatment of CM

Generic treatment	Doses
Anticonvulsants	
Divalproex sodium[a]	500–1500 mg/day
Gabapentin[a]	300–3000 mg
Topiramate[a]	50–200 mg
Zonisamide	100–400 mg
Antidepressants	
Monoamine oxidase inhibitors	
Phenelzine	30–90 mg/day
Tricyclic antidepressants	
Amitriptyline[a]	30–150 mg
Nortriptyline	30–100 mg
Selective serotonin reuptake inhibitors	
Fluoxetine	10–40 mg
Venlafaxine	37.5–225 mg
Mirtazapine	15–45 mg
Beta-blockers	
Atenolol[a]	25–100 mg
Metoprolol	50–200 mg
Nadolol	20–240 mg
Propranolol[a]	30–240 mg
Timolol[a]	10–30 mg
Calcium channel antagonists	
Verapamil[a]	120–720 mg
Nimodipine	40 mg three times a day
Diltiazem	30–60 mg three times a day
Amlodipine	2.5–10 mg every day
Serotonergic agents	
Methysergide[a]	2–12 mg
Cyproheptadine	2–16 mg
Pizotifen[a]	1.5–3 mg
Miscellaneous	
Lisinopril	10–40 mg
Botulinum toxin A injection[a]	155–195 units (intramuscular)
Feverfew	50–82 mg/day
Magnesium gluconate	400–600 mg/day
Riboflavin	400 mg/day
Petasites 75 mg[a]	75 mg twice a day

[a]Evidence for moderate efficacy from at least two well-designed placebo-controlled trials.

Table 10.4. Possible reasons leading to treatment failure

1. **The diagnosis is incomplete or incorrect**
   A secondary headache disorder goes undiagnosed
   A primary headache disorder present is misdiagnosed
   The number of headache disorders is not clear

2. **Important exacerbating factors have been missed**
   Acute headache medication or caffeine overuse
   Hormonal triggers
   Dietary or lifestyle triggers
   Psychosocial factors
   Other medications

3. **Pharmacotherapy has been inadequate**
   Ineffective drug
   Excessive initial doses
   Inadequate final doses
   Inadequate duration of treatment
   Combination therapy required
   Poor absorption
   Noncompliance

4. **Nonpharmacologic treatment has been inadequate**
   Physical medicine
   Cognitive-behavioral therapy

5. **Other factors**
   Unrealistic expectations
   Comorbid and concomitant conditions
   Inpatient treatment required

the patient has both CM and hemicrania continua and only one is being treated) (Table 10.5).

2. Reassess whether exacerbating factors have been missed

Medication overuse, caffeine overuse, dietary or lifestyle triggers, hormonal triggers, psychosocial factors, or the use of other medications that trigger headaches, such as nitroglycerin, may lead to intractability. In the search for exacerbating factors, we begin by asking about factors the patient may have identified, and then probe for common and uncommon exacerbating factors, especially those that are subject to modification or intervention. It is also important to notice that in patients with multiple conditions, medications used to treat other diseases may have headache as an adverse event. Some of these medications are listed in Table 10.6.

3. Reassess whether pharmacotherapy has been inadequate

Inadequate pharmacotherapy may occur if inappropriate treatments are selected, if excessive initial doses are used, if final doses are inadequate, if the duration of treatment is too short, if combination treatment is required, if the patient fails to absorb the drug, or if the patient is noncompliant. Medications appropriate for the patient's diagnosis or diagnoses should be carefully reviewed. It is important to determine the dosage and duration of treatment with prior therapies.

When patients report that acute treatment is unsuccessful, it is important to understand what they mean: (1) Was there no response or was there an incomplete response to treatment? (2) Did the treatment response take too long? (3) Did the headache respond well initially but then recur? (4) Did the treatment cause too many side effects? By understanding the type of treatment failure, corrective strategies can be developed.

There are also common reasons why preventive treatment fails. Unsuccessful treatment is often the result of incorrect dosing strategies. Short-acting propranolol given once a day may be ineffective. Treatment is often discontinued prematurely, if one or two breakthrough headaches occur before an effective dose is established. Preventive treatment is often incompletely effective if taken when the patient is overusing acute medications.

Preventive medications must be given at an adequate dose for an adequate duration. It is best to start preventive agents at a low dose and then gradually increase the dose until therapeutic effects, treatment limiting side effects, or the ceiling dose for the agent in question have been reached. At least several weeks are required to evaluate the success or failure of a treatment. Further increases beyond the ceiling dose may be necessary if there is a partial response at the ceiling dose without side effects but the headaches remain disabling. Some patients may take appropriate doses of a drug but not achieve the necessary blood levels for response due to difficulty with absorption.

Table 10.5. Secondary headaches that mimic chronic benign headache syndromes

Headache associated with vascular disorders
Cerebrovascular disease including carotid artery dissection and arteriovenous malformation Arteritis including giant cell arteritis
Headache associated with nonvascular intracranial disorders
Low CSF pressure syndrome (spontaneous or posttraumatic CSF "leak") High CSF pressure without papilledema Intracranial: Lyme disease, HIV, encephalitis, fungal meningitis, etc.
Headache associated with substances or their withdrawal
Overuse of acute headache medications (rebound or toxic drug overuse syndromes)
Headache associated with the cranium, neck, eyes, ears, nose, sinuses, teeth, mouth, or other facial or cranial structures
Otolaryngologic disease, including chronic sphenoid sinusitis (or other sinus disease) Nasopharyngeal disorders, including carcinoma Disorders of the trigeminal nerve, including dental and oral disease, jaw pathology Subacute angle-closure glaucoma, optic neuritis, and other ocular disorders Occipitocervical disease including Arnold–Chiari malformation type I, upper cervical joint, root, or nerve (neuralgic) syndromes
Headache associated with non-cephalic infection, metabolic or systemic disturbances
Hepatitis, renal disease, vitamin B_{12} deficiency, anemia, exposure to carbon monoxide and other toxins Hormonal disturbances/endocrinologic disease (estrogen, thyroid disease, hyperprolactinemia, etc.) Vasculitis, rheumatic and connective tissue disorders
Miscellaneous
Mediastinal and thoracic processes including angina, mass lesions, superior vena cava syndrome

CSF, cerebrospinal fluid.

Table 10.6. Selected medications reported to cause headaches

Amantadine	Monoamine oxidase inhibitors
Calcium channel blockers	Nonsteroidal anti-inflammatory agents
Caffeine	Nitrates
Corticosteroids	Nicotinic acid
Cyclophosphamide	Phenothiazines
Dipyridamole	Ranitidine
Estrogens	Sympathomimetics
Ethanol	Tamoxifen
Hydralazine	Tetracyclines
Indomethacin	Theophylline
L-Dopa	Trimethoprim

Rational polytherapy

Although monotherapy is usually recommended, rational combination therapy is sometimes necessary, especially in the setting of comorbid illness. For the depressed or anxious migraine sufferer, antidepressants are usually a rational choice, but the addition of an antiepileptic medication (divalproex sodium), a beta-blocker, or a calcium channel blocker may be useful. For the patient with truly refractory headache and refractory depression, a monoamine oxidase inhibitor is sometimes the only effective treatment option. Methysergide, alone or in combination with a calcium channel blocker, may help to control refractory headache, particularly refractory chronic cluster headache [45].

Noncompliance with prescribed preventive medication or misuse of acute treatment is common [46]. Noncompliance with nonpharmacologic treatment can render treatment unsuccessful.

4. Nonpharmacologic treatment may be inadequate

Patients with occipital tenderness and trigger points often do not get relief of their headache disorder until they have a nerve block or trigger point injection [47]. Patients with intractable headache disorders sometimes are relieved by the use of trigger point injections into tender areas using a local anesthetic with or without a corticosteroid. Physical therapy is often a useful adjunct for these patients.

Patients who are tense and anxious and have trouble coping with their daily existence can have trouble getting their headaches under control. Cognitive training helps them decrease the stress they impose on themselves and may improve their headaches. In patients with intractable headache, it is useful to separate pain and ability to function. If pain does not improve, behavioral strategies should focus on optimizing function.

Conclusion

CM is a deleterious complication in a subset of patients with episodic migraine. The phenotype of CM may vary in comparison to the prior episodic attacks, and may also be heterogeneous across age groups. Key to its management is establishing the proper diagnosis. Thereafter, treatment should focus on multidisciplinary aspects including assessing for past treatment failures, minimizing exacerbating factors (especially medication overuse), and establishing the appropriate pharmacologic and nonpharmacologic strategies.

References

1. Eadie MJ. The pathogenesis of migraine—17th to early 20th century understandings. *J Clin Neurosci* 2005;**12**(4):383–8.
2. Haut SR, Bigal ME, Lipton RB. Chronic disorders with episodic manifestations: focus on epilepsy and migraine. *Lancet Neurol* 2006; **5**(2):148–57.
3. Bigal ME, Lipton RB. The prognosis of migraine. *Curr Opin Neurol* 2008;**21**(3): 301–8.
4. Mathew NT. Transformed migraine. *Cephalalgia* 1993;**13**(Suppl. 12):78–83.
5. Silberstein SD, Lipton RB, Sliwinski M. Classification of daily and near-daily headaches: field trial of revised IHS criteria. *Neurology* 1996;**47**(4):871–5.
6. Classification and diagnostic criteria for headache disorders, cranial neuralgias and facial pain. Headache Classification Committee of the International Headache Society. *Cephalalgia* 1988;**8**(Suppl. 7):1–96.
7. The International Classification of Headache Disorders. 2nd Edition. Headache Classification Subcommittee of the International Headache Society *Cephalalgia* 2004;**24**(Suppl. 1):9–160.
8. Mathew NT, Reuveni U, Perez F. Transformed or evolutive migraine. *Headache* 1987;**27**(2): 102–6.
9. Bigal ME, Rapoport AM, Sheftell FD, Tepper SJ, Lipton RB. Chronic migraine is an earlier stage of transformed migraine in adults. *Neurology* 2005;**65**(10):1556–61.
10. Bigal ME, Tepper SJ, Sheftell FD, Rapoport AM, Lipton RB. Field testing alternative criteria for chronic migraine. *Cephalalgia* 2006; **26**(4):477–82.
11. Bigal M, Rapoport A, Sheftell F, Tepper S, Lipton R. The International Classification of Headache Disorders revised criteria for chronic migraine—field testing in a headache specialty clinic. *Cephalalgia* 2007;**27**:230–4.
12. Olesen J, Bousser MG, Diener HC, et al. New appendix criteria open for a broader concept of chronic migraine. *Cephalalgia* 2006; **26**(6):742–6.
13. Bigal ME, Lipton RB, Tepper SJ, Rapoport AM, Sheftell FD. Primary chronic daily headache and its subtypes in adolescents and adults. *Neurology* 2004;**63**(5):843–7.
14. Bigal ME, Rapoport AM, Tepper SJ, Sheftell FD, Lipton RB. The classification of chronic daily headache in adolescents—a comparison between the second edition of the international classification of headache disorders and alternative diagnostic criteria. *Headache* 2005;**45**(5):582–9.
15. Bigal ME, Lipton RB. The differential diagnosis of chronic daily headaches: an algorithm-based approach. *J Headache Pain* 2007;**8**(5): 263–72.

16. Rapoport AM, Bigal ME. Hemicrania continua: clinical and nosographic update. *Neurol Sci* 2003;**24**(Suppl. 2):S118–21.

17. Bordini C, Antonaci F, Stovner LJ, Schrader H, Sjaastad O. "Hemicrania continua": a clinical review. *Headache* 1991;**31**(1):20–6.

18. Wang SJ, Juang KD, Fuh JL, Lu SR. Psychiatric comorbidity and suicide risk in adolescents with chronic daily headache. *Neurology* 2007;**68**(18):1468–73.

19. Scher AI, Stewart WF, Lipton RB. The comorbidity of headache with other pain syndromes. *Headache* 2006;**46**(9):1416–23.

20. Jette N, Patten S, Williams J, Becker W, Wiebe S. Comorbidity of migraine and psychiatric disorders—a national population-based study. *Headache* 2008;**48**(4):501–16.

21. Lipton RB, Silberstein SD. Why study the comorbidity of migraine? *Neurology* 1994; **44**(10 Suppl. 7):S4–5.

22. Bigal ME, Rapoport AM, Sheftell FD, Tepper SJ, Lipton RB. Transformed migraine and medication overuse in a tertiary headache centre—clinical characteristics and treatment outcomes. *Cephalalgia* 2004;**24**(6): 483–90.

23. Lake AE, 3rd, Lipchik GL, Penzien DB, Rains JC, Saper JR, Lipton RB. Psychiatric comorbidity with chronic headache: evidence-based clinical implications—introduction to the supplement. *Headache* 2006;**46**(Suppl. 3):S73–5.

24. Baskin SM, Lipchik GL, Smitherman TA. Mood and anxiety disorders in chronic headache. *Headache* 2006;**46**(Suppl. 3):S76–87.

25. Sheftell FD. Chronic daily headache. *Neurology* 1992;**42**(3 Suppl. 2):32–6.

26. Rapoport A, Stang P, Gutterman DL, et al. Analgesic rebound headache in clinical practice: data from a physician survey. *Headache* 1996;**36**(1):14–9.

27. Rapoport AM. Analgesic rebound headache. *Headache* 1988;**28**(10):662–5.

28. Lipton RB, Bigal ME. Migraine: epidemiology, *impact*, and risk factors for progression. *Headache* 2005;**45**(Suppl. 1):S3–13.

29. Bigal ME, Lipton RB. Modifiable risk factors for migraine progression. *Headache* 2006; **46**(9):1334–43.

30. Bigal ME, Lipton RB. Modifiable risk factors for migraine progression (or for chronic daily headaches)—clinical lessons. *Headache* 2006;**46**(Suppl. 3):S144–6.

31. Zeeberg P, Olesen J, Jensen R. Discontinuation of medication overuse in headache patients: recovery of therapeutic responsiveness. *Cephalalgia* 2006;**26**(10):1192–8.

32. Dodick DW, Mauskop A, Elkind AH, DeGryse R, Brin MF, Silberstein SD. Botulinum toxin type a for the prophylaxis of chronic daily headache: subgroup analysis of patients not receiving other prophylactic medications: a randomized double-blind, placebo-controlled study. *Headache* 2005;**45**(4): 315–24.

33. Diener HC, Dodick DW, Goadsby PJ, et al. Utility of topiramate for the treatment of patients with chronic migraine in the presence or absence of acute medication overuse. *Cephalalgia* 2009;**29**(10):1021–7.

34. Bigal ME, Sheftell FD, Tepper SJ, Rapoport AM. Discontinuation of medication overuse in headache patients: recovery of therapeutic responsiveness. *Cephalalgia* 2007;**27**(6):568; author reply 568–9.

35. Saper JR, Lake AE, 3rd. Continuous opioid therapy (COT) is rarely advisable for refractory chronic daily headache: limited efficacy, risks, and proposed guidelines. *Headache* 2008;**48**(6):838–49.

36. Mathew NT. Transformed migraine, analgesic rebound, and other chronic daily headaches. *Neurol Clin* 1997;**15**(1):167–86.

37. Rapoport AM. Medication overuse headache: awareness, detection and treatment. *CNS Drugs* 2008;**22**(12):995–1004.

38. Grazzi L, Andrasik F, Usai S, Bussone G. Headache with medication overuse: treatment strategies and proposals of relapse prevention. *Neurol Sci* 2008;**29**(2):93–8.

39. Bigal ME, Borucho S, Serrano D, Lipton RB. The acute treatment of episodic and chronic migraine in the USA. *Cephalalgia* 2009; **29**(8):891–7.

40. Meskunas CA, Tepper SJ, Rapoport AM, Sheftell FD, Bigal ME. Medications associated with probable medication overuse headache reported in a tertiary care headache center over a 15-year period. *Headache* 2006;**46**(5):766–72.

41. Tepper SJ. Debate: analgesic overuse is a cause, not consequence, of chronic daily

headache. Analgesic overuse is a cause of chronic daily headache. *Headache* 2002; **42**(6):543–7.

42. Sheftell FD, Bigal ME. Medication overuse headache. *Continuum (Am Acad Neurol)* 2006;**12**:147–63.

43. Freitag FG, Diamond S, Diamond M, Urban G. Botulinum toxin type A in the treatment of chronic migraine without medication overuse. *Headache* 2008;**48**(2):201–9.

44. Lipton RB, Silberstein SD, Saper JR, Bigal ME, Goadsby PJ. Why headache treatment fails. *Neurology* 2003;**60**(7):1064–70.

45. Krymchantowski AV, Bigal ME. Polytherapy in the preventive and acute treatment of migraine: fundamentals for changing the approach. *Expert Rev Neurother* 2006;**6**(3):283–9.

46. Bigal M, Krymchantowski AV, Lipton RB. Barriers to satisfactory migraine outcomes. What have we learned, where do we stand? *Headache* 2009;**49**(7):1028–41.

47. Ailani J, Young WB. The role of nerve blocks and botulinum toxin injections in the management of cluster headaches. *Curr Pain Headache Rep* 2009;**13**(2):164–7.

Part III

Tension-type Headache

Diagnosis, Subtypes, Epidemiology, Progression, Prognosis, and Comorbidity of Tension-type Headache

Sara C. Crystal[1], Uri Napchan[2,3], and Matthew S. Robbins[2]

[1]New York University Medical Center, New York, NY, USA
[2]Albert Einstein College of Medicine, Bronx, NY, USA
[3]Middletown Medical PC, Middletown, NY, USA

Introduction

Although research on tension-type headache (TTH) is scarce compared to that on migraine, TTH has the greatest socioeconomic impact of any primary headache type because it is so common. TTH is the most prevalent type of primary headache in all age groups worldwide. While the disease burden due to TTH is higher in those with the chronic compared to the episodic form, even episodic TTH (ETTH) can significantly impact quality of life. Medical and psychiatric comorbidities may contribute to the burden, conferring a worse prognosis. This review will focus on the diagnosis and classification of TTH, its epidemiology in different age groups, factors associated with its progression and remission, and associated comorbidities.

Historical aspects and classification

The general phenotype of the TTH attack is one of short or long duration, with a pressing or tightening (nonpulsating) pain quality, and with a bilateral location. The pain intensity is typically mild or moderate, without any aggravation by physical activity. Associated features that are commonly seen in migraine are typically absent or minimal, including nausea, vomiting, photophobia, and phonophobia.

In 1988, the International Headache Society published its first headache classification criteria and placed TTH under section 2 of the primary headache disorders [1]. The committee's goal was to establish operational diagnostic criteria by which individuals could be classified based on clinical features. The committee divided TTH into either episodic or chronic. In addition, the committee added an option to further subclassify both ETTH and chronic TTH (CTTH) as being associated or unassociated with a disorder of pericranial muscle as a way to stimulate research into the role of the muscle in TTH.

After the publication of the initial International Headache Society diagnostic criteria, Rasmussen et al. attempted to classify 740 individuals in the general population with headaches [2]. The authors found that the classification criteria were exhaustive—only two individuals of the 740 had headaches that were "not classifiable." The authors also found that individuals with TTH usually fulfilled three if not all four of the features of the diagnostic criteria, as well as the all the criteria for the associated symptoms. The character of the pain in the TTH attack was pressing in quality in 78%, mild to moderate in intensity in 99%, bilateral in location in 90%, and not aggravated by physical activity in 72% of individuals.

Following the suggestions proposed by the committee, studies were performed to further understand the role of pericranial muscles in TTH. One small study did not find a difference in the electromyographic (EMG) activity of the posterior neck and frontal muscles in subjects with or without ETTH [3]. Another study found a positive association between muscle tenderness and a diagnosis of TTH, but the EMG data were not helpful in assigning individual diagnoses [4]. In another study, the authors compared individuals with CTTH, ETTH, migraine, and controls using three modalities (EMG, pressure algometry, and manual palpation) [5]. The diagnostic capacity was increased when two or three modalities were used compared to just a single test. The authors also pointed out that the existence of headache at the time of testing should be taken into consideration as a different pattern could be seen. The overall data do not suggest the usefulness of EMG in the diagnosis of TTH.

Making the diagnosis

The second edition of the International Classification of Headache Disorders (ICHD-2) definitively divides TTH into three subtypes based on a patient's attack frequency: an infrequent episodic form in which headaches occur on 1 or fewer days per month on average (Table 11.1), a frequent episodic form in which headaches occur on between 1 and 14 days per month for at least 3 months (Table 11.2), and a chronic form, with 15 or more monthly headache days over a 3-month period (Table 11.3). Frequent ETTH and CTTH are further subdivided based on the presence or absence of pericranial tenderness [6].

The diagnostic criteria for all TTH subtypes include at least two of the following pain characteristics: bilateral location, nonpulsating quality, mild or moderate intensity, and lack of aggravation with routine physical activity. Infrequent and frequent TTH are both diagnoses of inclusion, as

Table 11.1. ICHD-2 diagnostic criteria for infrequent ETTH

A. At least 10 episodes occurring on <1 day/month (<12 days/year) and fulfilling criteria B–D
B. Headache lasting from 30 min to 7 days
C. Headache has ≥2 of the following characteristics:
   1. Bilateral location
   2. Pressing/tightening (nonpulsating) quality
   3. Mild or moderate intensity
   4. Not aggravated by routine physical activity
D. Both of the following:
   1. No nausea or vomiting (anorexia may occur)
   2. No more than one of photophobia or phonophobia
E. Not attributed to another disorder

Table 11.2. ICHD-2 diagnostic criteria for frequent ETTH

A. At least 10 episodes occurring on ≥1 but <15 days/month for ≥3 months (≥12 and <180 days/year) and fulfilling criteria B–D
B. Headache lasting from 30 min to 7 days
C. Headache has ≥2 of the following characteristics:
   1. Bilateral location
   2. Pressing/tightening (nonpulsating) quality
   3. Mild or moderate intensity
   4. Not aggravated by routine physical activity
D. Both of the following:
   1. No nausea or vomiting (anorexia may occur)
   2. No more than one of photophobia or phonophobia
E. Not attributed to another disorder

attacks may be accompanied by either photophobia or phonophobia, but not both, and diagnoses of exclusion in that nausea and vomiting must be absent. For CTTH, no more than one of three features of mild nausea, photophobia, and phonophobia may be present, and moderate or severe nausea or vomiting precludes the diagnosis [6].

Table 11.3. ICHD-2 diagnostic criteria for CTTH

A. Headache occurring on ≥15 days/month (≥180 days/year) for ≥3 months and fulfilling criteria B–D
B. Headache lasts hours or may be continuous
C. Headache has ≥2 of the following characteristics:
   1. Bilateral location
   2. Pressing/tightening (nonpulsating) quality
   3. Mild or moderate intensity
   4. Not aggravated by routine physical activity
D. Both of the following:
   1. Not >1 of photophobia, phonophobia, and mild nausea
   2. Neither moderate or severe nausea nor vomiting
E. Not attributed to another disorder

SCIENCE REVISITED

TTH in patients with migraine may have a different underlying pathophysiology than in patients with pure TTH. In migraineurs, ETTH and migraine likely occur on a continuum and are biologically related, while ETTH in individuals without migraine may have a distinct mechanism. This model is supported by several studies exploring the response of TTH to triptans in patients with and without ICHD-2-diagnosed migraine. Whereas migraineurs obtain pain relief from triptans for all their headache types including TTH, patients with pure TTH typically do not respond to triptans.

TIPS AND TRICKS

One potential treacherous area with the diagnostic category of "probable TTH" is that individuals may fit the criteria for both probable ETTH and probable migraine. A recent population study in three different regions in Germany attempted to analyze the 6-month prevalence of migraine, TTH, probable migraine, and probable TTH [7]. The authors found that using the new criteria resulted in headache categories that were not mutually exclusive, and questioned the need for the diagnosis of probable migraine and probable TTH. The diagnostic committee pointed out this limitation in the original publication and recommended that, in such cases, all other available information may be used to decide which diagnosis is more likely. For example, a family history of migraine, headaches associated with menses, and a positive response to a migraine-specific medication (such as a triptan) may suggest a diagnosis of probable migraine.

Compared to the episodic form, CTTH is more treatment-refractory, is associated with a higher prevalence of medication overuse, and has a greater impact on quality of life [8].

In the ICHD-2, the committee added probable infrequent ETTH and probable frequent ETTH for those who fulfill all but one criterion and do not fulfill the criteria for migraine without aura. The committee also added probable CTTH for those who fulfilled the criteria for CTTH but where there is or has been medication overuse for the previous 2 months.

Epidemiology of TTH in various age groups

TTH in adults

The epidemiology of TTH in different age groups within the population is summarized in Table 11.4. TTH, with a lifetime prevalence of 78% [9], is the most common primary headache disorder [10]. Its prevalence varies by age, gender, and continent [9, 11, 12]. In the USA, the 1-year prevalence is 38.3% in adults [12]. In both sexes, the prevalence peaks between 30 and 39 years of age, at 42.3% in men and 46.9% in women, subsequently declining with increasing age [12]. Prevalence of TTH is slightly higher in women in all age, race, and education groups, with a female:male ratio ranging from 1.16:1 to 3:1 [12, 13, 14, 15].

Table 11.4. Epidemiology of TTH in various age groups

	Children/adolescents	Adults	Elderly
Prevalence (ETTH/CTTH)	ETTH: 10%–25% Increases with age CTTH: 0%–1.5%	ETTH: 38% Peak prevalence 30–39 years; decreases with age CTTH: 2%–3%	ETTH: 25%–45% CTTH: 2%–3%
Female:male ratio	1:1 until age 12, 1.4:1 between 13 and 15 years	1.16–3:1	1–1.8:1
Factors associated with TTH	Divorced parents Fewer peer relationships Depressive symptoms Neck/shoulder pain Oromandibular dysfunction	Analgesic overuse Depression Anxiety TMD	Analgesic overuse History of migraine Depression Anxiety Other pain syndromes

Prevalence of TTH varies across continents. It is much more common in Europe, with a 1-year prevalence of up to 80%, than in Asia or the Americas, where the prevalence ranges from 20% to 30% [16]. A review of population-based epidemiologic studies reported a global prevalence of current headache in all ages of 47% for all headache, 38% for TTH, and 10% for migraine. In studies limited to adults, the numbers were similar: 46% for all headache, 42% for TTH, and 11% for migraine. The lifetime prevalence was not surprisingly higher, at 66% for all headaches, 46% for TTH, and 14% for migraine [16].

Only one study has addressed the incidence of TTH. In Denmark, subjects were followed over 12 years to capture the incidence of developing frequent TTH, found to be 14.2 per 1000 person–years. Incidence of TTH was highest at age 25–34 for both men and women, with a female:male ratio of 3:1, and declined with age. Risk factors for incident frequent TTH included poor self-related health and sleep, and difficulty with relaxation after work [17].

Chronic daily headache (CDH) is a heterogeneous group of primary headache disorders of long duration that includes CTTH, chronic migraine, hemicrania continua, and new daily persistent headache. The global prevalence of CDH is 3%–4% in adults [16, 18, 19, 20, 21, 22]. It is most common in Central and South America, affecting up to 5% of the population, and least common in Africa (1.7%) [16]. In the general population, CTTH represents the majority of CDH, with a prevalence of 2%–3%, whereas chronic migraine is the most common type of CDH treated in specialty centers. For CTTH, the overall 1-year period prevalence in the USA was 2.2%; the prevalence in women (2.8%) was twice that of men (1.4%) [12].

TTH in the elderly

Several studies have focused on the epidemiology of TTH in the elderly. While its prevalence declines with age, TTH continues to be relatively frequent in the elderly population [23]. In adults aged 60–65 years in the USA, the prevalence of ETTH was 25.6% for men and 27.1% for women [12]. Studies of the elderly (>65 years old) reported a 1-year prevalence of TTH of 44.5% in Italy and 33.1% in Brazil [18, 24]. While several studies of TTH in the elderly have found a decrease in prevalence with advancing age [18, 25], others have found no significant decline [15, 24, 26], in contrast to migraine, which decreased significantly. Because TTH can occasionally present for the first time in the elderly, it is important to exclude secondary causes, as headaches that begin after the age of 65 are more likely to be due to underlying pathology [23].

✋ CAUTION!

Although TTH is the most common primary headache disorder in the population, patients with both primary and secondary intracranial neoplasms are more likely to present with a headache phenotype consistent with TTH than with migraine.

The prevalence of CDH, including CTTH, remains fairly constant throughout adulthood, in contrast to ETTH, which may remit with advancing age. CTTH affects 2%–3% of both the general adult and elderly population [9, 12, 18, 20, 21].

TTH in children and adolescents

The prevalence of TTH in children and adolescents ranges from 10% to 25% in population-based studies, varying by continent and increasing with age. Some studies report an equal prevalence of TTH in boys and girls [27, 28], while one study found a female preponderance only after age 12 [29]. Headache episodes typically begin at age 7 years, with an average duration of 2 hours. Compared to migraine, the duration, frequency, intensity, and medication use associated with TTH episodes are typically all lower on average [30]. Diagnostic criteria for TTH in children and adolescents are the same as for adults [7], although TTH may be difficult to differentiate from migraine in this population as some of the symptoms overlap, and children may have difficulty describing their symptoms [27]. In addition, younger adolescents with ETTH may experience significantly more migraine-like symptoms than older adolescents with ETTH [31].

The prevalence of CDH, including CTTH, is lower in children than adults. In a population-based study of individuals aged 10 to over 60 years in rural Brazil, CDH prevalence was lowest in the youngest group, ages 10–19 (1.8%) [32]. In studies specifically exploring CTTH in children with CDH, the prevalence ranges from 0% to 1.5% [27, 28, 29, 33].

Progression and prognosis of TTH

Several studies have focused on the prognosis of TTH, exploring risk factors for progression from ETTH to CTTH and for developing headache persistence (Table 11.5). In patients with CDH, remission to less than 180 headaches per year is fairly common, ranging between one-third and two-thirds of subjects [21, 22, 34], but improvement to a "normal" frequency of less than one headache per week is rare. In a study of 62 patients with TTH, at 10-year follow-up 75% with ETTH continued to experience episodic headache, while 25% had progressed to the chronic form. In patients with baseline CTTH, 31% had headache that remained chronic, 21% developed medica-

Table 11.5. Factors associated with progression and remission of CDH

Risk factors for progression/persistence	Factors associated with remission
Analgesic overuse	Higher educational level
CDH onset after age 32 years	Older age
CDH duration of 6 years or more	
Baseline frequency of >2 headaches per month	
Body mass index ≥30 kg/m²	
Baseline CTTH	
Coexisting migraine	
Not being married	
Sleeping problems	
Depression	
Anxiety	

tion overuse, and the remaining 48% remitted to the episodic form, with or without the use of preventive treatments, over a 10-year period. Depression, anxiety, and medication overuse predicted a poor outcome [35]. A study of adults without headache at baseline found that low socioeconomic status predicted the development of CDH at 11-year follow-up [36]. In the elderly, risk factors for the development of CDH are similar to those in the adult population, and include analgesic overuse, depression, history of migraine, and other pain syndromes [21].

In a population-based study [34], prevalence of CDH decreased slightly with age, was more common in women and in previously married individuals, and was inversely associated with educational level. At follow-up 11 months later, 3% of controls (<104 headaches per year) developed CDH, and 6% had progressed to an intermediate headache frequency (105–179 headaches per year). Risk factors associated with the new onset of CDH included a baseline headache frequency of more than two headaches per month and obesity. Of patients with CDH at baseline, 44% continued to report 180 or more headaches per year, 43% improved to an intermediate frequency, and 14% remitted to fewer than 52 headaches per year. Remission to less than one headache per week was associated with increased educational level, elapsed time between interviews, and older age in women but not men [34].

As in adults, TTH in children is related to psychosocial factors. In one study, children with TTH were more likely to have divorced parents and had fewer peer relationships compared to children with migraine and headache-free controls [37]. Depressive symptoms, musculoskeletal pain, and oromandibular dysfunction are also more frequent in children with TTH compared to controls [28]. Predictably, depressive symptoms are more common in children with frequent ETTH than those with less frequent attacks [38]. Over 50% of children with CTTH may experience predisposing physical or emotional stress [39].

Comorbidity of TTH

TTH, and CTTH in particular, is associated with certain medical and psychiatric conditions (Figure 11.1). Several studies have reported an association between temporomandibular disorder (TMD) and headache [32, 40, 41], although the relationship may be confounded by the fact that headache may be a symptom manifestation of TMD. A recent study exploring the presence of migraine, ETTH, CDH, and TMD in an adult population [40] found that as reported symptoms of TMD increased, the prevalence of all three headache types increased. In the absence of TMD symptoms, headache prevalence was 38%, compared to 73% in subjects with three or more TMD symptoms. Da Silva et al. [32] reported a prevalence of TMD in 58% of patients with CDH. While individuals with CTTH were more likely to have TMD than were those with chronic migraine, the

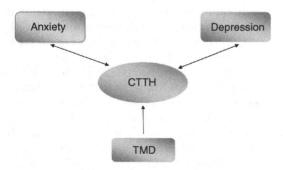

Figure 11.1. Comorbidities associated with CTTH.

difference did not reach statistical significance. In another study, headache was almost twice as prevalent in subjects with symptoms of TMD than without them, but headache frequency and subtype were not specified [41].

TMD may contribute to headache by involvement of the pericranial musculature. Deviations from normal temporomandibular function may activate pain receptors in the masticatory muscles, leading to a sensitization of pericranial and central nociceptors, which converge in the trigeminal nucleus caudalis. The development of central sensitization is thought to play an important role in the progression from episodic headaches to their chronic forms [8, 42].

The relationship between CDH and psychiatric disease has been well established [32, 43, 44, 45, 46, 47]. In a population-based study in Brazil, over two-thirds of subjects with CDH had psychiatric disorders [32]. Generalized anxiety was found to be the most frequent comorbidity (38.5%), followed by major depression (32.7%). Startlingly, suicidal ideation was reported by 17.3% of subjects.

Depression, anxiety, and panic disorder [47] occur more frequently in patients with CTTH than ETTH. In studies exploring psychiatric comorbidity by CDH subtype, some report a higher prevalence in CM versus CTTH [32, 47], while others suggest that headache frequency, not severity, has a more significant impact on psychological well-being [48, 49]. Psychiatric comorbidity likely contributes to an increased burden of accompanying headache symptoms [50].

Mechanisms proposed to explain the relationship between headache and psychiatric comorbidity are that CDH causes depression and anxiety, that depression and anxiety cause CDH, or that the relationship is bidirectional, with psychiatric disease leading to the development of CDH, and CDH contributing to depression and anxiety. One study suggested that the relationship may be bidirectional for migraine, but unidirectional for other severe nonmigraine headaches, in that they predict, but are not caused by, depression [51]. Depression and CDH may share a common pathophysiology.

It is important to identify and treat comorbid psychiatric disorders in patients with CDH, as they may confer a worse prognosis [21, 22, 52], and are associated with higher medical service-seeking behavior [43]. In addition, the presence of psychiatric disease may provide therapeutic opportunities, such as treating headache and depression with a single medication, or with nonpharmacologic approaches that have been found to be helpful for both conditions, such as stress management, biofeedback, and cognitive-behavioral therapy.

Conclusion

TTH is the most prevalent headache disorder in all age groups and regions of the world. It causes a significant burden, both to the individual and to society. Psychiatric and physical comorbidities are common, especially in CTTH, and likely confer a worse prognosis. Treatment needs to address both headache and associated comorbidities in order to be effective.

References

1. Classification and diagnostic criteria for headache disorders, cranial neuralgias and facial pain. Headache Classification Committee of the International Headache Society. *Cephalalgia*. 1988;**8**(Suppl. 7):1–96.
2. Rasmussen BK, Jensen R, Olesen J. A population-based analysis of the diagnostic criteria of the International Headache Society. *Cephalalgia* 1991;**11**(3):129–34.
3. Hatch JP, Prihoda TJ, Moore PJ, et al. A naturalistic study of the relationships among electromyographic activity, psychological stress, and pain in ambulatory tension-type headache patients and headache-free controls. *Psychosom Med* 1991;**53**(5):576–84.
4. Hatch JP, Moore PJ, Cyr-Provost M, Boutros NN, Seleshi E, Borcherding S. The use of electromyography and muscle palpation in the diagnosis of tension-type headache with and without pericranial muscle involvement. *Pain* 1992;**49**(2):175–8.
5. Sandrini G, Antonaci F, Pucci E, Bono G, Nappi G. Comparative study with EMG, pressure algometry and manual palpation in tension-type headache and migraine. *Cephalalgia* 1994;**14**(6):451–7; discussion 394–5.
6. The International Classification of Headache Disorders. 2nd edition. *Cephalalgia* 2004;**24**(Suppl. 1):9–160.
7. Pfaffenrath V, Fendrich K, Vennemann M, et al. Regional variations in the prevalence of

migraine and tension-type headache applying the new IHS criteria: the German DMKG Headache Study. *Cephalalgia*. 2009;**29**(1):48–57.
8. Bendtsen L, Jensen R. Tension-type headache: the most common, but also the most neglected, headache disorder. *Curr Opin Neurol* 2006;**19**(3):305–9.
9. Rasmussen BK, Jensen R, Schroll M, Olesen J. Epidemiology of headache in a general population—a prevalence study. *J Clin Epidemiol* 1991;**44**(11):1147–57.
10. Jensen R. Diagnosis, epidemiology, and impact of tension-type headache. *Curr Pain Headache Rep* 2003;**7**(6):455–9.
11. Gobel H, Petersen-Braun M, Soyka D. The epidemiology of headache in Germany: a nationwide survey of a representative sample on the basis of the headache classification of the International Headache Society. *Cephalalgia* 1994;**14**(2):97–106.
12. Schwartz BS, Stewart WF, Simon D, Lipton RB. Epidemiology of tension-type headache. *JAMA* 1998;**279**(5):381–3.
13. Lavados PM, Tenhamm E. Epidemiology of tension-type headache in Santiago, Chile: a prevalence study. *Cephalalgia* 1998;**18**(8):552–8.
14. Solomon GD, Kunkel RS, Jr., Frame J. Demographics of headache in elderly patients. *Headache* 1990;**30**(5):273–6.
15. Schwaiger J, Kiechl S, Seppi K, et al. Prevalence of primary headaches and cranial neuralgias in men and women aged 55–94 years (Bruneck Study). *Cephalalgia* 2009;**29**(2):179–87.
16. Stovner L, Hagen K, Jensen R, et al. The global burden of headache: a documentation of headache prevalence and disability worldwide. *Cephalalgia* 2007;**27**(3):193–210.
17. Lyngberg AC, Rasmussen BK, Jorgensen T, Jensen R. Incidence of primary headache: a Danish epidemiologic follow-up study. *Am J Epidemiol* 2005;**161**(11):1066–73.
18. Prencipe M, Casini AR, Ferretti C, et al. Prevalence of headache in an elderly population: attack frequency, disability, and use of medication. *J Neurol Neurosurg Psychiatry* 2001;**70**(3):377–81.
19. Scher AI, Stewart WF, Liberman J, Lipton RB. Prevalence of frequent headache in a

population sample. *Headache* 1998;**38**(7): 497–506.

20. Castillo J, Munoz P, Guitera V, Pascual J. Kaplan Award 1998. Epidemiology of chronic daily headache in the general population. *Headache* 1999;**39**(3):190–6.

21. Wang SJ, Fuh JL, Lu SR, et al. Chronic daily headache in Chinese elderly: prevalence, risk factors, and biannual follow-up. *Neurology* 2000;**54**(2):314–9.

22. Lu SR, Fuh JL, Chen WT, Juang KD, Wang SJ. Chronic daily headache in Taipei, Taiwan: prevalence, follow-up and outcome predictors. *Cephalalgia* 2001;**21**(10):980–6.

23. Crystal SC, Grosberg BM. Tension-type headache in the elderly. *Curr Pain Headache Rep* 2009;**13**(6):474–8.

24. Bensenor IM, Lotufo PA, Goulart AC, Menezes PR, Scazufca M. The prevalence of headache among elderly in a low-income area of Sao Paulo, Brazil. *Cephalalgia* 2008;**28**(4): 329–33.

25. Pascual J, Berciano J. Experience in the diagnosis of headaches that start in elderly people. *J Neurol Neurosurg Psychiatry* 1994; **57**(10):1255–7.

26. Camarda R, Monastero R. Prevalence of primary headaches in Italian elderly: preliminary data from the Zabut Aging Project. *Neurol Sci* 2003;**24**(Suppl. 2):S122–4.

27. Ozge A, Bugdayci R, Sasmaz T, et al. The sensitivity and specificity of the case definition criteria in diagnosis of headache: a school-based epidemiological study of 5562 children in Mersin. *Cephalalgia* 2003;**23**(2):138–45.

28. Anttila P, Metsahonkala L, Aromaa M, et al. Determinants of tension-type headache in children. *Cephalalgia* 2002;**22**(5):401–8.

29. Laurell K, Larsson B, Eeg-Olofsson O. Prevalence of headache in Swedish schoolchildren, with a focus on tension-type headache. *Cephalalgia* 2004;**24**(5):380–8.

30. Anttila P. Tension-type headache in childhood and adolescence. *Lancet Neurol* 2006; **5**(3):268–74.

31. Karli N, Akgoz S, Zarifoglu M, Akis N, Erer S. Clinical characteristics of tension-type headache and migraine in adolescents: a student-based study. *Headache* 2006;**46**(3):399–412.

32. da Silva Jr A, Costa EC, Gomes JB, et al. Chronic headache and comorbities: a

two-phase, population-based, cross-sectional study. *Headache* 2010;**50**:1306–12.

33. Abu-Arefeh I, Russell G. Prevalence of headache and migraine in schoolchildren. *BMJ* 1994;**309**:765–9.

34. Scher AI, Stewart WF, Ricci JA, Lipton RB. Factors associated with the onset and remission of chronic daily headache in a population-based study. *Pain* 2003;**106**(1–2):81–9.

35. Murk H JR. Prognosis of tension-type headache: a 10-year follow-up study of patients with frequent tension-type headache. *Cephalalgia* 2000;**20**:434.

36. Hagen K, Vatten L, Stovner LJ, Zwart JA, Krokstad S, Bovim G. Low socio-economic status is associated with increased risk of frequent headache: a prospective study of 22718 adults in Norway. *Cephalalgia* 2002;**22**(8): 672–9.

37. Karwautz A, Wober C, Lang T, et al. Psychosocial factors in children and adolescents with migraine and tension-type headache: a controlled study and review of the literature. *Cephalalgia*. 1999;**19**(1):32–43.

38. Anttila P, Sourander A, Metsahonkala L, Aromaa M, Helenius H, Sillanpaa M. Psychiatric symptoms in children with primary headache. *J Am Acad Child Adolesc Psychiatry* 2004;**43**(4):412–9.

39. Abu-Arafeh I. Chronic tension-type headache in children and adolescents. *Cephalalgia* 2001;**21**(8):830–6.

40. Goncalves DA, Bigal ME, Jales LC, Camparis CM, Speciali JG. Headache and symptoms of temporomandibular disorder: an epidemiological study. *Headache* 2010;**50**(2):231–41.

41. Ciancaglini R, Radaelli G. The relationship between headache and symptoms of temporomandibular disorder in the general population. *J Dent* 2001;**29**(2):93–8.

42. Chen Y. Advances in the pathophysiology of tension-type headache: from stress to central sensitization. *Curr Pain Headache Rep* 2009; **13**(6):484–94.

43. Wang SJ, Juang KD. Psychiatric comorbidity of chronic daily headache: impact, treatment, outcome, and future studies. *Curr Pain Headache Rep* 2002;**6**(6):505–10.

44. Mitsikostas DD, Thomas AM. Comorbidity of headache and depressive disorders. *Cephalalgia* 1999;**19**(4):211–7.

45. Puca F, Genco S, Prudenzano MP, et al. Psychiatric comorbidity and psychosocial stress in patients with tension-type headache from headache centers in Italy. The Italian Collaborative Group for the Study of Psychopathological Factors in Primary Headaches. *Cephalalgia* 1999;**19**(3):159–64.

46. Holroyd KA, Stensland M, Lipchik GL, Hill KR, O'Donnell FS, Cordingley G. Psychosocial correlates and impact of chronic tension-type headaches. *Headache* 2000;**40**(1):3–16.

47. Juang KD, Wang SJ, Fuh JL, Lu SR, Su TP. Comorbidity of depressive and anxiety disorders in chronic daily headache and its subtypes. *Headache* 2000;**40**(10):818–23.

48. Cassidy EM, Tomkins E, Hardiman O, O'Keane V. Factors associated with burden of primary headache in a specialty clinic. *Headache* 2003;**43**(6):638–44.

49. Marcus DA. Identification of patients with headache at risk of psychological distress. *Headache* 2000;**40**(5):373–6.

50. Mongini F, Rota E, Deregibus A, et al. Accompanying symptoms and psychiatric comorbidity in migraine and tension-type headache patients. *J Psychosom Res* 2006;**61**(4):447–51.

51. Breslau N, Schultz LR, Stewart WF, Lipton RB, Lucia VC, Welch KM. Headache and major depression: is the association specific to migraine? *Neurology* 2000 25;**54**(2):308–13.

52. Guidetti V, Galli F. Psychiatric comorbidity in chronic daily headache: pathophysiology, etiology, and diagnosis. *Curr Pain Headache Rep* 2002;**6**(6):492–7.

Pathophysiology and Genetics of Tension-type Headache

Sait Ashina[1] and Lars Bendtsen[2]

[1]Albert Einstein College of Medicine, Beth Israel Medical Center, New York, NY, USA
[2]University of Copenhagen, Glostrup Hospital, Glostrup, Copenhagen, Denmark

Introduction

Tension-type headache (TTH) is one of the most prevalent headache disorders, with substantial costs both for the individual and society [1]. The understanding of pathophysiology of TTH is less complete than that of migraine, possibly due to a lack of scientific interest. In its infrequent episodic form, TTH can be regarded as a common and minimally intrusive occurrence, making it less important than migraine. However, in its frequent form, TTH has a major impact on both the individual and the population level. The progress in basic and clinical neuroscience in the past two decades has increased our understanding of the pathophysiology of TTH. It has been suggested that abnormalities in peripheral and central nociceptive systems in combination with environmental and genetic factors are involved in the pathophysiology of TTH.

Pathophysiology

Environmental and psychological factors

Emotional factors have been implicated as risk factors for the development of TTH, but the relationship between cause and effect is not clear.

Stress and mental tension are the most common reportable precipitating factors of TTH, and a positive correlation between headache and stress has been reported in patients with TTH [2, 3]. It has recently been demonstrated that stress induces more headache in patients with chronic TTH (CTTH) than in healthy controls, possibly by hyperalgesic effects on already sensitized pain pathways [4, 5]. However, stress did not enhance the abnormal temporal summation of pain or modulate diffuse noxious inhibitory control mechanisms [6].

Depression is common in frequent TTH and may interact with pathophysiologic mechanisms in TTH [7]. There may be a bidirectional relationship between depression and frequent TTH. Psychological abnormalities in TTH may be viewed as secondary rather than primary. Janke et al. [8] demonstrated that depression increased vulnerability to TTH in patients with frequent headaches during and following the laboratory stress test, and was associated with increased pericranial muscle tenderness. Thus, depression may contribute to an increased excitability of central nociceptive pathways, i.e., central sensitization, in patients with CTTH [8, 9]. The neurobiologic mechanisms by which emotional factors influence TTH are unknown, and further studies are needed to explore the possible relation of the corticolimbic circuits to central sensitization in TTH. Further, maladaptive coping strategies, for example catastrophizing and avoidance, seem to be common in TTH [10].

Peripheral factors

Peripheral factors have long been considered to be of importance in the mechanism of TTH. Increased tenderness in the pericranial muscles during attacks and headache-free periods is a common clinical finding and is the best-documented abnormality in patients with episodic and chronic TTH [11, 12, 13, 14, 15]. Tenderness has been demonstrated to be uniformly increased throughout the pericranial region, and is positively associated with both the intensity and the frequency of TTH [11, 13, 14]. Tenderness and hardness have been found to be increased both on days with and without headache, indicating that hardness is not the consequence of actual headache [9, 16, 17].

Sustained pericranial muscle contraction has long been suggested to be an etiologic factor in TTH. Sustained experimental tooth-clenching was reported to induce more headaches in TTH patients than healthy controls [18], and these patients are more likely to develop shoulder and neck pain in response to static exercise than controls [19]. Several laboratory-based electromyography (EMG) studies have reported normal or only slightly increased muscle activity in TTH [20]. However, EMG activity has been reported to be increased at myofascial trigger points [21], and it is possible that continuous activity in a few motor units over a long time could be sufficient for excitation or sensitization of the peripheral nociceptors [22]. A recent series of pilot studies reported an increased number of active trigger points in both patients with frequent episodic TTH and patients with CTTH [23, 24, 25]. A microanalysis study in TTH demonstrated an increase in muscle blood flow during exercise that was lower in patients than in controls, but lactate levels in a tender site in the trapezius muscle did not differ between patients and controls [26]. It was suggested that the altered blood flow was caused by altered sympathetic outflow

to blood vessels in striated muscle secondary to a central sensitization of nociceptive pathways.

The increased myofascial pain sensitivity in TTH could be secondary to a release of inflammatory mediators resulting in the excitation and sensitization of peripheral sensory afferents. Infusion of a combination of endogenous substances into the trapezius muscle resulted in more pain in patients with frequent episodic TTH compared to controls [27]. The "inflammatory" hypothesis has been challenged by Ashina et al. [28], who demonstrated that the *in vivo* interstitial concentrations of adenosine 5-triphosphate, glutamate, glucose, pyruvate, urea, and prostaglandin E_2 in tender muscles during rest and static exercise did not differ between patients with CTTH and controls.

Overall, previous studies indicate that muscle pain in TTH is not caused by generalized excessive muscle contraction and muscle ischemia. It cannot be excluded that a locally increased muscle tone without EMG activity may result in microtrauma to muscle fibers and tendon insertions, or that excessive activity in a few motor units may excite or sensitize peripheral nociceptors. Pericranial myofascial pain sensitivity is increased in patients with TTH, and the peripheral activation or sensitization of myofascial nociceptors could play a role in the increased pain sensitivity.

Central factors

The increased myofascial pain sensitivity in TTH could also be due to central factors such as sensitization of second-order neurons at the level of the spinal dorsal horn/trigeminal nucleus, sensitization of supraspinal neurons, and decreased antinociceptive activity from supraspinal structures. Pain detection thresholds have been reported normal in patients with episodic TTH in studies performed before the separation between the infrequent and frequent form of TTH in the second edition of the International Classification of Headache Disorders [12, 29, 30, 31, 32]. Pain detection thresholds may be decreased in patients with frequent episodic TTH [27, 33], and both pain detection and tolerance thresholds were found to be decreased in patients with CTTH in studies performed with a sufficient or large sample size [11, 33, 34, 35, 36, 37, 38]. The

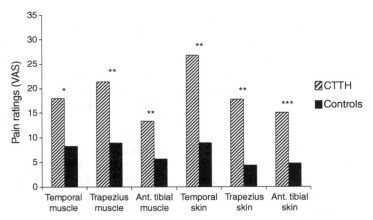

Figure 12.1. Pain perception study demonstrating pronounced generalized hyperalgesia in patients with CTTH. Pain ratings to suprathreshold single electrical stimulation (VAS, visual analog scale) of skin and muscle in patients with CTTH and healthy controls. *$P < 0.05$, **$P < 0.01$, ***$P < 0.001$. (Data from [37]. Reprinted with permission from Sage.)

difference in pain sensitivity is even more pronounced in the cephalic and extracephalic regions in CTTH when recording pain sensitivity to clinically relevant stimuli, i.e., suprathreshold stimuli (Figure 12.1) [37].

Hypersensitivity to various sensory stimulus modalities has been demonstrated in CTTH, including pressure [11, 34, 36], thermal [36], electrical [35, 37, 39, 40, 41], and inflammatory (intramuscular infusions of painful substances) [27, 33, 42, 43] stimuli. In addition, sensitivity to various stimulus modalities in various tissues, i.e., muscle, skin, tendons, and peripheral nerves, is increased both at cephalic and extracephalic sites, both during and outside a headache phase [11, 33, 34, 35, 36, 37, 42].

Increased temporal summation to pressure pain and a trend toward increased temporal summation to electrical pain in patients with CTTH compared to controls has been reported [6, 37]. These studies point toward the generalized increase in pain sensitivity in patients with frequent TTH. Widespread pain sensitivity in frequent and CTTH supports the role of central sensitization. A population-based study demonstrated a close relationship between altered pain perception and chronification of headache, and confirmed findings from experimental studies [44]. Further, it was demonstrated that the increase in TTH prevalence over a 12-year period was related to increased pain sensitivity [44].

Increased pain sensitivity is a consequence of frequent TTH, not a risk factor, and the results support the hypothesis that central sensitization plays an important role in the chronification of TTH [45].

In addition, the stimulus–response function for pressure versus pain in the pericranial muscles is not only quantitatively, but also qualitatively altered in patients with CTTH. The above hypothesis was further supported by a recent study demonstrating a decrease in volume of gray matter brain structures involved in pain processing in patients with CTTH [46]. This decrease was positively correlated with duration of headache, and is most likely a consequence of central sensitization generated by prolonged input from the pericranial myofascial structures [46]. However, generalized hypersensitivity and central sensitization can only partially account for the increased pericranial tenderness in patients with CTTH because of an incomplete correlation between general pain hypersensitivity and pericranial tenderness [11, 13].

Decreased antinociceptive activity from the supraspinal structures, i.e., deficient descending inhibition, may also contribute to the increased pain sensitivity in CTTH [6, 35, 39, 40, 47, 48]. A recent high-density brain electroencephalogram mapping study found an impaired inhibition of nociceptive input in CTTH [48]. Impaired descending inhibition could be the primary abnormality, or it could contribute to or be a consequence of central sensitization [22]. Further studies are needed to clarify this issue. Both central sensitization and deficient descending inhibition may contribute to the development of CTHH from its episodic form.

Mechanism-based treatment

The hypothesis of central sensitization in TTH is further supported by clinical pharmacologic studies. Amitriptyline, a tricyclic antidepressant medication that is the mainstay prophylactic agent in TTH, has been shown to reduce both headache and pericranial myofascial tenderness in patients with CTTH [49]. It was suggested that the reduction of myofascial tenderness during treatment with amitriptyline might be caused by a segmental reduction of central sensitization in combination with an enhanced efficacy of noradrenergic or serotonergic descending inhibition [49]. Findings of lower serotonin (5-hydroxytryptamine; 5-HT) reuptake inhibition and a higher analgesic efficacy of amitriptyline than citalopram, a selective serotonin reuptake inhibitor, suggest that 5-HT reuptake inhibition is not the major mechanism of action of amitriptyline in TTH [50].

Animal studies have shown that sensitization of pain pathways may be caused by or associated with activation of nitric oxide synthase (NOS) and the generation of nitric oxide. NOS inhibitors can reduce central sensitization in animal models of persistent pain [51]. Given this evidence, Ashina et al. demonstrated that infusion of the nitric oxide donor glyceryl trinitrate induces TTH-like headache attacks in patients with CTTH [52]. In addition, the analgesic effect of an NOS inhibitor was studied. This drug significantly reduced headache [53] as well as pericranial myofascial tenderness and hardness [54] in patients with CTTH. Sarchielli et al. [55] reported increased platelet NOS activity in patients with CTTH, possibly reflecting central upregulation of NOS. These pharmacologic data support the role of central sensitization in the pathophysiology of CTTH. Moreover, these findings suggest that inhibition of nitric oxide and thereby central sensitization may become a novel approach in the future treatment of CTTH.

The rationale for the use of botulinum toxin in pain conditions is the antinociceptive action of this drug in the peripheral and central nervous systems [56]. Randomized placebo-controlled trials have demonstrated that botulinum toxin has not been shown to be superior to placebo in the treatment of CTTH [57, 58]. The exact reason why botulinum toxin does not work for CTTH headache but works for chronic migraine is not clear.

Genetics

Due to the enormous prevalence and variability in the frequency and severity of TTH, any inheritance is almost certain to be polygenic in this headache condition. The population-relative risk in first- and second-degree relatives compared with normal controls has been calculated in a single Danish study. In CTTH, the risk was increased threefold, indicating a genetic predisposition [59, 60]. The mode of inheritance was investigated by complex segregation analysis, which indicated that CTTH has multifactorial inheritance and supported the view that CTTH has genetic components in pathophysiology because the multifactorial model had a better fit than the sporadic model [60]. Ulrich et al. [61] examined the relative importance of genetic and environmental influences for the development of TTH by analyses of twins. It was concluded that an environmental influence was of major importance for ETTH, and a genetic factor had minor contribution. At present, we adopt the view that the great majority of the population, perhaps all, has the potential to develop TTH if exposed to sufficiently strong environmental factors.

Conclusion

Pericranial myofascial mechanisms are probably of importance in episodic TTH, whereas sensitization of nociceptive pathways in the CNS due to prolonged nociceptive stimuli from pericranial myofascial tissues seems to be responsible for the conversion of episodic to CTTH (Figure 12.2 and Table 12.1). This hypothesis delineates two major targets for future treatment strategies: (1) to identify the source of peripheral nociception in order to prevent the development of central sensitization and thereby the transformation of episodic into CTTH; and (2) to reduce established central sensitization [20, 22, 62, 63].

Chronic tension-type headache

Continuous painful input from pericranial myofascial tissues

induce | and maintain

central sensitization such that normally innocuous stimuli
become painful

Conversion from episodic to chronic tension-type headache

Figure 12.2. The proposed pathophysiologic model of CTTH delineates two major aims for future research: (1) to identify the source of peripheral nociception in order to prevent the development of central sensitization in patients with episodic TTH, and (2) to reduce established central sensitization in patients with CTTH. (Modified from Bendtsen L. Central sensitization in tension-type headache—possible pathophysical mechanisms. *Cephalalgia* 2000; 20: 23 [22]. Reprinted with permission from SAGE.)

Table 12.1. Pathophysiology of TTH

Localization		Mechanisms	Therapeutic implications
Peripheral			
	Pericranial muscle and nociceptors (Aδ-fibers and C-fibers)	Peripheral sensitization Increased muscle hardness Increased muscle tenderness	Acetaminophen Nonsteroidal anti-inflammatory drugs Physical therapy
Central			
	Cervical spinal dorsal horn/trigeminal spinal nucleus	Central sensitization	Amitriptyline NOS inhibition
	Periaqueductal gray (midbrain) and rostral ventral medulla	Deficient descending inhibition	
	Thalamus	Central sensitization	Amitriptyline NOS inhibition
	Limbic system	Emotional control of pain	Biofeedback Relaxation therapy
	Cerebral cortex	Central sensitization	Amitriptyline NOS inhibition

References

1. Schwartz BS, Stewart WF, Lipton RB. Lost workdays and decreased work effectiveness associated with headache in the workplace. *J Occup Environ Med* 1997;**39**:320–7.
2. Spierings EL, Ranke AH, Honkoop PC. Precipitating and aggravating factors of migraine versus tension-type headache. *Headache* 2001;**41**:554–8.
3. Rasmussen BK. Migraine and tension-type headache in a general population: precipitating factors, female hormones, sleep pattern and relation to lifestyle. *Pain* 1993;**53**: 65–72.

4. Cathcart S, Petkov J, Pritchard D. Effects of induced stress on experimental pain sensitivity in chronic tension-type headache sufferers. *Eur J Neurol* 2008;**15**:552–8.

5. Cathcart S, Winefield AH, Lushington K, Rolan P. Effect of mental stress on cold pain in chronic tension-type headache sufferers. *J Headache Pain* 2009;**10**:367–73.

6. Cathcart S, Winefield AH, Lushington K, Rolan P. Noxious inhibition of temporal summation is impaired in chronic tension-type headache. *Headache* 2010;**50**:403–12.

7. Holroyd KA, Stensland M, Lipchik GL, Hill KR, O'Donnell FS, Cordingley G. Psychosocial correlates and impact of chronic tension-type headaches. *Headache* 2000;**40**:3–16.

8. Janke EA, Holroyd KA, Romanek K. Depression increases onset of tension-type headache following laboratory stress. *Pain* 2004; **111**:230–8.

9. Lipchik GL, Holroyd KA, O'Donnell FJ, et al. Exteroceptive suppression periods and pericranial muscle tenderness in chronic tension-type headache: effects of psychopathology, chronicity and disability. *Cephalalgia* 2000;**20**:638–46.

10. Heckman BD, Holroyd KA. Tension-type headache and psychiatric comorbidity. *Curr Pain Headache Rep* 2006;**10**:439–47.

11. Bendtsen L, Jensen R, Olesen J. Decreased pain detection and tolerance thresholds in chronic tension-type headache. *Arch Neurol* 1996;**53**:373–6.

12. Jensen R, Rasmussen BK, Pedersen B, Olesen J. Muscle tenderness and pressure pain thresholds in headache. A population study. *Pain* 1993;**52**:193–9.

13. Jensen R, Bendtsen L, Olesen J. Muscular factors are of importance in tension-type headache. *Headache* 1998;**38**:10–7.

14. Langemark M, Olesen J. Pericranial tenderness in tension headache. A blind, controlled study. *Cephalalgia* 1987;**7**:249–55.

15. Lipchik GL, Holroyd KA, Talbot F, Greer M. Pericranial muscle tenderness and exteroceptive suppression of temporalis muscle activity: a blind study of chronic tension-type headache. *Headache* 1997;**37**:368–76.

16. Sakai F, Ebihara S, Akiyama M, Horikawa M. Pericranial muscle hardness in tension-type headache. A non-invasive measurement method and its clinical application. *Brain* 1995;**118**(Pt 2):523–31.

17. Ashina M, Bendtsen L, Jensen R, Sakai F, Olesen J. Muscle hardness in patients with chronic tension-type headache: relation to actual headache state. *Pain* 1999;**79**:201–5.

18. Jensen R, Olesen J. Initiating mechanisms of experimentally induced tension-type headache. *Cephalalgia* 1996;**16**:175–82.

19. Christensen MB, Bendtsen L, Ashina M, Jensen R. Experimental induction of muscle tenderness and headache in tension-type headache patients. *Cephalalgia* 2005;**25**: 1061–7.

20. Jensen R. Pathophysiological mechanisms of tension-type headache: a review of epidemiological and experimental studies. *Cephalalgia* 1999;**19**:602–21.

21. Hubbard DR, Berkoff GM. Myofascial trigger points show spontaneous needle EMG activity. *Spine (Phila Pa 1976)* 1993;**18**:1803–7.

22. Bendtsen L. Central sensitization in tension-type headache – possible pathophysiological mechanisms. *Cephalalgia* 2000;**20**:486–508.

23. Fernandez-de-Las-Penas C, Cuadrado ML, Pareja JA. Myofascial trigger points, neck mobility, and forward head posture in episodic tension-type headache. *Headache* 2007;**47**:662–72.

24. Fernandez-de-Las-Penas C, Alonso-Blanco C, Cuadrado ML, Pareja JA. Myofascial trigger points in the suboccipital muscles in episodic tension-type headache. *Man Ther* 2006;**11**:225–30.

25. Fernandez-de-Las-Penas C, Alonso-Blanco C, Cuadrado ML, Gerwin RD, Pareja JA. Myofascial trigger points and their relationship to headache clinical parameters in chronic tension-type headache. *Headache* 2006;**46**: 1264–72.

26. Ashina M, Stallknecht B, Bendtsen L, et al. In vivo evidence of altered skeletal muscle blood flow in chronic tension-type headache. *Brain* 2002;**125**:320–6.

27. Mork H, Ashina M, Bendtsen L, Olesen J, Jensen R. Induction of prolonged tenderness in patients with tension-type headache by means of a new experimental model of myofascial pain. *Eur J Neurol* 2003;**10**:249–56.

28. Ashina M, Stallknecht B, Bendtsen L, et al. Tender points are not sites of ongoing

inflammation -in vivo evidence in patients with chronic tension-type headache. *Cephalalgia* 2003;**23**:109–16.

29. Jensen R. Mechanisms of spontaneous tension-type headaches: an analysis of tenderness, pain thresholds and EMG. *Pain* 1996;**64**:251–6.

30. Gobel H, Weigle L, Kropp P, Soyka D. Pain sensitivity and pain reactivity of pericranial muscles in migraine and tension-type headache. *Cephalalgia* 1992;**12**:142–51.

31. Bovim G. Cervicogenic headache, migraine, and tension-type headache. Pressure-pain threshold measurements. *Pain* 1992;**51**:169–73.

32. The International Classification of Headache Disorders. 2nd edition. Headache Classification Subcommittee of the International Headache Society. *Cephalalgia* 2004;**24**(Suppl. 1):9–160.

33. Schmidt-Hansen PT, Svensson P, Bendtsen L, Graven-Nielsen T, Bach FW. Increased muscle pain sensitivity in patients with tension-type headache. *Pain* 2007;**129**:113–21.

34. Schoenen J, Bottin D, Hardy F, Gerard P. Cephalic and extracephalic pressure pain thresholds in chronic tension-type headache. *Pain* 1991;**47**:145–9.

35. Langemark M, Bach FW, Jensen TS, Olesen J. Decreased nociceptive flexion reflex threshold in chronic tension-type headache. *Arch Neurol* 1993;**50**:1061–4.

36. Langemark M, Jensen K, Jensen TS, Olesen J. Pressure pain thresholds and thermal nociceptive thresholds in chronic tension-type headache. *Pain* 1989;**38**:203–10.

37. Ashina S, Bendtsen L, Ashina M, Magerl W, Jensen R. Generalized hyperalgesia in patients with chronic tension-type headache. *Cephalalgia* 2006;**26**:940–8.

38. Sandrini G, Antonaci F, Pucci E, Bono G, Nappi G. Comparative study with EMG, pressure algometry and manual palpation in tension-type headache and migraine. *Cephalalgia* 1994;**14**:451–7.

39. Lindelof K, Jung K, Ellrich J, Jensen R, Bendtsen L. Low-frequency electrical stimulation induces long-term depression in patients with chronic tension-type headache. *Cephalalgia* 2010;**30**:860–7.

40. Sandrini G, Rossi P, Milanov I, Serrao M, Cecchini AP, Nappi G. Abnormal modulatory influence of diffuse noxious inhibitory controls in migraine and chronic tension-type headache patients. *Cephalalgia* 2006;**26**:782–9.

41. Ashina S, Babenko L, Jensen R, Ashina M, Magerl W, Bendtsen L. Increased muscular and cutaneous pain sensitivity in cephalic region in patients with chronic tension-type headache. *Eur J Neurol* 2005;**12**:543–9.

42. Lindelof K, Ellrich J, Jensen R, Bendtsen L. Central pain processing in chronic tension-type headache. *Clin Neurophysiol* 2009;**120**:1364–70.

43. Mork H, Ashina M, Bendtsen L, Olesen J, Jensen R. Experimental muscle pain and tenderness following infusion of endogenous substances in humans. *Eur J Pain* 2003;**7**:145–53.

44. Buchgreitz L, Lyngberg AC, Bendtsen L, Jensen R. Frequency of headache is related to sensitization: a population study. *Pain* 2006;**123**:19–27.

45. Buchgreitz L, Lyngberg AC, Bendtsen L, Jensen R. Increased pain sensitivity is not a risk factor but a consequence of frequent headache: a population-based follow-up study. *Pain* 2008;**137**:623–30.

46. Schmidt-Wilcke T, Leinisch E, Straube A, et al. Gray matter decrease in patients with chronic tension type headache. *Neurology* 2005;**65**:1483–6.

47. Pielsticker A, Haag G, Zaudig M, Lautenbacher S. Impairment of pain inhibition in chronic tension-type headache. *Pain* 2005;**118**:215–23.

48. Buchgreitz L, Egsgaard LL, Jensen R, Arendt-Nielsen L, Bendtsen L. Abnormal pain processing in chronic tension-type headache: a high-density EEG brain mapping study. *Brain* 2008;**131**:3232–8.

49. Bendtsen L, Jensen R. Amitriptyline reduces myofascial tenderness in patients with chronic tension-type headache. *Cephalalgia* 2000;**20**:603–10.

50. Ashina S, Bendtsen L, Jensen R. Analgesic effect of amitriptyline in chronic tension-type headache is not directly related to serotonin reuptake inhibition. *Pain* 2004;**108**:108–14.

51. Meller ST, Gebhart GF. Nitric oxide (NO) and nociceptive processing in the spinal cord. *Pain* 1993;**52**:127–36.

52. Ashina M, Bendtsen L, Jensen R, Olesen J. Nitric oxide-induced headache in patients with chronic tension-type headache. *Brain* 2000;**123**(Pt 9):1830–7.

53. Ashina M, Lassen LH, Bendtsen L, Jensen R, Olesen J. Effect of inhibition of nitric oxide synthase on chronic tension-type headache: a randomised crossover trial. *Lancet* 1999; **353**:287–9.

54. Ashina M, Bendtsen L, Jensen R, Lassen LH, Sakai F, Olesen J. Possible mechanisms of action of nitric oxide synthase inhibitors in chronic tension-type headache. *Brain* 1999; **122**(Pt 9):1629–35.

55. Sarchielli P, Alberti A, Floridi A, Gallai V. L-Arginine/nitric oxide pathway in chronic tension-type headache: relation with serotonin content and secretion and glutamate content. *J Neurol Sci* 2002;**198**:9–15.

56. Guyer BM. mechanism of botulinum toxin in the relief of chronic pain. *Curr Rev Pain* 1999;**3**:427–31.

57. Padberg M, de Bruijn SF, de Haan RJ, Tavy DL. Treatment of chronic tension-type headache with botulinum toxin: a double-blind, placebo-controlled clinical trial. *Cephalalgia* 2004;**24**:675–80.

58. Silberstein SD, Gobel H, Jensen R, et al. Botulinum toxin type A in the prophylactic treatment of chronic tension-type headache: a multicentre, double-blind, randomized, placebo-controlled, parallel-group study. *Cephalalgia* 2006;**26**:790–800.

59. Ostergaard S, Russell MB, Bendtsen L, Olesen J. Comparison of first degree relatives and spouses of people with chronic tension headache. *BMJ* 1997;**314**:1092–3.

60. Russell MB, Ostergaard S, Bendtsen L, Olesen J. Familial occurrence of chronic tension-type headache. *Cephalalgia* 1999;**19**: 207–10.

61. Ulrich V, Gervil M, Olesen J. The relative influence of environment and genes in episodic tension-type headache. *Neurology* 2004;**62**(11):2065–9.

62. Ashina M. Neurobiology of chronic tension-type headache. *Cephalalgia* 2004;**24**:161–72.

63. Milanov I, Bogdanova D. Pain and tension-type headache: a review of the possible pathophysiological mechanisms. *J Headache Pain* 2004;**5**:4–11.

Treatment of Tension-type Headache

Sara C. Crystal and Katherine A. Henry

New York University School of Medicine, New York, NY, USA

Introduction

Tension-type headache (TTH) is the most common primary headache disorder, with a lifetime prevalence of 78% [1, 2]. TTH can be episodic or chronic. While the impact of TTH is higher with the chronic (CTTH) than the episodic (ETTH) form, both can affect quality of life and warrant treatment. Pharmacologic and nonpharmacologic treatments, including behavioral interventions, spinal manipulation, physical therapy, and acupuncture will be discussed in this chapter.

Diagnostic criteria

TTH is divided into three subtypes based on attack frequency: an *infrequent episodic* form in which headaches occur on average on 1 day or less per month, a *frequent episodic* form in which headaches occur on 1–14 days per month for at least 3 months, and a *chronic form*, with 15 or more headache days per month. Frequent episodic and chronic TTH is further subdivided based on the presence or absence of pericranial tenderness. Diagnostic criteria for all three subtypes include at least two of the following pain characteristics: bilateral location, nonpulsating quality, mild or moderate intensity, and lack of aggravation with routine physical activity. Infrequent and frequent TTH are both diagnoses of inclusion, as attacks may be accompanied by either photophobia or phonophobia, but not both, and diagnoses of exclusion in that nausea and vomiting must be absent. For CTTH, no more than one of three features of mild nausea, photophobia, and phonophobia may be present, and moderate or severe nausea or vomiting precludes the diagnosis [3].

Pathophysiology of TTH

Despite, or because of, its broad reach, TTH has stymied researchers in their efforts to characterize the physiologic underpinnings of the disease. Whether due to the varying patient populations, lack of patients presenting for treatment, or difficulty in obtaining samples of patients with discrete variants of TTH, TTH has proven difficult to study. A particular difficulty is the diagnostic overlap with migraine. Peripheral pain mechanisms (e.g., myofascial nociception) are generally believed to play a role in the pathogenesis of infrequent ETTH and frequent ETTH [4]. In the first edition of the International Classification of Headache Disorders (ICHD), TTH was classified into headaches with and without pericranial

Headache, First Edition. Edited by Matthew S. Robbins, Brian M. Grosberg, and Richard B. Lipton.
© 2013 John Wiley & Sons, Ltd. Published 2013 by John Wiley & Sons, Ltd.

tenderness, and tenderness to palpation and/or electromyography (EMG) were required to make a diagnosis. In addition, headaches without pericranial tenderness were suggested to be of potentially psychogenic origin [5]. Later studies did not support the notion that EMG was useful in the diagnosis of TTH; however, studies of pressure-controlled manual palpation have revealed the usefulness of this technique [6]. Therefore, the use of manual palpation to identify pericranial tenderness is used in the latest iteration of the ICHD (ICHD-2) in the diagnostic criteria for TTH [3].

Further research into the peripheral pain pathways in tension headache, such as muscle ischemia and inflammation, has yielded mixed results [7, 8, 9]. Overall, studies have found that pain thresholds are inversely associated with pain to pericranial muscle palpation in TTH, and the lower threshold in CTTH is suggestive of abnormalities in central processing [8].

SCIENCE REVISITED

Alterations in the descending inhibitory tracts that ameliorate pain have been implicated in the development of CTTH [9]. Structural studies using MRI voxel-based morphometry have shown atrophy in the areas of the brainstem important in the pathogenesis of headache pain [10].

Pharmacologic treatment of ETTH

Many studies in the literature have investigated the various degrees of efficacy using simple analgesics, nonsteroidal anti-inflammatory drugs (NSAIDs), and combination medications. The reader is directed to the extensively referenced European Federation of Neurological Societies guideline on the treatment of TTH [11]. The highlights of their recommendations for the treatment of ETTH are summarized below and in Table 13.1.

Simple analgesics

Several randomized, placebo-controlled trials have shown that acetaminophen is effective at 1000 mg, over placebo and equal to aspirin. Because of its greater gastrointestinal tolerability,

Table 13.1. Pharmacologic (acute) treatment of ETTH

Medication	Dose (mg)
Acetaminophen	1000
Aspirin	500–1000
Ibuprofen	200–800
Naproxen sodium	375–875
Ketoprofen	12.5–50
Caffeine (adjuvant)	65–200

it is best to start with acetaminophen, which has fewer gastrointestinal side effects.

Nonsteroidal anti-inflammatory agents

The pharmacologic mainstay of treatment for ETTH is the use of NSAIDs. Aspirin (500–1000 mg) is more effective than placebo, but NSAIDs have been more effective in a number of randomized trials. In terms of efficacy, the differences between various NSAIDs are marginal. Ibuprofen 200 mg, 400 mg, or 800 mg, should be tried first and, if ineffective, naproxen sodium, 375 mg, 500 mg, or 875 mg, should be used. There is also evidence to support the use of ketoprofen in doses of 12.5–50 mg. Ketorolac at a dose of 60 mg intramuscularly is a useful treatment in the emergency department. All patients prescribed NSAIDs should be cautioned about the risks of gastrointestinal bleeding.

Combination medications and opioids

The addition of caffeine, in doses of 65–200 mg, increases the efficacy of naproxen sodium and simple analgesics. Many of these combination medicines are available over the counter, and for that reason great caution should be exercised in their use due to the increased risk of medication overuse headache. Further, the addition of opioids to these combinations does not improve efficacy. Opioids have no place in the treatment of TTH.

Triptans

In general, triptans do not have a role in the treatment of TTH. The exception, however, is in the case of TTH in the migraineur. It has been shown that triptans may be effective for headaches in between migraines (interval headaches). It has

Table 13.2. Pharmacologic treatment for CTTH prevention

Medication	Dosage	Efficacy	Adverse effects
Amitriptyline	Start 10–25 mg at night Titrate to 75–100 mg over 2–4 weeks	High	Sedation, weight gain, dry mouth
Venlafaxine	37.5–75 mg/day	Moderate	Nausea, decreased libido
Mirtazapine	15–30 mg/day	Moderate	Sedation, dizziness, weight gain
Tizanidine	12–24 mg/day divided	Low	Sedation, dizziness

been postulated that while these headaches may meet the criteria for TTH, that they in fact may be mild migraine.

While many of the treatments described above may be effective in CTTH, they have been primarily studied in ETTH. The approach to the treatment of CTTH should focus on preventive treatment and the abortive treatment approach individualized to the patient's needs.

Pharmacologic treatment of CTTH

Symptomatic or acute treatment should be limited in patients with CTTH, to avoid the development of medication overuse headache and renal and hepatic toxicity. Further, acute treatment is often ineffective in CTTH [12]. Preventive therapy should be considered in patients with CTTH and frequent ETTH, because of its tendency to develop into the chronic form (Table 13.2) [12]. Comorbid conditions, such as obesity and depression, should be taken into account [11]. While the goal of preventive medications for headache is ideally a reduction of 50% or more in attack frequency, a goal of 30% reduction in CTTH is more realistic [12].

Although there are a number of trials of preventive drugs in TTH, interpretation of the results of many of them is limited by small sample size or the different outcome measures used. The guidelines for drug trials in TTH published by the International Headache Society [13] recommend that the primary outcomes measured should be the number of days with headache or the area under the headache curve (AUC). The AUC, calculated by multiplying the duration and the intensity of the headache, is also referred to as the headache index. However, many studies use other measures of efficacy, making comparisons between studies difficult.

Verhagen et al. [14] reviewed randomized controlled trials (RCTs) evaluating prophylactic drugs and nonpharmacologic treatments for TTH, rating trials based on the level of bias. The authors noted that most studies lacked the power to detect statistically significant differences between treatment arms due to their small sample sizes, and that the primary outcome of 50% improvement in headache, used in many studies, may be too high.

Antidepressants

Tricyclic antidepressants

Amitriptyline, a tricyclic antidepressant, should be the first drug of choice for CTTH prevention [15]. It was first shown to be effective for CTTH in 1964, by Lance and Curan [16], and several RCTs published since then have confirmed this result. Bendtsen et al. found that amitriptyline reduced the AUC by 30% compared to placebo [17].

The exact mechanism of action of amitriptyline in headache is unknown. Amitriptyline acts primarily as a serotonin and norepinephrine reuptake inhibitor, but also functions as an alpha-1-adrenergic, histamine, and acetylcholine receptor antagonist. Ashina et al. [18] demonstrated that the antinociceptive action of amitriptyline in CTTH is not directly related to serotonin reuptake inhibition. In this study, patients with CTTH were randomized to receive amitriptyline, citalopram, or placebo. Outcome measures included AUC and platelet serotonin (5-HT) levels. While citalopram was more effective than amitriptyline at inhibiting serotonin reuptake, as evidenced by lower 5-HT levels, amitriptyline was more effective than citalopram and placebo in headache reduction. The authors concluded that the effect of amitriptyline in the reduction of CTTH is not completely explained by its effect on serotonin reuptake inhibition, and that other mechanisms, including norepinephrine reuptake inhibition, NMDA receptor antagonism, and muscarinic blockade may play a role.

Amitriptyline may also be effective in CTTH by reducing pericranial muscle tenderness. In a double-blind, placebo-controlled three-way crossover study, Bendtsen and Jensen [19] demonstrated that amitriptyline reduced pericranial muscle tenderness in patients who had at least a 30% reduction in headache intensity in response to the drug. Amitriptyline did not affect the detection of painful pressure or electrical stimuli, implying that the drug reduces nociception from the pericranial musculature, rather than pain sensitivity in general. Citalopram, in contrast, had no effect on headache intensity or muscle tenderness.

In a recent meta-analysis by Jackson et al. [20] of trials of tricyclic agents for the treatment of migraine, TTH, and mixed headaches, tricyclics significantly reduced the number of days with TTH, by an average of 6.9 days per month. Tricyclics also reduced the number of doses of analgesics used for acute treatment. The effectiveness of tricyclic treatment appears to increase over time. While adverse effects were more frequently reported with tricyclics compared to placebo, only dry mouth and drowsiness occurred statistically more significantly. Amitriptyline was the most frequently studied tricyclic, used in 13 out of 17 studies. One study used nortriptyline (when amitriptyline was not tolerated), and the remainder of the studies used amitriptylinoxide, clomipramine and mianserin, and desipramine.

Selective serotonin reuptake inhibitors

The rationale behind the use of selective serotonin reuptake inhibitors (SSRIs) for headache is that serotonin modulates descending pain signals from the brainstem [12]. Moja et al. [21] published a Cochrane analysis concluding that SSRIs are less effective than tricyclics for CTTH, and that the SSRI citalopram was no more effective than placebo. Although side effects were more common with tricyclics than SSRIs, dropout rates were similar. Analgesic use was lower in patients receiving tricyclics compared to an SSRI or placebo. Jackson et al. [20] similarly reported that tricyclics were more likely than SSRIs to produce an improvement of at least 50% in TTH. Paroxetine was studied in an open-label trial of CTTH patients who failed amitriptyline, and was found to be ineffective [22]. In studies comparing tricyclics with tetracyclic antidepressants and buspirone, there were no statistically significant differences [20].

Mirtazapine

Like amitriptyline, mirtazapine has effects on noradrenergic and serotonergic receptors, but its mode of action is more selective than that of amitriptyline [23]. While amitriptyline inhibits the presynaptic reuptake of 5-HT and noradrenaline in the central nervous system, mirtazapine increases noradrenergic and serotonergic transmission through a blockade of presynaptic alpha-2-receptors, and is selective to $5\text{-}HT_2$ and $5\text{-}HT_3$ receptors. In a placebo-controlled, double-blind trial [23], mirtazapine at a dose of 30 mg per day reduced the AUC by 34% compared to placebo. These patients had all failed to respond to other treatments, including amitriptyline. The authors concluded that the therapeutic gain for mirtazapine was similar to that of amitriptyline, and recommended it as a second-line treatment for patients who cannot tolerate or fail to respond to amitriptyline. No studies to date have compared amitriptyline with mirtazapine. Low-dose mirtazapine in combination with ibuprofen was not effective for CTTH prophylaxis [24]. Side effects of mirtazapine include drowsiness, dizziness, and weight gain.

Venlafaxine

The extended-release form of venlafaxine, a serotonin and norepinephrine reuptake inhibitor, was found to reduce the average days of headache per month from 15 to 12 in patients with either frequent ETTH or CTTH, but did not improve the headache intensity [25]. Side effects of venlafaxine include nausea, vomiting, dizziness, and loss of libido.

Muscle relaxants

Tizanidine is an alpha-2-agonist with antinociceptive and muscle relaxant properties [26]. Two of three placebo-controlled trials for CTTH showed significant benefit, but the usefulness of the results is limited by sample size or outcome measures [27, 28, 29]. An open-label RCT [26] involving 18 patients evaluated the efficacy and impact on quality of life of a combined treatment with tizanidine and amitriptyline, to determine whether the combination would have a faster onset of action than amitriptyline alone. Patients treated with the combination of amitriptyline 20 mg daily for 3 months with tizanidine 4 mg daily for the first 3 weeks had an improved frequency, intensity, and duration of headaches in the first 4 weeks of treatment, although there were no significant differences at the end of the 90-day treatment period.

Botulinum toxin type A

The rational for use of botulinum toxin in TTH is the combination of its muscle relaxant and antinociceptive actions in the central and peripheral nervous systems [30]. While benefits have been reported in an open-label study [31] and one placebo-controlled trial [32], other double-blind placebo-controlled trials have reported mostly negative results [33, 34, 35, 36].

Nonpharmacologic treatments

Nonpharmacologic treatments should be considered for all patients with CTTH, although evidence is lacking for some of these modalities. Trigger identification and avoidance is important; the most common triggers of TTH are physical and mental stress, excessive caffeine use, inadequate or inappropriate food intake, dehydration, too much or too little sleep, and hormonal changes [11]. Nonpharmacologic treatments include behavioral interventions such as biofeedback, cognitive-behavioral therapy (CBT) and other stress management techniques, physical therapy/spinal manipulation, exercise, and acupuncture. Several trials have compared pharmacologic and nonpharmacologic treatments [37, 38, 39], while others have compared various nonpharmacologic modalities to each other and to placebo [40, 41, 42].

Behavioral treatments

Holroyd et al. [38] conducted a randomized, placebo-controlled trial in which patients with CTTH received either tricyclic antidepressants (amitriptyline up to 100 mg per day or nortriptyline up to 75 mg per day), placebo medication, stress management techniques (relaxation and cognitive coping skills) plus placebo, or stress management plus antidepressant medication.

The authors found that tricyclics and stress management therapy were both more effective than placebo in reducing headache activity, analgesic use, and headache-related disability, but antidepressants had a quicker onset of action. Patients treated with stress management and antidepressants were more likely to experience a 50% or greater reduction in headache index scores than those receiving placebo or either treatment alone [38].

In a separate prospective randomized trial, Holroyd et al. [37] compared CBT with amitriptyline in patients with CTTH, and found that both approaches produced clinically significant improvements in headache activity, as measured both by patients and by clinicians. In some measures, CBT was slightly more effective than amitriptyline.

In 2000, the US Headache Consortium [43] published evidence-based guidelines on behavioral and physical treatments for migraine. The panel recommended that relaxation training, thermal biofeedback combined with relaxation training, EMG biofeedback, and CBT may be considered for migraine prevention (Grade A evidence), and that behavioral therapy may be combined with preventive drug therapy to achieve greater improvement (Grade B). The panel concluded that evidence-based treatment recommendations were not yet possible regarding acupuncture, cervical manipulation, transcutaneous electric nerve stimulation, occlusal adjustment, and hyperbaric oxygen as preventive or acute migraine treatment (Grade C).

Similarly, a meta-analysis of behavioral treatments for TTH reviewed over 100 articles published between 1966 and 1999, including 35 RCTs [44]. The authors found that behavioral treatments were significantly more effective than control conditions, but not more effective than amitriptyline. Improvement with various behavioral treatment methods ranged from 35% to 55%. In a recent meta-analysis of biofeedback for headache, Nestoriuc et al. [45] found that, for TTH, biofeedback produced a medium to large effect size compared to the untreated control groups, and a medium effect size compared to placebo, both of which were statistically significant.

In another meta-analysis of behavioral treatments of TTH, Verhagen et al. [46] reviewed 44

RCTs, and concluded that there was insufficient evidence to conclude that relaxation training, EMG biofeedback, and CBT were more beneficial than placebo or no treatment. They found limited evidence that relaxation with EMG biofeedback training might be more effective than placebo. The authors noted that the outcome measure of at least a 50% improvement in headache used in most studies may be too strict to detect clinically significant differences, in contrast to studies of shoulder pain, in which an improvement of 15% is considered significant.

Spinal manipulation, physical therapy, and exercise

Lenssinck et al. [47] performed a systematic review of RCTs of physical therapy and spinal manipulation for TTH, and identified two studies as being of high quality. In one RCT [39], spinal manipulation provided by chiropractors was compared to amitriptyline 30 mg daily for CTTH. The primary outcomes measured were change in daily headache intensity, weekly headache frequency, analgesic use, and functional health status. After 6 weeks, there was a small but significant reduction in headache intensity with amitriptyline compared to spinal manipulation, although amitriptyline was associated with more side effects. There were no significant differences between groups in the other measures. However, 4 weeks after treatment cessation, patients who received spinal manipulation had sustained a significant improvement in all outcomes, while those in the amitriptyline group reverted to their baseline values. Spinal manipulation failed to show a benefit for ETTH in another RCT [42]. Based on a review of these two studies, Lenssinck et al. concluded that there was insufficient evidence to determine the effectiveness of physical therapy and spinal manipulation for TTH [47].

In an RCT comparing the effectiveness of exercise therapy/physical therapy combined with a craniocervical training program with physical therapy alone, the exercise group showed a significantly reduced frequency, intensity, and duration of headaches at the 6-month follow-up [40].

Patients with TTH, including ETTH, CTTH, and probable TTH, were evaluated in an RCT comparing osteopathic treatment plus progressive muscle relaxation with progressive muscle relaxation exercises alone [41]. While frequency of the headaches improved with the combined treatment, their intensity did not.

Acupuncture

A recent Cochrane analysis reviewed 11 trials that examined whether acupuncture is effective for TTH prophylaxis, compared to no treatment or routine care only, "sham" acupuncture, or other treatments including PT, massage, and relaxation [48]. Sham treatment mimicked true acupuncture, but differed in at least one aspect inherent to acupuncture theory, such as the correct needle location or depth of penetration. Two trials comparing acupuncture to routine care [49] or symptomatic treatment of acute headaches only [50] found that acupuncture significantly reduced the frequency and intensity of headaches. Effects were larger in the trial comparing acupuncture to acute treatment only, with 45% responders in the acupuncture group compared to 4% in the control group [50]. Data from six trials comparing acupuncture with sham treatment were pooled, finding a small but significant reduction in headache frequency with acupuncture. In the trials comparing acupuncture with PT, massage or exercise, acupuncture was not found to be superior. The authors concluded that acupuncture could be of benefit in patients with frequent ETTH or CTTH [48].

TTH in children

The challenge in the evaluation and treatment of TTH and other headache types in children is the difficulty of determining what the child is experiencing. Children do not experience headache in the same fashion as adults, with their headaches often being shorter in duration and relieved by rest or nonpharmacologic approaches. The initial approach to treatment should focus on behavioral approaches and identification of triggers. If headaches are not relieved with these approaches, simple analgesics or NSAIDs should be used. Biobehavioral approaches plus tricyclics are often used in children with frequent or CTTH. Unfortunately, randomized, placebo-controlled studies in the treatment of this age group are lacking.

TTH in the elderly

Headaches are not uncommon in the elderly, and 25% of men and 27% of women in their 60s experience TTH [51]. There are very few data in the literature to guide the clinician in the treatment of TTH in the elderly. Intercurrent medical illnesses and medications require that the clinician be cognizant of the side effects and interactions of various medications. The use of alternative approaches to treatment, such as lifestyle modification, physical therapy, and sleep hygiene may decrease the need for pharmacotherapy. When using medications, it is best to start with low doses and titrate slowly upwards to a minimum effective dose, and remain cognizant of interactions with the patient's other medications. Start with simple analgesics and move on to anti-inflammatory agents. Because of the increased risk of gastrointestinal bleeding in the elderly, it may be beneficial to initiate preventive treatment early, to avoid frequent abortive treatment with NSAIDs. Tricyclics should be used with caution in older adults due to their anticholinergic side effects. Anticonvulsants may be useful; however, the risks of the various medications should be reviewed from the perspective of use in the elderly.

> ✋ **CAUTION!**
>
> Older age is a "red flag" for secondary causes of headache. Other red flags that may signal a dangerous headache are the presence of systemic signs or illness, neurologic deficits, abrupt onset, and a progression or change in an existing headache.

References

1. Jensen R. Diagnosis, epidemiology, and impact of tension-type headache. *Curr Pain Headache Rep* 2003;**7**(6):455–9.
2. Rasmussen BK, Jensen R, Schroll M, Olesen J. Epidemiology of headache in a general population—a prevalence study. *J Clin Epidemiol* 1991;**44**(11):1147–57.
3. The International Classification of Headache Disorders: 2nd edition. *Cephalalgia* 2004;**24**(Suppl. 1): 9–160.
4. Fumal A, Schoenen J. Tension-type headache: current research and clinical management. *Lancet Neurol* 2008;**7**(1):70–83.
5. Classification and diagnostic criteria for headache disorders, cranial neuralgias and facial pain. Headache Classification Committee of the International Headache Society. *Cephalalgia* 1988;**8**(Suppl. 7):1–96.
6. Jensen R, Rasmussen BK, Pedersen B, Olesen J. Muscle tenderness and pressure pain thresholds in headache. A population study. *Pain* 1993;**52**(2):193–9.
7. Mork H, Ashina M, Bendtsen L, Olesen J, Jensen R. Possible mechanisms of pain perception in patients with episodic tension-type headache. A new experimental model of myofascial pain. *Cephalalgia* 2004;**24**(6): 466–75.
8. Ashina M, Stallknecht B, Bendtsen L, et al. Tender points are not sites of ongoing inflammation—in vivo evidence in patients with chronic tension-type headache. *Cephalalgia* 2003;**23**(2):109–16.
9. Ashina S, Bendtsen L, Ashina M. Pathophysiology of tension-type headache. *Curr Pain Headache Rep* 2005;**9**(6):415–22.
10. Schmidt-Wilcke T, Leinisch E, Straube A, et al. Gray matter decrease in patients with chronic tension type headache. *Neurology* 2005;**65**(9):1483–6.
11. Bendtsen L, Evers S, Linde M, Mitsikostas DD, Sandrini G, Schoenen J. EFNS guideline on the treatment of tension-type headache—report of an EFNS task force. *Eur J Neurol* 2010;**17**(11):1318–25.
12. Lenaerts ME. Pharmacotherapy of tension-type headache (TTH). *Expert Opin Pharmacother* 2009;**10**(8):1261–71.
13. Bendtsen L, Bigal ME, Cerbo R, et al. Guidelines for controlled trials of drugs in tension-type headache: second edition. *Cephalalgia* 2010;**30**(1):1–16.
14. Verhagen AP, Damen L, Berger MY, Passchier J, Koes BW. Lack of benefit for prophylactic drugs of tension-type headache in adults: a systematic review. *Fam Pract* 2010;**27**(2): 151–65.
15. Jensen R, Torelli P. Treatment of tension-type headache. *Handb Clin Neurol* 2010;**97**: 377–86.
16. Lance JW, Curan DA. Treatment of chronic tension headache. *Lancet* 1964;**1**:1236–9.
17. Bendtsen L, Jensen R, Olesen J. A non-selective (amitriptyline), but not a selective

(citalopram), serotonin reuptake inhibitor is effective in the prophylactic treatment of chronic tension-type headache. *J Neurol Neurosurg Psychiatry* 1996;**61**(3):285–90.

18. Ashina S, Bendtsen L, Jensen R. Analgesic effect of amitriptyline in chronic tension-type headache is not directly related to serotonin reuptake inhibition. *Pain.* 2004; **108**(1–2):108–14.

19. Bendtsen L, Jensen R. Amitriptyline reduces myofascial tenderness in patients with chronic tension-type headache. *Cephalalgia* 2000;**20**(6):603–10.

20. Jackson JL, Shimeall W, Sessums L, et al. Tricyclic antidepressants and headaches: systematic review and meta-analysis. *BMJ* 2010;**341**:c5222.

21. Moja PL, Cusi C, Sterzi RR, Canepari C. Selective serotonin re-uptake inhibitors (SSRIs) for preventing migraine and tension-type headaches. *Cochrane Database Syst Rev* 2005;(3):CD002919.

22. Holroyd KA. Treating chronic tension-type headache not responding to amitriptyline hydrochloride with paroxetine hydrochloride: a pilot evaluation. *Headache* 2003;**43**: 999–1004.

23. Bendtsen L, Jensen R. Mirtazapine is effective in the prophylactic treatment of chronic tension-type headache. *Neurology* 2004; **62**(10):1706–11.

24. Bendtsen L, Buchgreitz L, Ashina S, Jensen R. Combination of low-dose mirtazapine and ibuprofen for prophylaxis of chronic tension-type headache. *Eur J Neurol* 2007;**14**(2): 187–93.

25. Zissis NP, Harmoussi S, Vlaikidis N, et al. A randomized, double-blind, placebo-controlled study of venlafaxine XR in out-patients with tension-type headache. *Cephalalgia* 2007;**27**(4):315–24.

26. Bettucci D, Testa L, Calzoni S, Mantegazza P, Viana M, Monaco F. Combination of tizanidine and amitriptyline in the prophylaxis of chronic tension-type headache: evaluation of efficacy and impact on quality of life. *J Headache Pain* 2006;**7**:34–6.

27. Fogelhom R, Murros K. Tizanidine in chronic tension-type headache: a placebo-controlled double-blind cross-over study. *Headache* 1992;**32**:509–13.

28. Saper JR, Lake AE, 3rd, Cantrell DT, Winner PK, White JR. Chronic daily headache prophylaxis with tizanidine: a double-blind, placebo-controlled, multicenter outcome study. *Headache* 2002;**42**(6):470–82.

29. Murros K, Kataja M, Hedman C, et al. Modified-release formulation of tizanidine in chronic tension-type headache. *Headache* 2000;**40**(8):633–7.

30. Mauskop A. Botulinum neurotoxin in the treatment of headache disorders. *Handb Clin Neurol* 2010;**97**:217–32.

31. Porta M. Botulinum toxin type A injections for myofascial pain syndrome and tension-type headache. *Eur J Neurol* 1999;**6**(Suppl. 4):S103–9.

32. Smuts J, Baker MK, Smuts HM. Prophylactic treatment of chronic tension-type headache using botulinum toxin type A. *Eur J Neurol* 1999;**6**(Suppl. 4):S99–102.

33. Gobel H, Lindner V, Krack PK, et al. Treatment of chronic tension-type headache with botulinum toxin. *Cephalalgia* 1999;**19**:455.

34. Silberstein SD, Gobel H, Jensen R, et al. Botulinum toxin type A in the prophylactic treatment of chronic tension-type headache: a multicentre, double-blind, randomized, placebo-controlled, parallel-group study. *Cephalalgia* 2006;**26**(7):790–800.

35. Straube A, Empl M, Ceballos-Baumann A, Tolle T, Stefenelli U, Pfaffenrath V. Pericranial injection of botulinum toxin type A (Dysport) for tension-type headache— a multicentre, double-blind, randomized, placebo-controlled study. *Eur J Neurol* 2008; **15**(3):205–13.

36. Rollnik JD, Tanneberger O, Schubert M, Schneider U, Dengler R. Treatment of tension-type headache with botulinum toxin type A: a double-blind, placebo-controlled study. *Headache* 2000;**40**(4):300–5.

37. Holroyd KA, Nash JM, Pingel JD, Cordingley GE, Jerome A. A comparison of pharmacological (amitriptyline HCL) and nonpharmacological (cognitive-behavioral) therapies for chronic tension headaches. *J Consult Clin Psychol* 1991;**59**(3):387–93.

38. Holroyd KA, O'Donnell FJ, Stensland M, Lipchik GL, Cordingley GE, Carlson BW. Management of chronic tension-type headache with tricyclic antidepressant medication,

stress management therapy, and their combination: a randomized controlled trial. *JAMA* 2001;**285**(17):2208–15.

39. Boline PD, Kassak K, Bronfort G, Nelson C, Anderson AV. Spinal manipulation vs. amitriptyline for the treatment of chronic tension-type headaches: a randomized clinical trial. *J Manipulative Physiol Ther* 1995; **18**(3):148–54.

40. van Ettekoven H, Lucas C. Efficacy of physiotherapy including a craniocervical training programme for tension-type headache; a randomized clinical trial. *Cephalalgia* 2006; **26**(8):983–91.

41. Anderson RE, Sensical C. A comparison of selected osteopathic treatment and relaxation for tension-type headaches. *Headache* 2006;**46**(8):1273–80.

42. Bove G, Nilsson N. Spinal manipulation in the treatment of episodic tension-type headache. *JAMA* 1998;**280**:1576–9.

43. Campbell JK, Penzien DB, Wall EM. Evidenced-based guidelines for migraine treatment: behavioral and physical treatments. Available at: http://www.aan.com/professionals/practice/pdfs/gl0089.pdf (accessed December 16, 2010_.

44. McCrory DC, Penzien DB, Gray RN, Hasselblad V. *Behavioral and Physical Treatments for Tension-type and Cervicogenic Headache.* Prepared for the Foundation for Chiropractic Education and Research; DesMoines, Iowa: 2001, No 2085.

45. Nestoriuc Y, Martin A, Rief W, Andrasik F. Biofeedback treatment for headache disorders: a comprehensive efficacy review. *Appl Psychophysiol Biofeedback* 2008;**33**: 125–40.

46. Verhagen AP, Damen L, Berger MY, Passchier J, Koes BW. Behavioral treatments of chronic tension-type headache in adults: are they beneficial? *CNS Neurosci Ther* 2009;**15**(2): 183–205.

47. Lenssinck ML, Damen L, Verhagen AP, Berger MY, Passchier J, Koes BW. The effectiveness of physiotherapy and manipulation in patients with tension-type headache: a systematic review. *Pain* 2004;**112**(3):381–8.

48. Linde K, Allais G, Brinkhaus B, Manheimer E, Vickers A, White AR. Acupuncture for tension-type headache. *Cochrane Database Syst Rev* 2009;(1):CD007587.

49. Jena S, Witt CM, Brinkhaus B, Wegscheider K, Willich SN. Acupuncture in patients with headache. *Cephalalgia* 2008;**28**(9):969–79.

50. Melchart D, Streng A, Hoppe A, et al. Acupuncture in patients with tension-type headache: randomised controlled trial. *BMJ* 2005;**331**:376–82.

51. Schwartz BS, Stewart WF, Simon D, Lipton RB. Epidemiology of tension-type headache. *JAMA* 1998;**279**(5):381–3.

Part IV

Trigeminal Autonomic Cephalalgias Including Cluster Headache

Diagnosis and Subtypes of Trigeminal Autonomic Cephalalgias

Arne May

Universitäts-Krankenhaus Eppendorf (UKE), Hamburg, Germany

Introduction and classification

Trigeminal autonomic cephalalgia (TAC) is now an accepted clinical term [1], first proposed by Goadsby and Lipton [2] for a group of primary headaches with pain and autonomic involvement in the facial area of the trigeminal nerve. All these headache syndromes have two features in common: they are short-lasting, unilateral, severe headache attacks accompanied by typical autonomic symptoms. The clinical features of the TACs at presentation are highly characteristic when typical. To date, the following syndromes belong to the TACs:

- episodic and chronic cluster headache (see Table 14.2);
- episodic and chronic paroxysmal hemicrania (see Table 14.3);
- short-lasting unilateral neuralgiform headache with conjunctival injection and tearing (SUNCT syndrome) (see Table 14.4).

Why is it important to know and recognize all the different types of TAC, given that they are relatively rare? First of all, these disabling conditions are easy to recognize. Second, in most cases a subclassification is possible and reasonable, as the therapeutic regimen and response differ. For neurologists, despite the diagnostic challenges, the short-lasting primary headaches are important to recognize because of their excellent, but highly selective response to treatment. In 1997, Peter Goadsby and Richard Lipton documented a nosologic analysis and definition of a group of short-lasting headache syndromes [2]. These paroxysmal hemicranias are characterized by frequent, short-lasting attacks of unilateral pain usually in the orbital, supraorbital, or temporal region. The pain is severe and associated with autonomic symptoms such as conjunctival injection, lacrimation, nasal congestion, rhinorrhea, ptosis, and eyelid edema.

Goadsby and Lipton divided these short-lasting primary headache syndromes into those exhibiting marked autonomic activation and those without autonomic activation. Table 14.1 below summarizes a list of short-lasting headaches with autonomic symptoms. The former group comprise chronic and episodic paroxysmal hemicrania, SUNCT syndrome, and cluster headache [1]. These headache syndromes are compared with other short-lasting headache disorders, such as hypnic headache, and a chronic headache syndrome with milder autonomic

Headache, First Edition. Edited by Matthew S. Robbins, Brian M. Grosberg, and Richard B. Lipton.
© 2013 John Wiley & Sons, Ltd. Published 2013 by John Wiley & Sons, Ltd.

features, hemicrania continua. Although not currently classified as a TAC, recent imaging data, however, place hemicrania continua nearer to the TACs [3], and future work will probably do the same with hypnic headache. Idiopathic stabbing headache, cough headache, exertional headache, sexual headache, and trigeminal neuralgia are not part of these syndromes as these short-lasting disorders have no autonomic component [1, 4].

Cluster headache

Cluster headache is certainly the most prominent and most common of the TACs and is considered to be one of the most severe pain syndromes in humans—female patients describe each attack as being worse than childbirth [5]. Despite the fact that a recent health-related quality of life study in 56 patients suggests that cluster headache has a marked functional consequence, even when appropriate treatments are used [6], cluster headache is still underdiagnosed and suboptimally managed in primary care [7].

The diagnosis of cluster headaches is exclusively a clinical task. The International Classification of Headache Disorders [1] uses explicit diagnostic criteria, which are "unambiguous, precise and with as little room for interpretation as possible." The fact that at least 14 synonyms for cluster headache have been used in the past underlines the former lack of etiologic understanding and importance of operational, hence explicit diagnostic criteria for research and clinical practice (see also http://www.i-h-s.org/). Cluster headache, in its typical form, is unmistakable. However, no single instrumental examination is able to define, ensure, or differentiate idiopathic headache syndromes [8]. Nevertheless, in the clinical setting, the use of neuroimaging (CT, MRI, magnetic resonance angiography, etc.) in headache patients varies widely. Electrophysiologic and laboratory examinations including examination of the cerebrospinal fluid are not helpful. For the initial diagnosis and in the case of an abnormal neurologic examination, a cranial CT scan and a cranial MRI should be considered in order to exclude abnormalities of the brain [9, 10]. Particularly in older patients, mass lesions or malformations in the midline have been described as being associated with symptomatic cluster headache [11, 12].

Clinical appearance

The stereotypical attacks may strike up to eight times a day, are relatively short-lived, and are characterized by strictly unilateral severe head pain accompanied by autonomic phenomena [1]. Only in approximately 15% of cases is a shift in side mentioned [13]. In contrast to migraineurs, cluster patients are restless and prefer to pace about or sit and rock back and forth. Some patients will exert pressure on the painful area with a hand over the affected eye and temple. Many will isolate themselves during the attack or leave the house to get into the cold or fresh air, and tend to become aggressive during an attack.

The unilateral autonomic symptoms such as ptosis, miosis, lacrimation, conjunctival injection, rhinorrhea, and nasal congestion occur only during the pain attack, and are ipsilateral to the pain, indicating parasympathetic hyperactivity and sympathetic impairment. In some patients, the signs of sympathetic paralysis (miosis and ptosis) persist indefinitely [14] but intensify during attacks. Sweating and cutaneous blood flow also increase on the painful side, particularly in areas of sympathetic deficit [15]. About 3% of all patients lack autonomic symptoms [16], and in rare cases sympathetic disturbances persist on the previously affected side of the face in patients whose cluster headache has switched sides [17].

It seems that there is no typical form of pain in these syndromes; it may be throbbing, sharp, or stabbing, and this may even vary from bout to bout and indeed between attacks. The pain, although usually involving the ophthalmic division of the trigeminal nerve, may also involve any part of the head as well, and may very occasionally not involve the ophthalmic division at all [18].

Another clinical landmark of the syndrome is the circadian rhythmicity of the relatively short-lived (15–180 minutes) painful attacks. In the episodic form, attacks occur daily for some weeks followed by a period of remission. In the chronic form, attacks occur without significant periods of remission or with annual remission periods shorter than 1 month in duration. On average, a cluster period lasts 6–12 weeks, while remissions can last up to 12 months. While circadian and circannual rhythmicity are characteristic of the episodic variant, little is known on rhythmicity in chronic cluster headache. A recent case report in a secondary chronic cluster headache showed, even in the chronic form, a distinct circadian and semi-circannual rhythmicity over time [19]. Infra- and supra-annual exacerbations over several weeks occurred independently of a 12-month cycle.

> ★ TIPS AND TRICKS
>
> One of the unique hallmarks of cluster headache is its periodicity. Patients often report attacks repeatedly occurring at a stereotyped time of the day or evening, particularly at night. Attacks often coincide with the onset of the rapid eye movement (REM) phase of sleep, although this association is not universal. In clinical practice, cluster headache patients are often advised not to take long naps for the fear that a REM sleep-triggered attack might occur.

Recognition of the periodicity of cluster headache is important for clinicians, as depending on the level of activity of the disease, a preventive medication may be efficient at some times and not at others. This implies that missing effects of preventives should not be misinterpreted as a failure—the prophylactic drugs may well be efficient again when the activity of the disease levels out again. In addition, a "clock-wise" circadian rhythmicity of attacks and an individual circannual preponderance should be considered as a hallmark for cluster headache. Sjaastad [20] suggested that episodic CH and secondary chronic CH have only minute differences and display smooth transitions, while primary chronic CH is a separate entity lacking the criterion of clustered attacks. A primary cluster headache is defined as not being related to any morphologic cause (e.g., the history and physical and neurologic diagnosis are normal), whereas a secondary cluster headache is defined as a headache with all features of a cluster headache but due to another disorder that is a known cause for this headache [1]. Primary chronic cluster headache seems to be more often medically intractable [5]. When chronic cluster headache is unresponsive to medical treatments, it becomes a serious problem, and even surgical options may have to be considered (see Chapter 17).

> ★ TIPS AND TRICKS
>
> The cluster period is another hallmark of episodic cluster headaches, which usually lasts 1–3 months at a time. These periods often exhibit a circannual periodicity, occurring at the same month or season year after year. Cluster periods are often grouped around the spring and autumn, but other patients may have their attack periods occur after the longest (summer solstice) and shortest (winter solstice) days of the year. If a patient has an established circannual periodicity of attacks, it may provide a therapeutic opportunity to start a prophylactic medication seasonally, pre-empting the predicted start of the attack period.

Differential diagnosis

All headache syndromes with short-lasting, unilateral, severe headache attacks and typical autonomic accompanying symptoms (e.g., paroxysmal hemicrania and short-lasting unilateral neuralgiform headache attacks with cranial autonomic features [SUNA]/SUNCT) need to be considered. However, these syndromes differ in the duration, frequency, and rhythmicity of the attacks [2] and in the intensity of the pain and autonomic symptoms, as well as in terms of treatment options (Table 14.1 and Chapter 17]). There are reports of aura in cluster headache [21] and even a "hemiplegic cluster" [22]. There also seem to be some cases of cluster headache without headache [23], cluster headache without autonomic symptoms [16, 24], and even bilateral cases [17]. In a series of well-observed case reports presenting three atypical cluster headaches, the authors suggests that as more cluster patients are seen by headache specialists, new forms of this well-defined primary headache syndrome will be identified (Table 14.2) [25]. However, the concept of trigemino-autonomic syndromes is certainly useful for clinicians seeking a pathophysiologic understanding of the primary *neuro*-vascular headaches and allowing us to place the various treatments aimed at treating or preventing these headaches into context.

The prevalence of cluster headache is approximately 0.1%, and the condition mostly affects

Table 14.1. Comparison of cluster headache with related headache syndromes

	Cluster headache	Paroxysmal hemicrania	SUNCT syndrome	Hemicrania continua	Hypnic headache
Epidemiology					
Gender (male:female)	3:1	1:3	8:1	1:1.8	1:1.8
Prevalence	0.9%	0.02%	Very rare	Rare	Very rare
Age of onset	28–30 years	20–40 years	20–50 years	20–30 years	40–70 years
Pain					
Quality	Boring, throbbing	Boring	Stabbing	Pressing	pulsating
Intensity	Extremely high	High	Moderate to high	Moderate	Moderate
Localization	Periorbital	Orbital, temporal	Orbital, temporal	Unilateral, temporal	Bifrontal, median
Duration of attack	15–120 min	2–45 min	5–250 sec	fluctuating, constant, with superimposed attacks	30–12 min
Frequency of attack	1–8 per day	1–40 per day	3–200 per day		1–2 per day
Autonomic symptoms	++	++	+	(+)	–
Circadian rhythmicity	+	(–)	–	–	+
Alcohol trigger	++	(+)	(–)	–	–
Therapy					
Treatment of choice	*Acute:* 100% oxygen, 15 L/min Intranasal lidocaine Sumatriptan subcutaneously *Preventive:* Verapamil Lithium carbonate Corticosteroids Topiramate Methysergide	*Acute:* Acetylsalicylic acid (naproxen and diclofenac) *Preventive:* Indomethacin	*Acute:* None *Preventive:* Lamotrigine	*Acute:* Diclofenac *Preventive:* Indomethacin	*Acute:* Caffeine *Preventive:* Verapamil Lithium carbonate
Second-line treatment and occasional reports	Valproic acid Ergotamine Melatonin Pizotifen Indomethacin	Corticosteroids Verapamil Acetazolamide Celecoxib	Gabapentin Carbamazepine Valproic acid Topiramate	Beta-cyclodextrin Naproxen Caffeine Corticosteroids	Flunarizine Atenolol Indomethacin

Table 14.2. Diagnostic criteria of cluster headache

A. At least five headache attacks fullfilling criteria B–D
B. Severe or very severe unilateral orbital, supraorbital, and/or temporal headache attacks, which last untreated for 15–180 min. During part (but less than half) of the time course of the cluster headache, attacks may be less severe, less frequent, or of shorter or longer duration
C. The headache is accompanied by at least 1 of the following symptoms ipsilateral to the pain:
   1. Conjunctival injection or lacrimation
   2. Nasal congestion and/or rhinorrhea
   3. Eyelid edema
   4. Forehead and facial sweating
   5. Miosis and/or ptosis
   6. A sense of restlessness and agitation
D. The attacks have a frequency from one every other day to 8 per day
E. History or physical and neurologic examination do not suggest any other disorder, and/or they are ruled out by appropriate investigations

Episodic cluster headache: At least two cluster periods lasting from 7 days to 1 year separated by pain-free periods lasting ≥1 month

Chronic cluster headache: Attacks occur for more than 1 year without remission or with remission <1 month

Probable cluster headache: Attacks fulfilling all but one criteria for cluster headache

Table 14.3. Diagnostic criteria of paroxysmal hemicrania

A. At least 20 attacks fulfilling criteria B–D
B. Attacks of severe unilateral orbital, supraorbital or temporal pain lasting 2–30 min
C. Headache is accompanied by at least one of the following:
   1. Ipisilateral conjunctival injection and/or lacrimation
   2. Ipsilateral nasal congestion and/or rhinorrhea
   3. Ipsilateral eyelid edema
   4. Ipsilateral forehead and facial sweating
   5. Ipsilateral miosis and/or ptosis
D. Attacks have a frequency above 5 per day for more than half the time, although periods with lower frequency may occur
E. Attacks are prevented completely by therapeutic doses of indomethacin
F. Not attributed to another disorder

Melatonin in particular is a marker of the circadian system, and a blunted nocturnal peak melatonin level and complete loss of circadian rhythm have been reported in cluster headache patients [29].

Although for hemicrania continua, it is clear that there is pain between worsenings, this interictal pain feature is now well recognized in the other TACs [18]. In a cohort of 52 patients with SUNCT/SUNA, 22 had interparoxysmal pain [30]. It may be that interparoxysmal pain and allodynia in TACs represent the coexistence of TAC biology with migraine [18]. The clinical importance is that one needs to be aware of these overlaps so as to identify the major presenting problem that requires treatment.

Paroxysmal hemicrania

Clinical appearance

Paroxysmal hemicrania was first described by Sjaastad [31] (for a review see Dodick [32]) and is characterized by relatively short bouts of severe unilateral pain in the orbital and temporal areas (Table 14.3). The typical attack duration is 10–20 minutes and the typical attack frequency is over five per day, but there are reports of between one

men. The attacks occur regularly, and their timing seems to be related to the sleep–wake cycle. Attacks most commonly appear in cluster periods (episodic cluster headache) lasting from a week to several months. The periods are separated by clinical remissions of at least 2 weeks. About 15%–20% of patients suffer from chronic symptoms (without remissions, i.e., chronic cluster headache). The most salient feature of cluster headache is the reported seasonal variation and the clock-wise regularity of the headache attacks [26]. Consequently, a whole range of circadian irregularities in hormone levels have been reported in cluster headache patients [27, 28].

and 40 attacks per day. The age of onset is usually in the 20s, with a 3:1 female:male ratio. Similar to cluster headache, a chronic and an episodic form have been described, and the syndrome also conveys a distinctive temporal pattern [33]. The pain is associated with at least one autonomic symptom, such as ipsilateral conjunctival injection and tearing with nasal congestion and rhinorrhea. Typically described as a problem of women, this seems incorrect from a substantial cohort that has recently been reported [34].

The syndrome is also characterized by its complete response to indomethacin. Although this response is exceptional and long-lasting, patients who develop gastrointestinal problems, notably peptic ulcer disease, on indomethacin are a substantial challenge. Some of these patients have responded to cyclooxygenase II inhibitors, and others seem to benefit from gabapentin.

Differential diagnosis

Again, all headache syndromes with short-lasting, unilateral, severe headache attacks und typical autonomic accompanying symptoms (e.g., cluster headache and SUNCT/SUNA) need to be considered. The hallmarks in differential diagnosis are the duration of the attacks and the complete response to indomethacin.

SUNCT syndrome

Clinical appearance

SUNCT is among the rarest idiopathic headache syndromes and is characterized by an extremely high frequency of attacks (up to 200 attacks a day) with less severe pain but marked autonomic activation during attacks (Table 14.4). It has been

Table 14.4. Diagnostic criteria of SUNCT syndrome

A. At least 5 attacks fulfilling criteria B–D
B. Attacks of unilateral orbital, supraorbital, or temporal stabbing or pulsating pain lasting 5–240 seconds
C. Pain is accompanied by ipsilateral conjunctival injection and lacrimation
D. Attacks occur with a frequency from 3–200 per day
E. Not attributed to another disorder

suggested that the SUNCT syndrome may be a subset of SUNA [30, 35]. Even though there are distinct clinical differences—such as the frequency and duration of attacks, and the different approach to treatment—many of the basic features of SUNCT, such as episodicity, autonomic symptoms, and unilaterality, are shared by other headache types, including cluster headache and chronic paroxysmal hemicrania. This suggests a pathophysiologic similarity to those syndromes, and prompted the suggestion to unify them on clinical grounds as TACs.

The paroxysms of pain usually last between 5 and 250 seconds, although longer, duller interictal pains have been reported. Patients can have up to 30 episodes per hour, although it is more usual to have five or six an hour. The frequency may also vary in bouts. The conjunctival injection seen with SUNCT is often the most prominent autonomic feature, and tearing may also be very obvious.

Differential diagnosis

Its major differential diagnosis is from trigeminal neuralgia. The most important clinical signs pointing towards SUNCT/SUNA and against trigeminal neuralgia include the prominent distribution of pain in the ophthalmic division of the trigeminal nerve, the triggering of attacks from cutaneous stimuli, and a lack of a refractory period for these triggers. In contrast to paroxysmal hemicrania, there is no reproducible effect of indomethacin in SUNCT/SUNA, and, in contrast to cluster headache, no important effect of oxygen, sumatriptan, or verapamil. For practical reasons, indomethacin should be tried in all extremely short-lasting headaches, before lamotrigine or carbamazepine is tried (see Chapter 17).

Hemicrania continua

Hemicrania continua is currently not recognized as belonging to the TAC, but has been grouped into Section 4 of the International Headache Society classification [1]. However, as many clinical signs as well as functional imaging point toward the inclusion of hemicrania continua in the TAC section, it is mentioned here for completeness. Hemicrania continua is characterized by a continuous, unilateral headache that varies in intensity, waxing and waning without disappearing completely [36]. The International Headache Society definition includes the criterion that the headache is side-locked, i.e. does not change sides. Usually, there are mild autonomic symptoms such as lacrimation, conjunctival injection, nasal symptoms, and ptosis/miosis, and the syndrome typically responds well to indomethacin [1].

★ TIPS AND TRICKS

Many authors advocate for an indomethacin trial for any TAC, in case the patient actually has either hemicrania continua with underrating of the continuous background pain, or paroxysmal hemicrania. In particular, paroxysmal hemicrania and cluster headache can have a significant overlap in terms of the frequency and duration of attacks, so patients with a TAC in which the attack frequency is at least five per day and/or the duration of attacks is shorter than 30 minutes should certainly be offered a trial of indomethacin.

Hemicrania continua is sometimes misdiagnosed as half-sided tension-type headache or chronic migraine. Hemicrania continua is probably underdiagnosed, but the absolute requirement for an effect of indomethacin is helpful in distinguishing it from other primary headaches. However, cases with bilateral pain have been reported [18], and, interestingly, typical migraine features of nausea, photophobia, and phonophobia in addition to the ipsilateral cranial autonomic symptoms may arise with exacerbations. In general terms, the background pain of hemicrania continua is more severe than the interparoxysmal pain of the other TACs, and the worsenings in hemicrania continua are longer than the paroxysms of the other TACs [18]. This is particularly important in differentiating hemicrania continua from paroxysmal hemicrania.

⟡ SCIENCE REVISITED

Hemicrania continua is not classified by the International Headache Society as a TAC, but functional imaging has demonstrated overlapping areas of attack-related activation with both TACs and migraine. Positron-emission tomography has revealed activation of the contralateral posterior hypothalamus and ipsilateral dorsal rostral pons and ventrolateral midbrain. In the TACs, hypothalamic activation may be seen ipsilateral to the side of the pain. In migraine, pontine activation may be seen contralateral to the side of the pain. The overlapping functional imaging patterns are not surprising, considering that hemicrania continua has clinical features of both TACs (strictly unilateral pain and prominent ipsilateral autonomic features) and migraine (long-duration attacks and frequent similar associated features such as nausea, photophobia, and phonophobia).

Conclusion

The TACs are a group of primary headache disorders that are distinctly recognizable by their shared features of short attacks featuring strictly unilateral pain in the first division of the trigeminal nerve that are accompanied by ipsilateral cranial autonomic features. Despite being rare in comparison to migraine or tension-type headache, they should not be unrecognized by the practitioner as they have such distinctive clinical manifestations, and each TAC may respond individually to specific therapies.

Acknowledgment

This work was supported by grants from the DFG (MA 1862/2-3) and BMBF (NeuroImageNord).

References

1. The International Classification of Headache Disorders. 2nd edition. Headache Classification Committee of the International Headache Society. *Cephalalgia* 2004;**24**(Suppl. 1): 1–160.

2. Goadsby PJ, Lipton RB. A review of paroxysmal hemicranias, SUNCT syndrome and other short-lasting headaches with autonomic feature, including new cases. *Brain* 1997;**120**(Pt 1):193–209.

3. Matharu MS, Cohen AS, McGonigle DJ, Ward N, Frackowiak RS, Goadsby PJ. Posterior hypothalamic and brainstem activation in hemicrania continua. *Headache* 2004;**44**(8): 747–61.

4. Olesen J, Tfelt-Hansen P, Welch K. *The Headaches* (2nd edn.). Philadelphia, PA: Lippincott Williams & Wilkins; 1999.

5. May A. Cluster headache: pathogenesis, diagnosis, and management. *Lancet* 2005;**366**: 843–55.

6. D'Amico D, Rigamonti A, Solari A, et al. Health-related quality of life in patients with cluster headache during active periods. *Cephalalgia* 2002;**22**(10):818–21.

7. Geweke LO. Misdiagnosis of cluster headache. *Curr Pain Headache Rep* 2002;**6**(1):76–82.

8. Sandrini G, Friberg L, Janig W, et al. Neurophysiological tests and neuroimaging procedures in non-acute headache: guidelines and recommendations. *Eur J Neurol* 2004;**11**(4): 217–24.

9. Favier I, Haan J, Ferrari MD. Cluster headache: to scan or not to scan. *Curr Pain Headache Rep* 2008;**12**(2):128–31.

10. Favier I, van Vliet JA, Roon KI, et al. Trigeminal autonomic cephalalgias due to structural lesions: a review of 31 cases. *Arch Neurol* 2007;**64**(1):25–31.

11. Hannerz J. A case of parasellar meningioma mimicking cluster headache. *Cephalalgia* 1989;**9**(4):265–9.

12. Purdy RA, Kirby S. Headaches and brain tumors. *Neurol Clin* 2004;**22**(1):39–53.

13. Manzoni GC, Terzano MG, Bono G, Micieli G, Martucci N, Nappi G. Cluster headache—clinical findings in 180 patients. *Cephalalgia* 1983;**3**(1):21–30.

14. Drummond PD. Dysfunction of the sympathetic nervous system in cluster headache. *Cephalalgia* 1988;**8**(3):181–6.

15. Drummond PD. Sweating and vascular responses in the face: normal regulation and dysfunction in migraine, cluster headache and harlequin syndrome. *Clin Auton Res* 1994;**4**(5):273–85.

16. Ekbom K. Evaluation of clinical criteria for cluster headache with special reference to the classification of the International Headache Society. *Cephalalgia* 1990;**10**(4): 195–7.

17. Sjaastad O (ed.). *Cluster Headache Syndrome.* London: WB Saunders; 1992.

18. Goadsby PJ, Cittadini E, Burns B, Cohen AS. Trigeminal autonomic cephalalgias: diagnostic and therapeutic developments. *Curr Opin Neurol* 2008;**21**(3):323–30.

19. Jurgens TP, Koch HJ, May A. Ten years of chronic cluster—attacks still cluster. *Cephalalgia* 2010;**30**(9):1123–6.

20. Sjaastad O. *Cluster Headache Syndrome.* London: WB. Saunders; 1992.

21. Silberstein SD, Niknam R, Rozen TD, Young WB. Cluster headache with aura. *Neurology* 2000;**54**(1):219–21.

22. Siow HC, Young WB, Peres MF, Rozen TD, Silberstein SD. Hemiplegic cluster. *Headache* 2002;**42**(2):136–9.

23. Leone M, Rigamonti A, Bussone G. Cluster headache sine headache: two new cases in one family. *Cephalalgia* 2002;**22**(1): 12–4.

24. Vigl M, Zebenholzer K, Wessely P. Cluster headache without autonomic symptoms? *Cephalalgia* 2001;**21**(9):926–7.

25. Rozen TD. Atypical presentations of cluster headache. *Cephalalgia* 2002;**22**(9):725–9.

26. Waldenlind E, Drummond PD. Synthesis of cluster headache pathophysiology. In Olesen J, Tfelt Hansen P, Welch KM (eds.). *The Headaches.* Philadelphia, PA: Lippincott Williams & Wilkins; 1999.

27. Leone M, Attanasio A, Croci D, et al. Neuroendocrinology of cluster headache. *Ital J Neurol Sci* 1999;**20**(7):S18–20.

28. Goadsby PJ. Pathophysiology of cluster headache: a trigeminal autonomic cephalalgia. *Lancet Neurol* 2002;**1**(4):251–7.

29. Waldenlind E, Gustafsson SA, Ekbom K, Wetterberg L. Circadian secretion of cortisol and melatonin in cluster headache during active cluster periods and remission. *J Neurol Neurosurg Psychiatry* 1987;**50**:207–13.

30. Cohen A, Matharu M, Goadsby P. Revisiting the International Headache Society Criteria for SUNCT and SUNA: a case series of 52 patients. *Cephalalgia* 2005;**25**:1194.

31. Sjaastad O, Dale I. Evidence for a new, treatable headache entity. *Headache* 1974;**14**(2): 105–8.

32. Dodick DW. Indomethacin-responsive headache syndromes. *Curr Pain Headache Rep* 2004;**8**(1):19–26.

33. Sjaastad O, Apfelbaum R, Caskey W, et al. Chronic paroxysmal hemicrania (CPH). The clinical manifestations. A review. *Ups J Med Sci Suppl* 1980;**31**:27–33.

34. Cittadini E, Matharu MS, Goadsby PJ. Paroxysmal hemicrania: a prospective clinical study of 31 cases. *Brain* 2008;**131**(Pt 4): 1142–55.

35. Cohen AS, Matharu MS, Goadsby PJ. Short-lasting unilateral neuralgiform headache attacks with conjunctival injection and tearing (SUNCT) or cranial autonomic features (SUNA) –a prospective clinical study of SUNCT and SUNA. *Brain* 2006;**129**(Pt 10): 2746–60.

36. Sjaastad O, Spierings EL. "Hemicrania continua": another headache absolutely responsive to indomethacin. *Cephalalgia* 1984; **4**(1):65–70.

Epidemiology, Progression, Prognosis, and Comorbidity of Trigeminal Autonomic Cephalalgias

Matthew S. Robbins[1] and Jessica Ailani[2]

[1]Albert Einstein College of Medicine, Bronx, NY, USA
[2]Georgetown University Hospital, Washington, DC, USA

Introduction

The trigeminal autonomic cephalalgias (TACs) are a group of three distinctive primary headache disorders that all feature repetitive, short-duration attacks of unilateral head pain in the distribution of the first division of the trigeminal nerve, and manifest accompanying ipsilateral cranial autonomic symptoms (lacrimation, conjunctival injection, rhinorrhea, nasal congestion, ptosis, or miosis) [1]. Cluster headache (CH) is the best characterized TAC, but the other two disorders, paroxysmal hemicrania (PH) and short-lasting unilateral neuralgiform headache attacks with conjunctival injection and tearing (SUNCT), are important clinical and epidemiologic entities as well. Table 15.1 compares and contrasts their basic epidemiologic profiles.

Even when taken together, the TACs are a rare group of headache disorders in any population. In this chapter, we will briefly describe the clinical features of CH, PH, and SUNCT, and then review in greater detail their epidemiologic characteristics, including comorbidity and progression.

Cluster headache

Overview of the clinical disorder

CH is a notoriously painful primary headache disorder, with short, severe episodes of unilateral head pain often centered around the orbit or temple, and with prominent ipsilateral signs of cranial parasympathetic activation. The attacks are typically accompanied by a prominent sense of restlessness or agitation. CH attacks have the longest duration of the TACs, ranging from 15–180 minutes, with the majority of patients having headache lasting 60 minutes. However, they also have the lowest attack frequency, ranging from one attack on alternate days to eight daily attacks [1]. Cluster attacks can be stereotyped in not only their attack characteristics, but also their timing, occurring at the same time of day, and more often during the rapid eye movement phase of sleep (60–90 minutes after falling asleep) [2].

In most patients, CH attacks typically group together during an attack period or cycle, which often lasts between 2 and 12 weeks. In 90% of patients with CH, remission periods occur between cluster cycles. This group of patients is

Headache, First Edition. Edited by Matthew S. Robbins, Brian M. Grosberg, and Richard B. Lipton.

Table 15.1. Epidemiologic profile of the TACs

Feature	CH	PH	SUNCT/SUNA
1-year prevalence	0.02%–0.1% (several studies)	0.05% (one study)	0.1% (one study)
1-year incidence	0.002%–0.01%	Unknown	Unknown
Female:male	1:4.3	1.6–2.4:1	1.5:1 (SUNCT) 2:1 (SUNA)
Peak age of onset	Third decade	Third to fourth decades	Fifth decade
Episodic:chronic subform	6–9:1	1:4	1:1–9 (SUNCT) Nearly all chronic (SUNA)

Table 15.2. One-year prevalence and incidence studies of CH

Reference	Prevalence or Incidence	Region	Number of subjects surveyed	CH cases per 100,000 (95% confidence interval)
[4]	Prevalence	Malaysia	595	0 (0–618)
[5]	Prevalence	Ethiopia	15,500	32 (10–75)
[6]	Prevalence	Germany	3,336	119 (3–238)
[7]	Prevalence	Germany	1,312	15 (10–550)
[8]	Incidence	USA	6,476	9.8 (6.0–13.6)
[9]	Incidence	USA	9,837	2.07 (0.01–4.1)
[10]	Incidence	Italy	26,628	2.5 (1.14–4.75)

deemed to have episodic CH (ECH), in which remission periods of 1 or more months occur on an annual basis. The 10% of CH patients who lack annual remission periods or experience remissions for less than 1 month annually are categorized as having chronic CH (CCH), which can be an intractable condition therapeutically [1].

Epidemiology

Although it is the most common TAC, CH is quite rare when compared to the more prevalent primary headache disorders of migraine and tension-type headache.

Prevalence and incidence

Overall, the lifetime prevalence of CH translates to one individual in 1000 having the disorder. A recent meta-analysis pooling population studies from the USA, Italy, Germany, Sweden, Norway, Portugal, Denmark, Greece, Malaysia, and Ethiopia revealed a lifetime prevalence of 124 per 100,000 persons and a 1-year prevalence of 53 per 100,000 persons [3]. One-year prevalence studies

of CH are rare [4, 5, 6, 7], and are summarized in Table 15.2. The practical utility of ascertaining the 1-year prevalence of CH may be limited by the fact that many patients with CH experience remission periods lasting over a year.

The incidence of CH has been captured by only three studies [8, 9, 10] (Table 15.2). Two of these studies were performed at the Mayo Clinic, with one of the same lead investigators and using identical methodology [8, 9]. Interestingly, the 1-year incidence of CH in Olmstead County, Minnesota, declined significantly, from 9.8 in 1980 to 2.07 in 1990 per 100,000 subjects. One postulated explanation is the population decline in smoking, with may be a risk factor for CH.

Gender

Unlike the majority of primary headache disorders, CH is a male-predominant disorder, with an overall male:female ratio in pooled prevalence studies of 4.3:1. The male:female ratio of CCH is 15:1, significantly higher than the 3.8:1 ratio encountered in ECH [3].

★ TIPS AND TRICKS

CH has traditionally been thought to be an overwhelmingly male-predominant disorder, but historically the initially described steep male:female ratio has dwindled over the decades, from 6.2:1 in the 1960s to 2.1:1 in the 1990s. This decrease could be related to a growing prevalence of CH among women because of changing lifestyle factors such as smoking, or a lack of reasonable ascertainment of CH among women in the past because of bias or decreased healthcare-seeking behavior [11]. In addition, women with CH are more likely to have migrainous symptoms such as nausea, vomiting, photophobia, and phonophobia with their attacks, which may also lead the practitioner to falsely recognize the condition as migraine [12].

Age

The older, clinic-based studies suggest that the onset of CH most commonly occurs between age 26 and 30 years [13]. However, of the three incidence studies, only one captured new male and female cases [8]. In this study, the peak incidence was age 40–49 years in men and 60–69 years in women. The earlier age of onset in CH patients seen in tertiary care may reflect an earlier selective consultation of more severe cases. On the whole, onset of CH seems to most commonly occur in middle age, although numerous childhood-onset cases have been reported, including patients presenting as young as age 1–3 years [14, 15, 16, 17]. Elderly patients can also occasionally present with CH, even in their eighth [18], ninth [19], and 10th [20] decades.

Race and geography

No clear racial or geographical disparities in prevalence of CH are known, as too few studies have addressed either these demographics, and population-based studies of CH have largely been restricted to white populations within Europe and the USA.

Comorbidity

Little is known regarding comorbidity of CH outside large case series from tertiary care centers. Obstructive sleep apnea seems to be more common in CH patients, and in a subset of these patients treatment of the sleep disorder has beneficial effects on their CH [21]. Peptic ulcers and coronary artery disease may occur more commonly in patients with CH, but this comorbidity may be simply because of the high prevalence of cigarette smoking in the CH population, [11] since as many as 72% of CH patients are active smokers and 14% are prior smokers [22].

Studies regarding the psychiatric comorbidity of CH have been somewhat inconsistent. One small single-center study documented an anxiety disorder in 23.8% of patients (14.3% generalized anxiety disorder and 9.5% panic disorder), and no patient had a mood disorder [23]. Personality studies of CH have shown that CH patients are more prone to anxiety, hypochondriasis, and hysteria, but not depression [24]. In a large survey of CCH patients in France, 75.7% were diagnosed with an anxiety disorder and 43.0% were diagnosed with depression [25]. However, one tertiary care study found that moderate to severe anxiety or depression in ECH and CCH patients was equally uncommon, and ECH and CCH patients did not significantly differ in their anxiety or depression profiles [26].

Regarding coexisting primary headache disorders, migraine may not actually be a true comorbidity, with a lower than expected prevalence of migraine in CH patients compared to the general population [27, 28], although no recent study has addressed this relationship. Other TACs can rarely coexist with CH, and CH can even evolve to another TAC spectrum disorder [29]. Like other primary headache disorders, CH patients commonly have primary stabbing headache as well [30].

Progression

A minority of patients with CH develop CCH, which can begin unremitting at the onset (CCHU) or evolve in patients who previously had ECH (CCHE). Overall, the ratio of ECH to CCH patients among prevalence studies is 6:1 [3]. Unfortunately, no population-based study has assessed the risk factors for progression of CH, and all data reported so far have been derived from tertiary care centers.

In one large Italian cohort, over a 10-year period ECH in 13% of patients evolved to CCH.

The risk factors for this progression were a longer history of CH (>20 years) and a later age of onset. About one-third of baseline CCH patients remitted to ECH over the 10-year period [31]. Patients who have more than one period of CH annually and short remission periods may also be at risk [32].

Despite the strikingly higher male:female ratio of CCH in comparison to ECH, no longitudinal study has confirmed that male gender is a risk factor for CH progression. In the 10-year study, too few female cases were captured to demonstrate a significant predictive effect by male gender [31]. Cigarette smoking, alcohol intake, and head trauma still remain unproven factors in CH progression [33].

★ TIPS AND TRICKS

Medication overuse is a notorious factor in migraine progression from its episodic to its chronic form. However, it is not a commonly reported phenomenon in patients with CH. In a small series of CH patients, 88% of those who developed medication overuse headache had a personal and/or family history of migraine. The medication overuse headache was distinctly separate from their CH attacks, did not necessarily contribute to any increased frequency of CH attacks, and resembled chronic daily headache of long duration [34].

Paroxysmal hemicrania

Overview of the clinical disorder

PH is an uncommon TAC first described by Sjaastad and Dale in 1974 [35]. It is a disorder characterized by repetitive attacks of severe unilateral head pain of short duration, accompanied by very prominent ipsilateral cranial autonomic features. The attacks of PH are shorter than those of CH but longer than those of SUNCT. The most distinctive feature of PH is its definitive response to the nonsteroidal anti-inflammatory agent indomethacin, unlike CH and SUNCT. PH can be divided into chronic PH (CPH), an unremitting form with a protracted course, and episodic PH (EPH), where painful attack periods are inter-spersed with temporary or permanent remission periods [1].

Epidemiology

The epidemiology of PH is difficult to capture not only because of the rarity of the disorder, but also because a fundamental requirement of the diagnostic criteria is its complete response to indomethacin, and any condition defined by its therapy may evade prevalence studies. Therefore, nearly all epidemiologic information generated to date derives from clinic-based, and not population-based, studies (Table 15.3).

Prevalence and incidence

The population prevalence and incidence of PH are not known. Only one population-based study has potentially captured a patient with PH in its prevalence data. Among 1838 individuals aged 18–65 years in Norway, one potential case was encountered, although a trial of indomethacin was not attempted, and the patient shared some features of neck–tongue syndrome [36]. However, assuming this patient did in fact have PH, the prevalence would be 0.05%. In the same cohort, the prevalence of CH was 0.3%, consistent with other studies of CH previously discussed [37].

Gender

Two of the three large clinical series have found a gender prevalence that is slightly skewed towards women, with a female:male ratio of 1.6–2.4:1 [38, 39]. However, the most recent series of 31 patients with PH showed a nearly equal gender ratio [40]. In one series of children with PH, five of the eight patients were male [41].

Age

The mean age of PH onset seems to be consistent across studies, ranging from 34 to 41 years [38, 39, 40]. The median onset may be slightly younger, in the third decade of life, and EPH may begin earlier than CPH [38]. A wide range of onset age has been reported, from 1 [42] to 81 [38] years, and one small series of eight children with PH has been described [41].

Race and geography

No known racial or geographic predilections for PH are known. The disorder has been reported to

Table 15.3. Patient characteristics in the clinical series of CPH

Reference	Antonaci and Sjaastad, 1989 [38]	Boes and Dodick, 2002 [39]	Cittadini et al., 2008 [40]
Cohort	Literature review + new cases	Single center	Single center
n	84	74	31
Years conducted	1974–1989	1976–1996	1995–2007
Female:male	2.4:1	1.6:1	1:1.2
Median age of onset (years)	21–30	NR	NR
Mean age of onset (years)	34.1	41	37
Mean age of diagnosis (years)	47.4	NR	NR
Age range (years)	11–81	6–75	4–68
Family history	Migraine 24% CH 1%	Migraine 15% Unclassified 4% CH 1% Trigeminal neuralgia 1%	Migraine and/or unclassified 58% PH 3%
Other headache disorders	Migraine 4%	Migraine 15% Tension-type headache 7% Unclassified 5%	Migraine 51%
Prior head or neck trauma	22%	23%	6%
Remission experienced	42%	12%	39%

CPH, chronic paroxysmal hemicrania; NR, not reported.

occur in patients in the USA [39], Europe [38, 40], India [43], Brazil [44], and South Africa [45].

Comorbidity

Little is known about the comorbidity of PH. In Antonaci and Sjaastad's large series, many coexisting medical and neurologic disorders were listed, but no particular disorder was noted to occur frequently [38]. No known psychiatric comorbidity has yet been identified, although in the pediatric series impairment of daily activities from PH was very high [41].

Other primary headache disorders frequently coexist in patients with PH. The most recent study demonstrated coexisting migraine in half of all PH sufferers [40], but tension-type headache, CH, and even trigeminal neuralgia may also be present [38, 39, 40]. Three of the eight children in the pediatric PH series had coexisting tension-type headache [41].

⚠ CAUTION!

Coexisting headache disorders can occur in patients with PH, and conversely PH can occur in patients with other primary headache disorders, including TACs. The practitioner should have a low threshold for initiating an indomethacin trial in a patient with CH when the attacks become more frequent or shorter in duration, or autonomic symptoms become more prominent. PH can occasionally evolve gradually from CH or even occur *de novo* and abruptly in CH patients [29].

Progression

Unlike other primary headache disorders such as migraine, tension-type headache, and CH, PH exists much more often in its chronic subform, where attacks occur for over 1 year without remission, or where remissions are shorter than 1 month at a time [1]. CPH seems to be present in 80% of all PH patients, whereas the remaining 20% have EPH [38, 40]. Although EPH is very uncommon, remission periods can still be experienced by 12%–42% of patients at some point in the course of the condition [38, 39, 40].

About 60% of PH patients have CPH at the onset [38, 40]. Among those patients that have EPH at the onset, about half will transition to CPH at some point in their clinical course, whereas the remainder will stay in the remitting stage. No known risk factors or differences between EPH patients progressing to CPH versus those remaining as EPH are known; the two groups seem to have a similar female:male ratio, age of disease onset, attack frequency, and attack duration. The transition from EPH to CPH is not usually abrupt, but occurs in a gradual fashion [38]. CPH tends to cease completely more often than remit to EPH; such a remission is a rare clinical scenario [40].

Short-lasting unilateral neuralgiform headache attacks with conjunctival injection and tearing

Overview of the clinical disorder

SUNCT is another rare TAC that was also first described by Sjaastad and colleagues in the late 1970s [46]. Like CH and PH, unilateral pain is centered in the first division of the trigeminal nerve, but the ipsilateral cranial autonomic symptoms are more prominent, the attacks are ultrashort and more frequent, and there is no consistent therapeutic benefit from indomethacin use. As the name implies, the autonomic symptoms are mainly conjunctival injection and lacrimation. When only one of these symptoms or other cranial autonomic symptoms are instead present, the disorder is classified as short-lasting unilateral neuralgiform headache attacks with cranial autonomic symptoms (SUNA) [1]. Therefore, SUNCT may be considered to be a subset of SUNA [1, 47].

Epidemiology

Like PH, SUNCT is an extremely rare primary headache disorder, with most epidemiologic data derived from reviews of previously reported cases and one large tertiary care single-center case series (Table 15.4) [47, 48].

Prevalence and incidence

The prevalence and incidence of SUNCT are unknown, although a clue comes from the same population-based study in Norway. Two women and no men with suspected SUNCT were identified among 1838 individuals aged 18–65 years, giving a prevalence of 0.1% [36]. The prevalence was twice that of PH in this study, and many practitioners also feel that, at least in tertiary care clinical practice, SUNCT is more common than PH [40, 47, 49]. SUNCT seems to comprise 83% of all SUNA cases [47].

Table 15.4. Patient characteristics in the largest SUNCT/SUNA review and clinical series

Reference	Matharu et al., 2003 [48]	Cohen et al., 2006 [47]	
Cohort	Literature review	Single center	
n	50	52	
Years conducted	1978–2003	1995–2005	
Subtype	All SUNCT	43 SUNCT	9 SUNA
Female:male	1:1.3	1.9:1	0.5:1
Mean age of onset (years)	48	48	44
Age of onset (years)	10–77	19–75	2–28
Mean age of onset to diagnosis (age)	NR	6.7	7.1
Other headache disorders	NR	Migraine 35%	Migraine 67%
Remission experienced	86%	65%	11%

NR, not reported.

Gender

The aggregate of SUNCT cases reported up until the late 1990s demonstrated a significant male predominance, with a male:female ratio of 4.3:1 [50]. However, the most recent large series of SUNCT/SUNA countered this finding, with a female:male ratio of 1.5:1. SUNCT (excluding SUNA) specifically had an even higher female:male ratio, at 1.9:1. On the other hand, the small sample of SUNA patients (excluding SUNCT) demonstrated a 2:1 female:male ratio [47].

Age

SUNCT seems to have its onset most commonly in the fifth decade of life, and 68% of patients experience the onset of the disorder between age 35 and 65 years [47, 48]. Patients as young as 5 [51] and as old as 88 [52] years have been reported to experience SUNCT. It is common for patients to remain undiagnosed for years after their symptom onset, and in the elderly it may be mistaken for trigeminal neuralgia [47].

✋ CAUTION!

SUNCT is commonly reported to be misdiagnosed as trigeminal neuralgia [47], and this may be particularly problematic in elderly individuals [53]. Elderly patients previously diagnosed with trigeminal neuralgia should always be queried for associated signs of ipsilateral cranial autonomic activation. In addition, SUNCT should be considered in elderly patients with trigeminal neuralgia who are unresponsive to first-line agents such as carbamazepine.

Race and geography

Although patients with SUNCT have been reported from a variety of continents [47, 48], no known racial or geographic predilection has been identified.

Comorbidity

No known specific comorbid medical or psychiatric illnesses are known to occur in patients with SUNCT. Patients with SUNA seem to have coexisting migraine more often than SUNCT patients [47].

Progression

Although a major literature review in 2003 suggested that SUNCT is more often an episodic disorder with long remission periods [48], the recent large case series suggests that, like PH, SUNCT and SUNA are predominantly chronic disorders. In the largest series, all of the patients with SUNA had chronic SUNA at the onset, only one of whom remitted to an episodic form. At the onset of the disorder, 47% of SUNCT patients had the chronic form, and 53% had the episodic form. Of the patients starting out with episodic SUNCT, 43% evolved to chronic SUNCT, with a mean time from onset to reach the chronic form of 8.4 years. Of the patients starting out with chronic SUNCT, only 15% remitted to the episodic form [47]. No known differences between these SUNCT patients with different temporal profiles were reported.

Conclusion

The TACs are an uncommon but distinctive group of primary headache disorders that have heterogeneous epidemiologic profiles quite unlike those of migraine and tension-type headache. Population-based studies are uncommon and mostly restricted to CH, the most common TAC. Unlike PH and SUNCT, the majority of CH patients have the episodic rather than chronic subform, and the prognosis of the TACs is variable but largely unknown. Future population-based or multicenter studies for these rare disorders will be required to more definitively characterize their epidemiology.

References

1. The International Classification of Headache Disorders: 2nd edition. *Cephalalgia* 2004; **24**(Suppl. 1):9–160.
2. Halker R, Vargas B, Dodick DW. Cluster headache: diagnosis and treatment. *Semin Neurol* 2010;**30**(2):175–85.
3. Fischera M, Marziniak M, Gralow I, Evers S. The incidence and prevalence of cluster headache: a meta-analysis of population-based studies. *Cephalalgia* 2008;**28**(6):614–8.
4. Alders EE, Hentzen A, Tan CT. A community-based prevalence study on headache in Malaysia. *Headache* 1996;**36**(6):379–84.

5. Tekle Haimanot R, Seraw B, Forsgren L, Ekbom K, Ekstedt J. Migraine, chronic tension-type headache, and cluster headache in an Ethiopian rural community. *Cephalalgia* 1995;**15**(6):482–8.

6. Katsarava Z, Obermann M, Yoon MS, et al. Prevalence of cluster headache in a population-based sample in Germany. *Cephalalgia* 2007;**27**(9):1014–9.

7. Evers S, Fischera M, May A, Berger K. Prevalence of cluster headache in Germany: results of the epidemiological DMKG study. *J Neurol Neurosurg Psychiatry* 2007;**78**(11):1289–90.

8. Swanson JW, Yanagihara T, Stang PE, et al. Incidence of cluster headaches: a population-based study in Olmsted County, Minnesota. *Neurology* 1994;**44**(3 Pt 1):433–7.

9. Black DF, Swanson JW, Stang PE. Decreasing incidence of cluster headache: a population-based study in Olmsted County, Minnesota. *Headache* 2005;**45**(3):220–3.

10. Tonon C, Guttmann S, Volpini M, Naccarato S, Cortelli P, D'Alessandro R. Prevalence and incidence of cluster headache in the Republic of San Marino. *Neurology* 2002;**58**(9):1407–9.

11. Manzoni GC. Gender ratio of cluster headache over the years: a possible role of changes in lifestyle. *Cephalalgia* 1998;**18**(3):138–42.

12. Rozen TD, Niknam RM, Shechter AL, Young WB, Silberstein SD. Cluster headache in women: clinical characteristics and comparison with cluster headache in men. *J Neurol Neurosurg Psychiatry* 2001;**70**(5):613–7.

13. Matharu MS, Goadsby PJ. Trigeminal autonomic cephalalgias: diagnosis and management. In Silberstein SD, Lipton RB, Dodick DW (eds.), *Wolff's Headache and Other Head Pain* (8th edn.). New York: Oxford University Press USA; 2008: pp. 379–430.

14. Terzano MG, Manzoni GC, Maione R. Cluster headache in one year old infant? *Headache* 1981;**21**(6):255–6.

15. Manzoni GC. Cluster headache and lifestyle: remarks on a population of 374 male patients. *Cephalalgia* 1999;**19**(2):88–94.

16. Garrido C, Tuna A, Ramos S, Temudo T. [Cluster headache in a 3 year old child]. *Rev Neurol* 2001 2001;**33**(8):732–5.

17. Kacinski M, Nowak A, Kroczka S, Gergont A. Cluster headache in 2-year-old Polish girl. *Cephalalgia* 2009;**29**(10):1091–4.

18. Evers S, Frese A, Majewski A, Albrecht O, Husstedt IW. Age of onset in cluster headache: the clinical spectrum (three case reports). *Cephalalgia* 2002;**22**(2):160–2.

19. Fischera M, Anneken K, Evers S. Old age of onset in cluster-headache patients. *Headache* 2005;**45**(5):615.

20. Seidler S, Marthol H, Pawlowski M, Heckmann JG. Cluster headache in a ninety-one-year-old woman. *Headache* 2006;**46**(1):179–80.

21. Graff-Radford SB, Teruel A. Cluster headache and obstructive sleep apnea: are they related disorders? *Curr Pain Headache Rep* 2009;**13**(2):160–3.

22. Schurks M, Diener HC. Cluster headache and lifestyle habits. *Curr Pain Headache Rep* 2008;**12**(2):115–21.

23. Jorge R, Leston J, Arndt S, Robinson R. Cluster headaches: association with anxiety disorders and memory deficits. *Neurology* 1999;**53**(3):543–7.

24. Evers S. Cognitive processing in cluster headache. *Curr Pain Headache Rep* 2005;**9**(2):109–12.

25. Donnet A, Lanteri-Minet M, Guegan-Massardier E, et al. Chronic cluster headache: a French clinical descriptive study. *J Neurol Neurosurg Psychiatry* 2007;**78**(12):1354–8.

26. Robbins MS, Bronheim R, Lipton RB, et al. Depression and anxiety in episodic and chronic cluster headache. *Headache* 2011;**51**(Suppl. 1):24.

27. Ekbom K. Migraine in patients with cluster headache. *Headache* 1974;**14**(2):69–72.

28. Solomon S, Cappa KG. The time relationships of migraine and cluster headache when occurring in the same patient. *Headache* 1986;**26**(10):500–2.

29. Robbins M, Grosberg B, Lipton R. Coexisting trigeminal autonomic cephalalgias and hemicrania continua. *Headache* 2010;**50**(3):489–96.

30. Dodick D. Indomethacin-responsive headache syndromes. *Curr Pain Headache Rep* 2004;**8**(1):19–26.

31. Manzoni GC, Micieli G, Granella F, Tassorelli C, Zanferrari C, Cavallini A. Cluster

headache—course over ten years in 189 patients. *Cephalalgia* 1991;**11**(4):169–74.

32. Torelli P, Cologno D, Cademartiri C, Manzoni GC. Possible predictive factors in the evolution of episodic to chronic cluster headache. *Headache* 2000;**40**(10):798–808.

33. Torelli P, Manzoni GC. What predicts evolution from episodic to chronic cluster headache? *Curr Pain Headache Rep* 2002;**6**(1): 65–70.

34. Paemeleire K, Bahra A, Evers S, Matharu MS, Goadsby PJ. Medication-overuse headache in patients with cluster headache. *Neurology* 2006;**67**(1):109–13.

35. Sjaastad O, Dale I. A new (?) Clinical headache entity "chronic paroxysmal hemicrania" 2. *Acta Neurol Scand* 1976;**54**(2):140–59.

36. Sjaastad O, Bakketeig L. The rare, unilateral headaches. Vågå study of headache epidemiology. *J Headache Pain* 2007;**8**(1):19–27.

37. Sjaastad O, Bakketeig L. Cluster headache prevalence. Vågå study of headache epidemiology. *Cephalalgia* 2003;**23**(7):528–33.

38. Antonaci F, Sjaastad O. Chronic paroxysmal hemicrania (CPH): a review of the clinical manifestations. *Headache* 1989;**29**(10): 648–56.

39. Boes C, Dodick D. Refining the clinical spectrum of chronic paroxysmal hemicrania: a review of 74 patients. *Headache* 2002;**42**(8): 699–708.

40. Cittadini E, Matharu M, Goadsby P. Paroxysmal hemicrania: a prospective clinical study of 31 cases. *Brain* 2008;**131**(Pt 4): 1142–55.

41. Blankenburg M, Hechler T, Dubbel G, Wamsler C, Zernikow B. Paroxysmal hemicrania in children—symptoms, diagnostic criteria, therapy and outcome. *Cephalalgia* 2009; **29**(8):873–82.

42. de Almeida D, Cunali P, Santos H, Brioschi M, Prandini M. Chronic paroxysmal hemicrania in early childhood: case report. *Cephalalgia* 2004;**24**(7):608–9.

43. Chakravarty A, Mukherjee A, Roy D. Trigeminal autonomic cephalalgias and variants: clinical profile in Indian patients. *Cephalalgia* 2004;**24**(10):859–66.

44. Veloso G, Kaup A, Peres M, Zukerman E. Episodic paroxysmal hemicrania with seasonal variation: case report and the EPH-cluster headache continuum hypothesis. *Arq Neuropsiquiatr* 2001;**59**(4):944–7.

45. Joubert J, Powell D, Djikowski J. Chronic paroxysmal hemicrania in a South African black. A case report. *Cephalalgia* 1987;**7**(3):193–6.

46. Sjaastad O, Russell D, Horven I, Bunaes U. Multiple neuralgiform unilateral headache attacks associated with conjunctival injection and appearing in clusters. A nosological problem. *Proc Scand Migraine Soc* 1978:31.

47. Cohen A, Matharu M, Goadsby P. Short-lasting unilateral neuralgiform headache attacks with conjunctival injection and tearing (SUNCT) or cranial autonomic features (SUNA)—a prospective clinical study of SUNCT and SUNA. *Brain* 2006;**129**(Pt 10): 2746–60.

48. Matharu M, Cohen A, Boes C, Goadsby P. Short-lasting unilateral neuralgiform headache with conjunctival injection and tearing syndrome: a review. *Curr Pain Headache Rep* 2003;**7**(4):308–18.

49. Larner A. Trigeminal autonomic cephalalgias: frequency in a general neurology clinic setting. *J Headache Pain* 2008;**9**(5):325–6.

50. Pareja J, Sjaastad O. SUNCT syndrome. A clinical review. *Headache* 1997;**37**(4):195–202.

51. Sékhara T, Pelc K, Mewasingh L, Boucquey D, Dan B. Pediatric SUNCT Syndrome. *Pediatr Neurol* 2005;**33**(3):206–7.

52. Vikelis M, Xifaras M, Mitsikostas D. SUNCT syndrome in the elderly. *Cephalalgia* 2005; **25**(11):1091–2.

53. Cohen A, Matharu M, Goadsby P. SUNCT syndrome in the elderly. *Cephalalgia* 2004; **24**(6):508–9.

Pathophysiology and Genetics of Trigeminal Autonomic Cephalalgias

Peter J. Goadsby

University of California, San Francisco, San Francisco, CA, USA

Introduction

The trigeminal autonomic cephalalgias (TACs) are a group of primary headache disorders characterized by unilateral head pain that occurs in association with prominent ipsilateral cranial autonomic features, such as lacrimation, conjunctival injection, or nasal symptoms [1, 2]. The TACs include cluster headache (CH), paroxysmal hemicrania (PH), and short-lasting unilateral neuralgiform headache attacks with conjunctival injection and tearing/cranial autonomic features (SUNCT/SUNA). The TACs are grouped into section three of the revised International Classification of Headache Disorders (ICHD-2) [3]. Whether hemicrania continua (HC) should be included is moot, and although the ICHD-2 did not include HC, this may have been an error [4]; HC is covered elsewhere (see Chapter 19).

The TACs, while having many similarities, differ in attack duration and frequency as well as their response to therapy. CH has the longest attack duration and a relatively low attack frequency. PH has an intermediate duration and intermediate attack frequency. SUNCT has the shortest attack duration and the highest attack frequency (Table 16.1). Fundamental to progress in any area is to understand its pathophysiology.

CH is by far the best understood, probably since it has been recognized for much longer [5] and, in some related part, because it is very much more common. CH will be dealt with in detail as the archetypal TAC, and the other syndromes contrasted for illustration and understanding.

Genetics of TACs

It seems likely from principle that TACs are genetically determined and in some way triggered to expression as we see them. An example of this is TAC-like syndromes triggered by trauma, such as dental [6] and ocular trauma [7] in CH, and head trauma in PH [8]. Certainly, larger analyses suggest the inheritance of susceptibility genes [9], just as is considered likely for migraine. Kudrow [10] studied 495 patients with CH; of the males (405), 27% were found to have at least one affected first-degree relative, and for the females (90), the figure was 37%. Of the 990 parents of these patients, 1.8% had CH, which is considerably more than the population prevalence. Kudrow's finding of a probable genetic component to CH has been corroborated in studies reporting between a 14-fold [11] and 39-fold [12] increase in the risk of CH among first-degree relatives. Twins with CH have been identified [13,

Headache, First Edition. Edited by Matthew S. Robbins, Brian M. Grosberg, and Richard B. Lipton.
© 2013 John Wiley & Sons, Ltd. Published 2013 by John Wiley & Sons, Ltd.

14, 15]. Most recently, two groups reported a lack of any correlation of *CACNA1A* gene polymorphisms in CH [16, 17].

For the other TACs, the situation is less clear. A family history has been reported in PH [18], although this may simply be a reporting bias of a rare event. Given the rarity, perhaps the expressivity is simply very modest in PH. For SUNCT/SUNA, the situation is even less clear.

Pathophysiologic features of TACs

The four major aspects of the pathophysiology of TACs (Table 16.1) are:

- the cranial distribution of the pain;
- the relative prominence of cranial autonomic features;
- the pattern of attacks, which offers the clinical signature for diagnosis;
- the distinct response to different therapies [19].

The cranial distribution of the pain is explained by an understanding of the trigeminovascular system, and the cranial autonomic features by a consideration of the trigeminal–autonomic reflex. These are somewhat generic to TACs, and indeed to many primary headache disorders. The pattern and therapies are distinct and will thus be explored separately for each TAC.

The trigeminovascular system

The trigeminovascular system is in a unique, indeed pivotal, position in terms of cerebrovascular physiology [20]. It is the sole sensory (afferent) innervation of the cerebral vessels and has, in addition, an efferent potential in pathophysiologic settings [21].

Table 16.1. Comparison of the TACs based on cohorts studied [92, 119, 123], and patients seen in practice

	CH	PH	SUNCT/SUNA
Sex (male:female)	3:1	1:1	1.5:1
Pain			
Quality	Sharp/stabbing/	Sharp/stabbing/	Sharp/stabbing/
Severity	throbbing	throbbing	throbbing
Distribution	Very severe	Very severe	Severe
	V1>C2>V2>V3	V1>C2>V2>V3	V1>C2>V2>V3
Attacks			
Frequency (/day)	1–8	11	100
Length (min)	30–180	2–30	1–10
Triggers			
Alcohol	+++	+	–
Nitroglycerin	+++	+	–
Cutaneous	–	–	+++
Agitation/restlessness	90%	80%	65%
Episodic versus chronic	90:10	35:65	10:90
Circadian/circannual periodicity	Present	Absent	Absent
Treatment effects			
Oxygen	70%	No effect	No effect
Sumatriptan 6 mg	90%	20%	<10%
Indomethacin	No effect	100%	No effect
Migraine features with attacks			
Nausea	50%	40%	25%
Photophobia/phonophobia	65%	65%	25%

C, cervical; V, trigeminal.

Anatomy: understanding the trigeminocervical complex

The trigeminovascular system consists of those neurons innervating the cerebral vessels and dura mater whose cell bodies are located in the trigeminal ganglion. The ganglion contains bipolar cells, the peripheral fiber making a synaptic connection with the vessels and other cranial structures, particularly the pain-producing large cranial vessels and dura mater [22, 23, 24, 25, 26], and the centrally projecting fiber synapsing in the caudal brainstem or high cervical cord [27, 28, 29]. Some projections have been noted to involve both cerebral (middle cerebral artery) and extracerebral (middle meningeal artery) vessels [30]. Activation of afferents in both the large venous sinuses [28] and intracranial arteries [29] leads to Fos production in neurons with the same anatomic distribution, the trigeminal nucleus caudalis and dorsal horns of C1 and C2—the *trigeminocervical complex* (TCC).

Transmitters

Several powerful vasodilatory peptides are to be found in cell bodies within the trigeminal ganglion that innervate blood vessels. These substances, calcitonin gene-related peptide (CGRP), substance P, and neurokinin A, are found in various combinations of neurons [31] so that virtually any combination may characterize any neuron. The functional consequences of these combinations are yet to be fully elucidated, but it seems likely that the trigemino-craniovascular innervation is homogenous at least in its vasodilation actions. Certainly, CGRP is elevated in both spontaneous [32] and nitroglycerin-provoked [33] CH, providing excellent evidence for trigeminovascular activation during acute attacks.

Physiology

Resting cerebral blood flow measured with iodoantipyrine and tissue autoradiography is not altered in the cat after section of the trigeminal ganglion. Indeed, after unilateral section, flow is identical to that in the homologous contralateral cortex [34]. Further, glucose utilization is not affected by section of the trigeminal ganglion. and thus the usual close relationship between flow and metabolism is not disturbed [34]. In contrast, stimulation of the trigeminal ganglion in humans by either thermocoagulation [35, 36] or injection of alcohol [37] can cause facial flushing, usually in the division or divisions appropriate to the manipulation. In addition, cerebral blood flow in humans is increased after trigeminal ganglion stimulation [38]. It has also been shown that facial flushing after trigeminal ganglion stimulation is accompanied by an increase in facial temperature of 1–2 °C [39]. Corresponding with this flush, there is an increase in the dilator peptides substance P and CGRP in the external jugular vein [40], even if the flush is cutaneously triggered [41], but this change is not seen in the peripheral circulation [42]. Such changes are also seen in the cat [40].

The trigeminal–autonomic reflex

Trigeminal ganglion stimulation in the cat [43] or monkey [44] leads to a diminution of carotid resistance, with increased flow and facial temperature predominantly through a reflex mechanism. The afferent limb of this arc is the trigeminal nerve, and the efferent limb is the facial/greater superficial petrosal nerve (parasympathetic) dilator pathway [45]. About 20% of the dilatation seen remains after facial nerve section, and is probably mediated directly by antidromic activation of the trigeminal system. The portion running through the parasympathetic outflow traverses the sphenopalatine (pterygopalatine) and otic ganglia [46], and employs vasoactive intestinal polypeptide (VIP) as its transmitter [47]. The cells of origin for the cranial parasympathetic autonomic vasodilator pathway are in the superior salivatory nucleus in the pons [48], which can be activated with stimulation of a trigeminovascular nociceptive input, such as that from the superior sagittal sinus [49]. This vasodilator reflex is the trigemino-parasympathetic or trigeminal–autonomic reflex [1], which is thus a normal physiologic reflex. Direct stimulation of the superior salivatory nucleus causes neuronal firing in the TCC [50], as well as enhancing the firing rate of light-responsive TCC neurons [51]. Activation of the facial nerve or stimulation of the sphenopalatine ganglion causes an increase in cerebral blood flow [52]. Further, the neurons projecting from the superior salivatory nucleus to the extracranial vessels release VIP as their primary transmitter [53]. It is known that VIP is released during CH and PH [54, 55], and may be the mediator of the symptoms associated with these conditions.

The trigeminal neural innervation of the cerebral circulation is somatotopically selective. Stimulation of the superior sagittal sinus increases cerebral blood flow as measured by laser Doppler flowmetry, but does not alter carotid flow in the same manner, in contrast to the effect of trigeminal ganglion stimulation, which increases both cerebral and non-cerebral cranial blood flow [56]. Similarly, in humans, painful stimuli, such as an injection of capsaicin, produce dilation of the internal carotid artery when administered into the skin innervated by the first (ophthalmic) division of the trigeminal nerve [57, 58]. However, when injected into the skin innervated by the third (mandibular) division or into the leg, there is no response in the ipsilateral carotid artery, despite the experience of pain [58]. It is thus clear that first (ophthalmic) division of trigeminal pain produces reflex activation of the cranial parasympathetic outflow. It is clear that this system can be activated in volunteers [59], so that what is exceptional in TACs is not the activation as much as its prominence.

Cluster headache

Ekbom and Greitz's classic observation during angiography of a patient suffering an acute CH, demonstrating localized narrowing of the internal carotid artery distal to the carotid canal [60], suggested a pathologic focus in the region of the cavernous sinus. The arguments for this locus for the disease [61] and for local inflammation [62] have been set out. There is no evidence for systemic inflammation as a basis for CH [63]. As has emerged in the last decade, a brain locus for the primary disorder is much more plausible [64] and will be set out here.

Cluster headache and the region of the posterior hypothalamic gray matter

Several lines of study suggest that central nervous mechanisms, particularly those involving the hypothalamus, play a role in CH. Data from clinical observations and neuroendocrine studies have suggested such a link, which has now been further investigated using functional imaging techniques. Taken together, the studies strongly suggest a role for this brain region. Indeed, there

is good basic science evidence for the link between the hypothalamus and TACs more broadly. The TCC also conveys somatosensory and visceral nociceptive information from the head and orofacial structures directly to the hypothalamus, along the trigeminohypothalamic tract [65, 66], and is activated by dural stimulation [67, 68].

Circadian timing and cluster headache

Kudrow [69] reported two significant peaks of bouts of in July and January. The general rise in frequency during the year was twice interrupted around the days when the clocks were altered for Daylight and Standard time. This alteration of CH onset with photoperiod changes significantly implicates hypothalamic mechanisms. About 50% of attacks of CH occur at night [70]: in a prospective study, it was shown that 39 of 77 spontaneous attacks of CH took place at night [71].

One area involved in human clock systems that is implicated by the clinical data on CH is the suprachiasmatic nucleus in the hypothalamic gray matter, which sits at the base of the third ventricle [72]. Melatonin is produced by the pineal gland, with a strong circadian rhythm regulated by the suprachiasmatic nucleus [73]. Connections between the retina and the hypothalamus are thought to provide light cues for the circadian rhythm [74]. The characteristic nocturnal peak of melatonin secretion is blunted during the active phase of CH [75], and the excretion of its metabolite abnormal [76]. There is an argument for using melatonin in the treatment of the condition [77], and two positive reports with small numbers of patients [78, 79] are encouraging.

Neuroendocrine changes in cluster headache

Kudrow [80, 81] was the first to point out that testosterone levels were altered in CH patients during the bout, and thus began to implicate hypothalamic dysfunction. This finding was, however, not reproduced [82]. Others have identified a reduction in mean testosterone levels during the acute attack compared to the period between attacks [83]. Serum estradiol levels did not differ in CH patients in and out of the bout [84]. Mean 24-hour cortisol levels are higher during an active bout compared to outside the bout [75]. A significant phase shift for cortisol secretion has also been shown for patients during a bout [85]. Similarly, circadian variations in prolactin secretion are not present in CH patients during a bout [86], although basal prolactin levels are no different from controls [87]. An increase in the secretion of prolactin has been reported during acute attacks of CH ([84, 86]; although this is disputed in [85]). Growth hormone shows a bimodal peak as a result of an advance in the evening peak in some patients [85]. Leone and colleagues [88] identified reduced responses to stimulation by thyrotropin-releasing releasing hormone. Taken together, these neuroendocrine changes have implicated the hypothalamus, particularly its neuroendocrine and chronobiologic functions, in CH.

Data from functional imaging in cluster headache

Using positron-emission tomography (PET) with the blood flow tracer $H_2^{15}O$, brain activation has been studied during acute CH. The areas activated fell into three categories: areas generally associated with pain, an area that seems specific to CH, and vascular structures [89].

Pain

The anterior cingulate gyrus was significantly activated, as would be expected, since in most human PET studies with pain, activation of the anterior cingulate is observed, perhaps as a part of the affective response [90]. Activation was also observed in the frontal cortex and insulae, and in the ventroposterior thalamus contralateral to the side of the pain. In addition, there was activation in the ipsilateral basal ganglia. This is not the first observation of basal ganglion changes associated with pain [90, 91], and may simply relate to movement, or the wish to move, that is common in patients with CH [92], or even to some deliberate inhibition of movement.

Cluster headache

The only activated area that is particular to CH, when compared to migraine in a triggered attack, is located at the base of the third ventricle in the posterior hypothalamic gray, or just posterior to it (Figure 16.1) [89]. Similarly, there is activation in the same region in a spontaneous attack [93,

94]. There is no such activation when patients with episodic CH move out of their bout and are studied [93]. Moreover, there is no comparable posterior change in migraine [95]. In one patient with both CH and migraine, whose attack was captured by a PET scanner, the phenotype of the attack, migraine without aura, matched the functional activation result, pontine change, without any hypothalamic activation [96].

In a provocative report, structural changes in the posterior hypothalamic gray matter were identified using the automated unbiased whole brain technique known as voxel-based morphometry (VBM) [97]. The study suggested that posterior hypothalamic gray matter was increased in volume, whereas the white matter was not [98]. Such a change does not seem to occur in migraine [99]. Indeed, using higher resolution MRI techniques, the finding is less clear. In reality, only anatomic histopathologic studies of this brain region will determine, what, if any, structural changes can be found.

> ### ⚗ SCIENCE REVISITED
>
> Functional neuroimaging and VBM have linked CH to activation and structural changes within the posterior hypothalamus. As such, posterior hypothalamic deep brain stimulation has been employed in patients with refractory chronic CH, with significant efficacy in some cases.

Vascular change

PET scans of capsaicin-induced pain in the ophthalmic (first) division of the trigeminal nerve [57] showed no hypothalamic activation, and provide an important negative control for the CH studies. Despite the fact that severe first division pain results from capsaicin injection, there is no posterior hypothalamic activation. The capsaicin experiment did demonstrate flow changes in an area consistent with the cavernous sinus/carotid artery, in the same way as there are flow changes in the vessels in CH, as would be predicted from the anatomic/physiologic arguments above. Using magnetic resonance angiography, it has been shown that the activation observed in the PET studies is due to dilatation of the internal

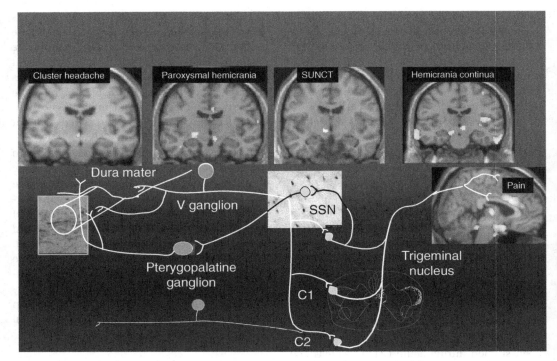

Figure 16.1. TACs are characterized pathophysiologically by facilitation of the trigeminal–autonomic reflex. The reflex has its afferent in fibers from the ophthalmic (first) division of the trigeminal nerve, and efferent pathway from cell bodies in the superior salivatory nucleus (SSN), whose outflow is through the VIIth cranial nerve synapses in the pterygopalatine ganglion, and thence projects through the greater superficial petrosal nerve. The regional of the posterior hypothalamic area seems crucial for the expression of the disorder since it is seen on imaging studies of each of the TACs: CH [89], PH [111], SUNCT [115], and HC [113].

carotid artery [100], and is specific to first division of trigeminal activation, in contrast to third division trigeminal or nontrigeminal pain [58]. Again, this vascular change is seen with migraine [96]. It must be concluded that the change in diameter of the internal carotid artery is an epiphenomenon, occurring as it does in migraine, CH, and experimental head pain, in the same distribution and to the same degree. Trigeminovascular activation is in fact a normal concomitant of nociceptive activation of the ophthalmic (first) division of the trigeminal nerve.

Is any peripheral drive necessary for cluster headache, or is it entirely a brain disorder?

A recognized treatment for intractable chronic CH is to section the trigeminal root proximal to the ganglion [101]. Unfortunately, not all patients respond to this treatment [102]. Cushing [22] observed many years ago that, after trigeminal root section, in addition to total facial anesthesia, the ipsilateral dura mater was insensitive. A patient with a complete trigeminal root section whose CH attacks have continued has been reported. While being completely anesthetic on the face, and without a corneal reflex or electrical blink reflexes, he continued to experience typical and unaltered headache that responded to sumatriptan injections [103].

There is no doubt that headache may arise purely from the brain, as in epileptic events [104, 105], or as migraine-like headaches being generated from the stimulation of brainstem regions [106, 107], or local brainstem lesions [108, 109]. Perhaps in CH the brain mechanisms are preeminent, and normal afferent traffic is perceived as painful, from time to time, rather than the primary driver being a peripheral nociceptive input. It is clear from animal experimental work that the cranial parasympathetic autonomic outflow can be driven from brainstem areas [110]. If CH drives the cranial parasympathetic outflow as a component of the acute attack, this might trigger the trigeminal autonomic reflex, but that reflex may not be absolutely necessary for the expression of an attack.

Paroxysmal hemicrania

The pathophysiologic mechanisms responsible for pain in PH are much less clear than for CH.

The most important recent finding for PH is activation on PET in the posterior hypothalamic region [111], as seen in other TACs [112], and in the ventral midbrain, as seen in HC [113]. A case of a patient in the Arctic region with less troublesome attacks in the light season reinforces hypothalamic mechanisms in this disorder [114].

SUNCT/SUNA

Of the TACs, indeed of all primary headache disorders, SUNCT/SUNA stands out in clinical terms for the simple observation that attacks may be triggered by cutaneous stimuli. Certainly, a similar brain area to that for CH and PH in the posterior hypothalamic gray region is active in SUNCT [115]. It may be unilateral, as with other TACs, or bilateral in some cases [116]. It would be instructive to see well-characterized, typical cases of trigeminal neuralgia imaged for comparison. From a clinical perspective, the classic cases of SUNCT do seem very different from those of trigeminal neuralgia, although one can see complexities, especially in SUNA when there is comorbid migraine, and more particularly in the expected patients who would have both trigeminal neuralgia and migraine.

Therapeutics and the TACs

The therapeutics of TACs seem particular to the syndromes (see Table 16.1). Their exploration will no doubt provide both insights into the uniqueness of the syndromes and directions for therapeutic developments.

Oxygen and cluster headache

The effect of oxygen in CH is well established [117]. Most recently, it has been shown that there are neurons in the TCC of the rat that respond to stimulation of the superior salivatory nucleus and are inhibited by 100% oxygen, but not air [50]. Given that HC [118] and SUNCT/SUNA [119] do not respond to oxygen in any substantial way, this population of neurons may be very informative in terms of discovering new treatments for CH.

Indomethacin and paroxysmal hemicrania

The mechanism behind the absolute responsiveness to indomethacin appears to be independent of the drug's effect on prostaglandin synthesis, since other nonsteroidal anti-inflammatory agents have little [120] or no [121, 122, 123] effect on PH, although certainly Sjaastad's first case (personal communication), and cases this author has seen, respond rather well to aspirin.

Most recently, the *in vivo* technique of intravital microscopy in rats has been utilized as a model of trigeminovascular nociception to study the potential mechanism of action of indomethacin. Dural vascular changes were produced using electrical (neurogenic) dural vasodilation (NDV), CGRP-induced dural vasodilation, and nitric oxide-induced dural vasodilation using nitric oxide donors. In each of these settings, the effect of intravenously administered indomethacin (5 mg/kg), naproxen (30 mg/kg), and ibuprofen (30 mg/kg) was tested. All of the tested drugs significantly inhibited NDV between 30% and 52%). While none of them was able to inhibit CGRP-induced dural vasodilation, only indomethacin reduced nitric oxide-induced dural vasodilation (by 35% ± 7%, 10 minutes post administration). The study concluded that nonsteroidal anti-inflammatory drugs inhibit the release of CGRP after NDV without a direct effect on CGRP. Further, a differentiating effect of indomethacin on inhibiting nitric oxide-induced dural vasodilation was reported, offering the exciting possibility that a nitric oxide-based mechanism is behind the unique effect of indomethacin on PH and hemicranias continua [124].

Lidocaine and SUNCT

Intravenous lidocaine is a very effective treatment for SUNCT/SUNA [119, 125]. This raises the question of how it may work. It can be shown in experimental animals that intravenous lidocaine inhibits durally induced activation of trigemi-nocervical neurons [126]. This can be achieved at doses comparable to those used in clinical practice. However, some effect of intravenous lidocaine is also seen in migraine. Given that topiramate is clearly useful in SUNCT [127], and similarly lamotrigine is very often effective, it can be speculated that a sodium channel may turn out to be important in therapeutics for SUNCT/SUNA. Much work needs to be done in this area to follow such leads.

References

1. Goadsby PJ, Lipton RB. A review of paroxysmal hemicranias, SUNCT syndrome and other short-lasting headaches with autonomic features, including new cases. *Brain* 1997;**120**:193–209.

2. Goadsby PJ, Cohen AS, Matharu MS. Trigeminal autonomic cephalalgias— diagnosis and treatment. *Curr Neurol Neurosci Rep* 2007;**7**:117–25.

3. Headache Classification Committee of the International Headache Society. The International Classification of Headache Disorders (second edition). *Cephalalgia* 2004; **24**(Suppl. 1):1–160.

4. Goadsby PJ, Cittadini E, Burns B, Cohen AS. Trigeminal autonomic cephalalgias— diagnostic and therapeutic developments. *Curr Opin Neurol* 2008;**21**:323–30.

5. Koehler PJ. Prevalence of headache in Tulp's Observationes Medicae (1641) with a description of cluster headache. *Cephalalgia* 1993;**13**:318–20.

6. Soros P, Frese A, Husstedt IW, Evers S. Cluster headache after dental extraction: implications for the pathogenesis of cluster headache? *Cephalalgia* 2001;**21**:619–22.

7. Evers S, Soros P, Brilla R, Gerding H, Husstedt I-W. Cluster headache after orbital exenteration. *Cephalalgia* 1997;**17**:680–2.

8. Matharu MS, Goadsby PJ. Post-traumatic chronic paroxysmal hemicrania (CPH) with aura. *Neurology* 2001;**56**:273–5.

9. Russell MB, Andersson PG, Iselius L. Cluster headache is an inherited disorder in some families. *Headache* 1996;**36**:608–12.

10. Kudrow L. *Cluster Headache: Mechanisms and Management.* Oxford: Oxford University Press; 1980.

11. Russell MB, Andersson PG, Thomsen LL, Iselius L. Cluster headache is an autosomal dominantly inherited disorder in some families: a complex segregation analysis. *J Med Gen* 1995;**32**:954–6.

12. Leone M, Russell MB, Rigamonti A, et al. Increased familial risk of cluster headache. *Neurology* 2001;**56**:1233–6.

13. Roberge C, Bouchard JP, Simard D, Gagne R. Cluster headache in twins. *Neurology* 1992;**42**:1255–6.

14. Sjaastad O, Shen JM, Stovner LJ, Elsas T. Cluster headache in identical twins. *Headache* 1993;**33**:214–7.

15. Couturier EG, Hering R, Steiner TJ. The first report of cluster headache in identical twins. *Neurology* 1991;**21**:761.

16. Haan J, van Vliet JA, Kors EE, et al. No involvement of calcium channel gene (CACNA1A) in a family with cluster headache. *Cephalalgia* 2001;**21**:959–62.

17. Sjostrand C, Giedratis V, EKbom K, Waldenlind E, Hillert J. CACNA1A gene polymorphisms in cluster headache. *Cephalalgia* 2001;**21**:953–8.

18. Cohen AS, Matharu MS, Goadsby PJ. Paroxysmal hemicrania in a family. *Cephalalgia* 2006;**26**:486–8.

19. Lance JW, Goadsby PJ. *Mechanism and Management of Headache* (6th edn.). London: Butterworth-Heinemann; 1998.

20. Goadsby PJ, Duckworth JW. Effect of stimulation of trigeminal ganglion on regional cerebral blood flow in cats. *Am J Physiol* 1987;**253**:R270–4.

21. May A, Goadsby PJ. The trigeminovascular system in humans: pathophysiological implications for primary headache syndromes of the neural influences on the cerebral circulation. *J Cereb Blood Flow Metab* 1999;**19**:115–27.

22. Cushing H. The sensory distribution of the fifth cranial nerve. *Bull Johns Hopkins Hosp* 1904;**15**:213–32.

23. Penfield W, McNaughton FL. Dural headache and the innervation of the dura mater. *Arch Neurol Psychiatry* 1940;**44**:43–75.

24. McNaughton FL. The innervation of the intracranial blood vessels and dural sinuses. *Proc Assoc Res Nerv Ment Dis* 1938;**18**: 178–200.

25. McNaughton FL, Feindel WH. Innervation of intracranial structures: a reappraisal. In Rose FC (ed.), *Physiological Aspects of Clinical Neurology*. Oxford: Blackwell Scientific Publications; 1977: pp. 279–93.

26. Feindel W, Penfield W, McNaughton F. The tentorial nerves and localization of intracranial pain in man. *Neurology* 1960;**10**: 555–63.

27. Kaube H, Keay KA, Hoskin KL, Bandler R, Goadsby PJ. Expression of c-*Fos*-like immunoreactivity in the caudal medulla and upper cervical cord following stimulation of the superior sagittal sinus in the cat. *Brain Res* 1993;**629**:95–102.

28. Goadsby PJ, Hoskin KL. The distribution of trigeminovascular afferents in the nonhuman primate brain *Macaca nemestrina*: a c-fos immunocytochemical study. *J Anat* 1997;**190**:367–75.

29. Hoskin KL, Zagami A, Goadsby PJ. Stimulation of the middle meningeal artery leads to Fos expression in the trigeminocervical nucleus: a comparative study of monkey and cat. *J Anat* 1999;**194**:579–88.

30. O'Connor TP, van der Kooy D. Pattern of intracranial and extracranial projections of trigeminal ganglion cells. *J Neurosci* 1986; **6**:2200–7.

31. Edvinsson L, MacKenzie ET, McCulloch J. *Cerebral Blood Flow and Metabolism*. New York: Raven Press; 1993.

32. Goadsby PJ, Edvinsson L. Human *in vivo* evidence for trigeminovascular activation in cluster headache. *Brain* 1994;**117**: 427–34.

33. Fanciullacci M, Alessandri M, Figini M, Geppetti P, Michelacci S. Increase in plasma calcitonin gene-related peptide from extracerebral circulation during nitroglycerin-induced cluster headache attack. *Pain* 1995; **60**:119–23.

34. Edvinsson L, McCulloch J, Kingman TA, Uddman R. On the functional role of the trigemino-cerebrovascular system in the regulation of cerebral circulation. In Owman C, Hardebo JE (eds.), *Neural Regulation of the Cerebral Circulation*. Stockholm: Elsevier; 1986: pp. 407–18.

35. Sweet WM, Wepsic JG. Controlled thermocoagulation of V ganglion and rootlets for differential destruction of pain fibres. Part I. V. Neuralgia. *J Neurosurg* 1974;**40**: 143–56.

36. Onofrio BM. Radiofrequency percutaneous Gasserian ganglion lesions. Results in 140 patients with trigeminal pain. *J Neurosurg* 1975;**42**:132–43.

37. Oka M. Experimental study on the vasodilator innervation of the face. *Med J Osaka Univ* 1950;**2**:109–16.

38. Tran-Dinh YR, Thurel C, Cunin G, Serrie A, Seylaz J. Cerebral vasodilation after the thermocoagulation of the trigeminal ganglion in humans. *Neurosurgery* 1992;**31**: 658–62.

39. Drummond PD, Gonski A, Lance JW. Facial flushing after thermocoagulation of the gasserian ganglion. *J Neurol Neurosurg Psychiatry* 1983;**46**:611–6.

40. Goadsby PJ, Edvinsson L, Ekman R. Release of vasoactive peptides in the extracerebral circulation of man and the cat during activation of the trigeminovascular system. *Ann Neurol* 1988;**23**:193–6.

41. Goadsby PJ, Edvinsson L, Ekman R. Cutaneous stimulation leading to facial flushing and release of calcitonin gene-related peptide. *Cephalalgia* 1992;**12**:53–6.

42. Schon H, Thomas DT, Jewkes DA, Ghatei MA, Mulderry PK, Bloom SR. Failure to detect plasma neuropeptide release during trigeminal thermocoagulation. *J Neurol Neurosurg Psychiatry* 1987;**50**:642–3.

43. Lambert GA, Bogduk N, Goadsby PJ, Duckworth JW, Lance JW. Decreased carotid arterial resistance in cats in response to trigeminal stimulation. *J Neurosurg* 1984; **61**:307–15.

44. Goadsby PJ, Lambert GA, Lance JW. Stimulation of the trigeminal ganglion increases flow in the extracerebral but not the cerebral circulation of the monkey. *Brain Res* 1986; **381**:63–7.

45. Goadsby PJ. Effect of stimulation of the facial nerve on regional cerebral blood flow and glucose utilization in cats. *Am J Physiol* 1989;**257**:R517–21.

46. Goadsby PJ, Lambert GA, Lance JW. The peripheral pathway for extracranial vasodilatation in the cat. *J Auton Nerv Syst* 1984; **10**:145–55.

47. Goadsby PJ, Macdonald GJ. Extracranial vasodilatation mediated by VIP (vasoactive intestinal polypeptide). *Brain Res* 1985;**329**: 285–8.

48. Spencer SE, Sawyer WB, Wada H, Platt KB, Loewy AD. CNS projections to the pterygopalatine parasympathetic preganglionic neurons in the rat: a retrograde transneuronal viral cell body labeling study. *Brain Res* 1990;**534**:149–69.

49. Knight YE, Classey JD, Kowacs F, Goadsby PJ. FOS expression in the rostral medulla and caudal pons after periaqueductal gray stimulation: comparison with superior sagittal sinus stimulation. *Cephalalgia* 2001;**21**:401.

50. Akerman S, Holland PR, Lasalandra MP, Goadsby PJ. Oxygen inhibits neuronal activation in the trigeminocervical complex after stimulation of trigeminal autonomic reflex, but not via direct dural activation of trigeminal afferents. *Headache* 2009;**49**: 1131–43.

51. Okamoto K, Tashiro A, Chang Z, Bereiter DA. Bright light activates a trigeminal nociceptive pathway. *Pain* 2010;**149**:235–42.

52. Goadsby PJ. Effect of stimulation of facial nerve on regional cerebral blood flow and glucose utilization in cats. *Am J Physiol* 1989;**257**(3 Pt 2):R517–21.

53. Goadsby PJ, MacDonald GJ. Extracranial vasodilation mediated by vasoactive intestinal polypeptide (VIP). *Brain Res* 1985; **329**(1–2):285–8.

54. Goadsby PJ, Edvinsson L. Human in vivo evidence for trigeminovascular activation in cluster headache. Neuropeptide changes and effects of acute attacks therapies. *Brain* 1994;**117**(Pt 3):427–34.

55. Goadsby PJ, Edvinsson L. Neuropeptide changes in a case of chronic paroxysmal hemicrania—evidence for trigemino-parasympathetic activation. *Cephalalgia* 1996; **16**(6):448–50.

56. Goadsby PJ, Knight YE, Hoskin KL, Butler P. Stimulation of an intracranial trigeminally-innervated structure selectively increases cerebral blood flow. *Brain Res* 1997;**751**: 247–52.

57. May A, Kaube H, Buechel C, et al. Experimental cranial pain elicited by capsaicin: a PET-study. *Pain* 1998;**74**:61–6.

58. May A, Buchel C, Turner R, Goadsby PJ. MR-angiography in facial and other pain: neurovascular mechanisms of trigeminal sensation. *J Cereb Blood Flow Metab* 2001; **21**:1171–6.

59. Frese A, Evers S, May A. Autonomic activation in experimental trigeminal pain. *Cephalalgia* 2003;**23**:67–8.

60. Ekbom K, Greitz T. Carotid angiography in cluster headache. *Acta Radiol* 1970;**10**: 177–86.

61. Moskowitz MA. Cluster headache – evidence for a pathophysiologic focus in the superior pericarotid cavernous sinus plexus. *Headache* 1988;**28**:584–6.

62. Hardebo JE. How cluster headache is explained as an intracavernous inflammatory process lesioning sympathetic fibres. *Headache* 1994;**34**:125–31.

63. Remahl IN, Waldenlind E, Bratt J, Ekbom K. Cluster headache is not associated with signs of a systemic inflammation. *Headache* 2000;**40**(4):276–81.

64. Goadsby PJ. Pathophysiology of cluster headache: a trigeminal autonomic cephalalgia. *Lancet Neurol* 2002;**1**:37–43.

65. Malick A, Strassman AM, Burstein R. Trigeminohypothalamic and reticulohypothalamic tract neurons in the upper cervical spinal cord and caudal medulla of the rat. *J Neurophysiol* 2000;**84**:2078–112.

66. Malick A, Burstein R. Cells of origin of the trigeminohypothalamic tract in the rat. *J Comp Neurol* 1998;**400**:125–44.

67. Benjamin L, Levy MJ, Lasalandra MP, et al. Hypothalamic activation after stimulation of the superior sagittal sinus in the cat: a Fos study. *Neurobiol Dis* 2004;**16**(3):500–5.

68. Malick A, Jakubowski M, Elmquist JK, Saper CB, Burstein R. A neurohistochemical blueprint for pain-induced loss of appetite. *Proc Natl Acad Sci U S A* 2001;**98**(17): 9930–5.

69. Kudrow L. The cyclic relationship of natural illumination to cluster period frequency. *Cephalalgia* 1987;**7**(Suppl. 6):76–8.

70. Ekbom K. A clinical comparison of cluster headache and migraine. *Acta Neurol Scand* 1970;**46**(Suppl. 41):1+.

71. Russell D. Cluster headache: severity and temporal profile of attacks and patient

activity prior to and during attacks. *Cephalalgia* 1981;**1**:209–16.

72. Moore-Ede MC. The circadian timing system in mammals: two pacemakers preside over many secondary oscillators. *Fed Proc* 1983;**42**:2802–8.

73. Moore RY. Circadian rhythms: basic neurobiology and clinical applications. *Annu Rev Med* 1997;**48**:253–66.

74. Hofman MA, Zhou JN, Swaab DF. Suprachiasmatic nucleus of the human brain: an immunocytochemical and morphometric analysis. *J Comp Neurol* 1996;**305**:552–6.

75. Waldenlind E, Gustafsson SA, Ekbom K, Wetterberg L. Circadian secretion of cortisol and melatonin in cluster headache during active cluster periods and remission. *J Neurol Neurosurg Psychiatry* 1987;**50**:207–13.

76. Leone M, Lucini V, Damico D, et al. Abnormal 24-hour urinary excretory pattern of 6-sulphatoxymelatonin in both phases of cluster headache. *Cephalalgia* 1998;**18**:664–7.

77. Leone M, Bussone G. Melatonin in cluster headache – rationale for use and possible therapeutic potential. *CNS Drugs* 1998;**9**:7–16.

78. Leone M, D'Amico D, Moschiano F, Fraschini F, Bussone G. Melatonin versus placebo in the prophylaxis of cluster headache: a double-blind pilot study with parallel groups. *Cephalalgia* 1996;**16**:494–6.

79. Peres MFP, Rozen TD. Melatonin in the preventative treatment of chronic cluster headache. *Cephalalgia* 2001;**21**:993–5.

80. Kudrow L. Plasma testosterone levels in cluster headache preliminary results. *Headache* 1976;**16**:228–31.

81. Kudrow L. Plasma testosterone and LH levels in cluster headache. *Headache* 1977;**17**:91–2.

82. Nelson RF. Testosterone levels in cluster and non-cluster migrainous patients. *Headache* 1978;**18**:265–7.

83. Romiti A, Martelletti P, Gallo MF, Giacovazzo M. Low plasma testosterone levels in cluster headache. *Cephalalgia* 1983;**3**:41–4.

84. Waldenlind E, Gustafsson SA. Prolactin in cluster headache: diurnal secretion, response to thyrotropin-releasing hormone, and relation to sex steroids and gonadotropins. *Cephalalgia* 1987;**7**:43–54.

85. Chazot G, Claustrat B, Brun J, Jordan D, Sassolas G, Schott B. A chronobiological study of melatonin, cortisol, growth hormone and prolactin secretion in cluster headache. *Cephalalgia* 1984;**4**:213–20.

86. Polleri A, Nappi G, Murialdo G, Bono G, Martignoni E, Savoldi F. Changes in the 24-hour prolactin pattern in cluster headache. *Cephalalgia* 1982;**2**:1–7.

87. Bussone G, Frediani F, Leone M, Grazzi L, Lamperti E, Boiardi A. TRH test in cluster headache. *Headache* 1988;**28**:462–4.

88. Leone M, Partuno G, Vescovi A, Bussone G. Neuroendocrine dysfunction in cluster headache. *Cephalalgia* 1990;**10**:235–9.

89. May A, Bahra A, Buchel C, Frackowiak RS, Goadsby PJ. Hypothalamic activation in cluster headache attacks. *Lancet* 1998;**352**:275–8.

90. Derbyshire SWG, Jones AKP, Gyulai F, Clark S, Townsend D, Firestone LL. Pain processing during three levels of noxious stimulation produces differential patterns of central activity. *Pain* 1997;**73**:431–45.

91. Chudler EH, Dong WK. The role of the basal ganglia in nociception and pain. *Pain* 1995;**60**:33–8.

92. Bahra A, May A, Goadsby PJ. Cluster headache: a prospective clinical study in 230 patients with diagnostic implications. *Neurology* 2002;**58**:354–61.

93. May A, Bahra A, Buchel C, Frackowiak RSJ, Goadsby PJ. PET and MRA findings in cluster headache and MRA in experimental pain. *Neurology* 2000;**55**:1328–35.

94. Sprenger T, Boecker H, Tolle TR, Bussone G, May A, Leone M. Specific hypothalamic activation during a spontaneous cluster headache attack. *Neurology* 2004;**62**:516–7.

95. Sprenger T, Goadsby PJ. What has functional neuroimaging done for primary headache . . . and for the clinical neurologist? *J Clin Neurosci* 2010;**17**:547–53.

96. Bahra A, Matharu MS, Buchel C, Frackowiak RSJ, Goadsby PJ. Brainstem activation specific to migraine headache. *Lancet* 2001;**357**:1016–7.

97. Ashburner J, Friston KJ. Voxel-based mor-phometry—the methods. *NeuroImage* 2000; **11**:805–21.

98. May A, Ashburner J, Buchel C, et al. Correla-tion between structural and functional changes in brain in an idiopathic headache syndrome. *Nat Med* 1999;**5**:836–8.

99. Matharu MS, Good CD, May A, Bahra A, Goadsby PJ. Brain structure in migraine is normal: a voxel-based morphometric study. *Cephalalgia* 2001;**21**:403.

100. May A, Buchel C, Bahra A, Goadsby PJ, Frackowiak RSJ. Intra-cranial vessels in trigeminal transmitted pain: a PET Study. *NeuroImage* 1999;**9**:453–60.

101. Kirkpatrick PJ, O'Brien M, MacCabe JJ. Trigeminal nerve section for chronic migrainous neuralgia. *Br J Neurosurg* 1993; **7**:483–90.

102. O'Brien MD, Kirkpatrick PJ, McCabe JJ. Trigeminal nerve section for chronic migrainous neuralgia. In Olesen J, Goadsby PJ (eds.), *Cluster Headache and Related Con-ditions. Frontiers in Headache Research*, Vol. 9. Oxford: Oxford University Press; 1999: pp. 291–5.

103. Matharu MS, Goadsby PJ. Triptan response in a cluster headache patient with surgically section trigeminal sensory root. *Cephalal-gia* 2001;**21**:496.

104. Young GB, Blume WT. Painful epileptic sei-zures. *Brain* 1983;**106**:537–54.

105. Siegel AM, Williamson PD, Roberts DW. Localized pain associated with seizures originating in parietal lobe. *Epilepsia* 1999;**40**:845–55.

106. Raskin NH, Hosobuchi Y, Lamb S. Headache may arise from perturbation of brain. *Head-ache* 1987;**27**:416–20.

107. Veloso F, Kumar K, Toth C. Headache sec-ondary to deep brain implantation. *Head-ache* 1998;**38**:507–15.

108. Haas DC, Kent PF, Friedman DI. Headache caused by a single lesion of multiple sclero-sis in the periaqueductal gray area. *Head-ache* 1993;**33**:452–5.

109. Goadsby PJ. Neurovascular headache and a midbrain vascular malformation—evidence for a role of the brainstem in chronic migraine. *Cephalalgia* 2002;**22**:107–11.

110. Goadsby PJ, Lambert GA, Lance JW. Effects of locus coeruleus stimulation on carotid vascular resistance in the cat. *Brain Res* 1983;**278**:175–83.

111. Matharu MS, Cohen AS, Frackowiak RSJ, Goadsby PJ. Posterior hypothalamic activa-tion in paroxysmal hemicrania. *Ann Neurol* 2006;**59**:535–45.

112. Cohen AS, Goadsby PJ. Functional neu-roimaging of primary headache disorders. *Curr Neurol Neurosci Rep* 2004;**4**:105–10.

113. Matharu MS, Cohen AS, McGonigle DJ, Ward N, Frackowiak RSJ, Goadsby PJ. Poste-rior hypothalamic and brainstem activation in hemicrania continua. *Headache* 2004; **44**:747–61.

114. Bekkelund SI, Lilleng H. Impact of extreme light exposure during summer season in an Arctic area on patients with migraine and chronic paroxysmal hemicrania (CPH). *Cephalalgia* 2006;**26**:1153–6.

115. May A, Bahra A, Buchel C, Turner R, Goadsby PJ. Functional MRI in spontaneous attacks of SUNCT: short-lasting neuralgiform head-ache with conjunctival injection and tearing. *Ann Neurol* 1999;**46**:791–3.

116. Cohen AS, Matharu MS, Kalisch R, Friston K, Goadsby PJ. Functional MRI in SUNCT (short-lasting unilateral neuralgiform head-ache attacks with conjunctival injection and tearing) and SUNA (short-lasting unilateral neuralgiform headache attacks with cranial autonomic symptoms) shows differential hypothalamic activation with increasing pain. *Cephalalgia* 2006;**26**:1402–3.

117. Cohen AS, Burns B, Goadsby PJ. High flow oxygen for treatment of cluster headache. A randomized trial. *JAMA* 2009;**302**:2451–7.

118. Cittadini E, Goadsby PJ. Hemicrania con-tinua: a clinical study of 39 patients with diagnostic implications. *Brain* 2010;**133**:1973–86.

119. Cohen AS, Matharu MS, Goadsby PJ. Short-lasting unilateral neuralgiform headache attacks with conjunctival injection and tearing (SUNCT) or cranial autonomic fea-tures (SUNA). A prospective clinical study of SUNCT and SUNA. *Brain* 2006;**129**:2746–60.

120. Sjaastad O, Antonaci F. A piroxicam deriva-tive partly effective in chronic paroxysmal

hemicrania and hemicrania continua. *Headache* 1995;**35**:549–50.

121. Pareja J, Sjaastad O. Chronic paroxysmal hemicrania and hemicrania continua. Interval between indomethacin administration and response. *Headache* 1996;**36**:20–3.

122. Antonaci F, Pareja JA, Caminero AB, Sjaastad O. Chronic paroxysmal hemicrania and hemicrania continua. Parenteral indomethacin: the "Indotest". *Headache* 1998;**38**: 122–8.

123. Cittadini E, Matharu MS, Goadsby PJ. Paroxysmal hemicrania: a prospective clinical study of thirty-one cases. *Brain* 2008;**131**: 1142–55.

124. Summ O, Andreou AP, Akerman S, Goadsby PJ. A potential nitrergic mechanism of action for indomethacin, but not of other COX inhibitors – relevance to indomethacin-sensitive headaches. *J Headache Pain* 2010; **11**:477–83.

125. Matharu MS, Cohen AS, Goadsby PJ. SUNCT syndrome responsive to intravenous lidocaine. *Cephalalgia* 2004;**24**:985–92.

126. Kaube H, Hoskin KL, Goadsby PJ. Lignocaine and headache: an electrophysiological study in the cat with supporting clinical observations in man. *J Neurol* 1994;**241**:415–20.

127. Cohen A, Matharu MS, Goadsby PJ. Double-blind placebo-controlled trial of topiramate in SUNCT. *Cephalalgia* 2007;**27**:758.

Treatment of Trigeminal Autonomic Cephalalgias Including Cluster Headache

Sarah Vollbracht and Brian M. Grosberg

Albert Einstein College of Medicine, Bronx, NY, USA

Introduction

The cornerstones of cluster headache management include patient education, prompt administration of effective headache abortive agents, and institution of cluster prophylaxis.

Patient education

Patients should be advised to avoid potential triggers of cluster headache during the active cluster period. Recommendations should include refraining from taking daytime naps, drinking alcoholic beverages, and using medications such as nitroglycerin that are vasodilators and can trigger attacks. Because many of these patients are heavy cigarette smokers, smoking cessation should also be strongly recommended.

Acute therapy

Because of the sudden onset and short time to peak intensity of attacks, abortive agents for cluster headache must work quickly and effectively. Parenteral, nasal, or pulmonary routes of drug administration are necessary to ensure a rapid onset of relief. Of these, subcutaneous sumatriptan is the treatment of choice in patients for whom it is not contraindicated. Oxygen inhalation also is very effective.

Sumatriptan

Subcutaneous sumatriptan is considered to be the most effective abortive agent for acute attacks of cluster headache, acting agonistically on peripheral and central serotonin 5-HT$_{1B/1D}$ receptors. In a randomized-controlled trial (RCT) of 6 mg of sumatriptan administered subcutaneously, 74% of patients experienced relief by 15 minutes compared with 26% of patients treated with placebo [1]. Additional benefits of the treated group included improved functional ability and reduced autonomic symptomatology. Studies of the long-term efficacy and safety of subcutaneous sumatriptan show significant headache relief with repeated and prolonged use of this abortive agent, even at doses of 6 mg twice daily for many months, without the development of tachyphylaxis or more frequent attacks [2, 3]. However, pre-emptive treatment with sumatriptan is not effective in preventing an oncoming attack.

Although sumatriptan is generally well tolerated, transient adverse effects include, but are not limited to, pain at the injection site, nausea, dizziness, vertigo, malaise, fatigue, neck pain, paresthesias, and noncardiac chest discomfort. The triptans are contraindicated in patients with

Headache, First Edition. Edited by Matthew S. Robbins, Brian M. Grosberg, and Richard B. Lipton.
© 2013 John Wiley & Sons, Ltd. Published 2013 by John Wiley & Sons, Ltd.

poorly controlled hypertension, ischemic heart disease, variant angina, and cerebrovascular and peripheral vascular disease.

> ### ☆ TIPS AND TRICKS
>
> If a patient has more than two attacks of cluster headache in a 24-hour period, the 4 mg dose of the sumatriptan injection may be considered, to allow for a maximum of three 4 mg doses rather than two 6 mg doses in a 24-hour period.

Intranasal sumatriptan (20 mg) is effective, but is inferior to the subcutaneous preparation at aborting the pain from the cluster attack. In one study of patients who were treated intranasally, only seven of the 52 treatments resulted in complete relief of pain within 15 minutes. In another 18 of these treatments, the pain was reduced by a mean of 42.2% at 15 minutes [4]. A bitter taste after nasal delivery of sumatriptan is commonplace, with a reported prevalence of 73% [5].

> ### ☆ TIPS AND TRICKS
>
> The sumatriptan 20 mg nasal spray may offer a viable alternative to self-injection or for when subcutaneous administration is accompanied by intolerable side effects.

Oxygen

Oxygen inhalation was first described as an effective symptomatic therapy for cluster headache in the 1950s. Since then, oxygen has been regarded as a standard of care for the symptomatic relief of a cluster attack. Inhalation of 100% oxygen is most effective when administered with the patient in a sitting position, using a loose-fitting, nonrebreathing facial mask at a flow rate of 10–12 L/min for 15 minutes. The response usually is rapid, benefiting roughly 70% of patients within 15 minutes [6, 7, 8]. In some patients, flow rates of up to 15 L/min may be necessary to achieve relief [9]. Administering oxygen close to the onset of attack often aborts the pain rapidly and entirely, although some patients find oxygen to be completely effective if taken when the pain is at maximum intensity. In other patients,

however, oxygen inhalation may simply delay rather than completely abort the attack.

Oxygen is a medically safe treatment, but patients need to be cautioned that it greatly enhances combustion, and fire precautions need to be observed. It can be used in conjunction with other abortive and preventive treatments, and administered multiple times daily if necessary. The main limitation of oxygen relates to its accessibility, especially when patients are out of the house.

Dihydroergotamine

Dihydroergotamine (DHE) can be administered intravenously, intramuscularly, intranasally, or subcutaneously; an inhaled formulation is being evaluated. Of these options, the intravenous preparation works the most effectively, usually providing relief within 15 minutes [10]. The intramuscular, subcutaneous, and intranasal routes of administration of DHE are slower in their action. An RCT of intranasal DHE (1 mg) and placebo demonstrated a reduction in pain intensity in the treatment group [11]. Contraindications to treatment with ergotamine derivatives include triptan use within 24 hours of intended ergot use, pregnancy, breastfeeding, cardiac, cerebral, and peripheral vascular disease, variant angina, and uncontrolled hypertension.

Zolmitriptan

Zolmitriptan can be administered orally or intranasally. Because of its rapid delivery and fast onset of action, the intranasal formulation is a more effective treatment option for cluster headache than the oral preparation. A small study involving five patients with cluster headache demonstrated a pain-free response in 75% of the cluster attacks treated with zolmitriptan 5 mg nasal spray at 15 minutes [12]. In an RCT comparing zolmitriptan 5 mg and 10 mg nasal spray with placebo, pain relief at 30 minutes was found in 42%, 61%, and 23% of patients, respectively, while freedom from pain at 30 minutes was reported in 28%, 50%, and 16%, respectively [13]. Similar results were noted in another RCT [14].

Lidocaine

Intranasal lidocaine administered via a spray bottle or by dropping a 4% viscous solution into the nostril ipsilateral to the pain provided only moderate relief from pain in fewer than one-third of patients. It may be useful in some patients as adjunctive therapy for the relief of acute cluster attacks [15].

Preventive therapy

The importance of developing an effective preventive regimen for patients with cluster headache cannot be overstated. Repetitive treatments with acute medications will become an exhaustive and costly exercise in most cluster sufferers who experience daily or near-daily attacks, occurring sometimes multiple times per day. The primary goals of preventive therapy are to provide rapid suppression of the attacks and to maintain that suppression over the expected duration of the cluster period.

The best way to achieve these goals is with the use of transitional and maintenance prophylaxis (Table 17.1). Transitional prophylaxis refers to the short-term use of corticosteroids, ergotamine tartrate, DHE, or greater occipital nerve blockade to rapidly suppress attacks during the interval of time required for the longer acting maintenance prophylactic agents to take effect. A maintenance prophylactic drug should be started at the same time and continued throughout the anticipated duration of the cluster period in patients with episodic cluster headache (ECH). For patients with chronic cluster headache (CCH), preventive treatment is used for an indefinite period of time or until the patient has been in remission without attacks for 6 months.

Transitional prophylaxis

Corticosteroids

Corticosteroids (prednisone and dexamethasone) are the most rapidly acting of the prophylactic agents, with suppression of attacks generally occurring within the first few days of use. In an open-label study of patients treated with prednisone, marked relief of cluster headache occurred in 77% of 77 patients with ECH, and partial relief in another 12% [16]. Treatment is generally initiated with prednisone 60 mg daily for 3–5 days, and then decreased by 10 mg every 3 days over an 18-day period. Dexamethasone at a dose of 4 mg twice daily for 2 weeks followed by 4 mg daily for 1 week has also been shown to be

Table 17.1. Preventive treatment for cluster headache

Transitional
• Prednisone 60 mg daily for 3–5 days, then 10 mg decrements every 3 days to off
• Ergotamine tartrate 1–2 mg orally or by suppository daily (divided dosage)
• DHE-45 0.5–1 mg subcutaneously or intramuscularly every 8–12 hours
• Occipital nerve blockade (e.g., 3–5 cm^3 of 0.5% bupivacaine and 10–20 mg of methylprednisolone)

Maintenance
• First line Verapamil 80 mg three times a day or 240 mg sustained release; up to 720 mg daily
• Second line Valproic acid 500–2000 mg daily in divided dosages Topiramate 50–200 mg in divided daily dosages Gabapentin 300–3600 mg in divided daily dosages
• Third line Methysergide 2 mg three times a day; up to 12 mg daily Lithium carbonate 150–300 mg three times a day or 450 mg sustained release

Adjunctive
• Melatonin 10 mg daily

effective [17]. Regardless of the corticosteroid used, cluster attacks usually recur when the dose is tapered off. Because of the adverse effects associated with corticosteroids, long-term treatment should be avoided.

Ergotamine

Both ergotamine tartrate (2 mg) and DHE-45 (1 mg) are effective agents for achieving rapid suppression of attacks when administered daily for a short period of time. Both can be administered in divided daily doses, not exceeding 4 mg of ergotamine tartrate and 3 mg of DHE-45. In refractory cases, a consecutive 3-day course of combined intravenous and subcutaneous or intranasal administration of DHE was found to be effective for rapid suppression of attacks [18].

The use of ergotamine derivatives is contraindicated within 24 hours of taking sumatriptan and in patients with peripheral vascular disease, ischemic heart disease, or uncontrolled hypertension, and women who are pregnant.

Greater occipital nerve blockade

The use of a corticosteroid and lidocaine or xylocaine injection into the area of the greater occipital nerve ipsilateral to the pain is an effective short-term treatment option. One open-label study of 14 patients reported a good response in four patients, a moderate response in five patients, and no response in the remaining five patients [19]. A second open-label study of 22 injections reported that 13 injections resulted in complete or partial response for a median of 21 days [20]. An RCT of 23 patients (16 with ECH and 7 with CCH) reported that 92% of patients receiving injections with long- and rapid-acting betamethasone and 2% xylocaine experienced at least a 50% reduction of attack frequency within 1 week compared to placebo [21].

Maintenance prophylaxis

Verapamil

Verapamil is considered to be the first-line preventive therapy in the treatment of both ECH and CCH. It is well tolerated and can be used safely with acute treatments and other preventive therapies. One open-label study reported more than a 75% improvement in 69% of 48 patients [22]. An RCT comparing verapamil 360 mg to placebo over a 14-day period in patients with ECH showed a statistically significant reduction in attack frequency in the patients treated with verapamil. The effect was more pronounced in the second week [23].

Verapamil is initiated at a dose of 80 mg three times daily or 240 mg sustained release once daily. Total doses of 720 mg daily or higher may be required [24]. The most common adverse effects are constipation, edema, and bradycardia. Other potential side effects include, but are not limited to, dizziness, nausea, fatigue, hypotension, and cardiac arrhythmias. Periodic ECGs should be performed to determine whether there is atrioventricular conduction delay or block if and when the dose is escalated.

Valproic acid

Valproic acid is useful as an adjunctive therapy in refractory cases of cluster headache and in patients who are unable to tolerate or are unresponsive to high doses of verapamil. An open-label study of 15 patients treated with sodium valproate at a dose ranging from 600 mg to 2000 mg reported a 73% favorable response rate [25]. It has been suggested that patients whose cluster headaches are associated with migrainous features may preferentially respond to valproic acid [26].

An RCT using 1000–2000 mg daily of sodium valproate in the prophylaxis of 96 patients with cluster headache reported no difference between the treatment group and placebo group in terms of the primary end-point of the study. However, the high success rate observed in the placebo group (50%) was likely a result of the spontaneous remission of the cluster period [27].

The medication is usually started at 250 mg twice daily and titrated upward in 250 mg increments to as high as 2000 mg daily according to clinical response and tolerability. Pancreatitis, thrombocytopenia, and platelet and hepatic dysfunction have been described with this medication. More common potential adverse effects include, but are not limited to, nausea, weight gain, hair loss, tremor, lethargy, and neural tube defects. Blood counts and liver function tests should be monitored at baseline and periodically throughout therapy.

Topiramate

Three open-label trials have suggested that topiramate is effective as add-on maintenance prophylactic therapy for refractory cases. One study demonstrated remission in nine out of 10 patients within 1–3 weeks, including two patients with refractory CCH. A reduction in cluster period duration was seen in all 10 patients [28]. Another study of five patients treated with topiramate 75–200 mg daily reported that topiramate was effective in three of the patients [29]. A third study of 26 patients reported that topiramate started at 25 mg daily and titrated every 3–7 days to 200 mg daily rapidly induced remission in 15 patients, with a mean time to remission of 14 days. An additional six patients reported a reduction in the number of daily attacks by 50%, and

12 patients reported a reduction in the duration of their cluster period [30].

Another open-label study, however, found no significant change in headache frequency with the use of topiramate. Of 33 patients, 23 with ECH and 10 with CCH, only seven patients (21%) reported a 50% or greater reduction in the daily number of attacks. Of the seven patients with improvement, doses of 100–150 mg were used, and the seven patients on doses of 200 mg reported no benefit [31].

In light of the available data, topiramate is a reasonable option for add-on therapy in refractory patients who do not respond to verapamil. Side effects of topiramate include paresthesias, cognitive dysfunction, ataxia, dizziness, somnolence, and, rarely, renal calculi and glaucoma. The potential for these adverse events can be reduced if topiramate is initiated at a low dose, and small incremental increases are made every week until the patient reaches the lowest effective dose.

Gabapentin

There are limited data regarding the efficacy of gabapentin as a preventive therapy for cluster headache. Small open-label trials and a handful of case reports have demonstrated that gabapentin may be an effective add-on therapy for refractory cluster headache. One small open-label study of 12 patients treated with 900 mg daily of gabapentin reported that all patients became pain-free within 8 days of starting the medication [35]. Another open-label study of patients treated with 800–3600 mg daily of gabapentin reported that 75% of patients experienced at least a 50% reduction in attacks [36]. Gabapentin has minimal side effects and few drug interactions; it is thus a reasonable adjunctive treatment option.

Lithium carbonate

A 1981 literature review collected data from more than 28 clinical trials involving 468 patients with cluster headache. Good to excellent results were seen for 78% of the 304 patients with CCH. These results were stable up to 4 years. The results for ECH, while still positive, were less robust than for CCH. Sixty-three percent of the 164 patients with ECH attained good results [32, 33]. A double-blind study comparing verapamil 360 mg daily with lithium 900 mg daily in 30 patients found

that lithium was equally as effective as verapamil when used as a prophylactic therapy for cluster headache [34].

The starting dose of lithium is 300 mg two times daily or 450 mg sustained release once daily. The therapeutic serum concentration in cluster headache is 0.4–0.8 mEq/L, which is usually attained with doses ranging from 600 mg to 900 mg daily. Lithium levels must be monitored regularly as lithium has an extremely narrow therapeutic window and the potential for many side effects. The serum lithium level should not go beyond 1.0 mEq/L, and should be measured 12 hours after the last dose. Baseline kidney and thyroid function tests should be obtained before initiating treatment and should be periodically monitored. Side effects include tremor, diarrhea, weakness, nausea, vomiting, anorexia, confusion, nystagmus, ataxia, extrapyramidal signs, seizures, hypothyroidism, and nephrogenic diabetes insipidus; coma and death may occur with toxic levels.

Methysergide

Methysergide is an extremely effective medication for the treatment of ECH, with roughly 70% of patients demonstrating good to excellent results [10]. The usual daily dose is 6 mg administered in three divided doses, but doses as high as 12 mg can be used if tolerated. Its use is limited by its side effect profile, and the drug is no longer available for use in the USA. Long-term use can result in fibrosis of the retroperitoneum, pleural lining, cardiac valves, and pericardium. It is recommended that a baseline ECG, CT or MRI of the chest, abdomen, and pelvis, urinalysis, and sedimentation rate be obtained prior to initiating methysergide therapy and periodically monitored throughout the treatment course. Patients should have a 1-month drug holiday every 6 months. Long-term use reduces its efficacy in 20% of patients. Short-term side effects include nausea, abdominal pain, muscle cramps, and edema. The active metabolite of methysergide is methylergotamine; thus, it should not be used with other ergot derivatives or vasoconstrictive agents such as sumatriptan.

Melatonin

Melatonin is produced by the pineal gland under the control of the suprachiasmatic nucleus of the hypothalamus. Patients with cluster headache have reduced serum levels of melatonin, particularly during an attack [37]. Melatonin has been investigated as a potential preventive therapy in the treatment of cluster headache, with mixed results. In a double-blind study of 20 patients treated with melatonin 10 mg compared to placebo, five of the 10 patients treated with melatonin attained remission within 3–5 days compared to none of the 10 patients in the placebo group [38]. In a report of two patients with CCH poorly controlled by verapamil 640 mg daily, pain freedom was achieved with melatonin 9 mg used as adjunctive therapy [39]. A pilot study of nine patients found there was no statistically significant difference between melatonin and placebo [40]. Although the data are mixed, melatonin is, given its benign side effect profile, a reasonable option for adjunctive therapy in refractory cluster headache.

Treatments for refractory cluster headache

Approximately 15% of patients develop CCH that is unresponsive to monotherapy, 10% having evolved from ECH and 5% having arisen *de novo*. Prior to considering surgical treatment options in these patients, it is important to try combination medical therapy, as patients may require more than one agent. If combination therapy is ineffective and all medical treatments have been exhausted, surgery may be a reasonable option. Usually reserved for patients with intractable CCH, surgery may rarely be considered for those patients with ECH who have frequent debilitating cluster periods and are unable to tolerate or have contraindications to preventive and acute therapy (Table 17.2). Only those patients with a stable psychological profile and strictly unilateral headaches that are localized primarily to the ophthalmic division of the trigeminal nerve are candidates for surgery. If the patient has a history of attacks alternating sides, there is a high risk of recurrence on the side contralateral to the surgery [41].

Surgery targeting the sensory trigeminal nerve

Several surgical procedures target the sensory trigeminal nerve. These include radiofrequency trigeminal rhizotomy, retrogasserian glycerol injection, alcohol injection into the supraorbital

Table 17.2. Surgical procedures for cluster headache

Procedures directed toward the sensory trigeminal nerve:
• Radiofrequency trigeminal rhizotomy • Retrogasserian glycerol injection • Alcohol injection into the supra- or infraorbital nerve, or gasserian ganglion • Trigeminal nerve root section • Microvascular decompression (MVD) and/or section of the nervus intermedius
Procedures directed toward autonomic pathways:
• Section of the greater superficial petrosal nerve or nervus intermedius • Section or cocainization of the sphenopalatine ganglion
Gamma-knife radiosurgery
Deep brain stimulation
Occipital nerve stimulation

or infraorbital nerves, gamma-knife radiosurgery, microvascular decompression, and trigeminal nerve root sectioning.

Radiofrequency trigeminal rhizotomy is the most commonly used destructive procedure aimed at the sensory trigeminal ganglion in patients with cluster headache. The overall response is positive, with patients reporting good to excellent results that in some last for several years after the procedure [42, 43]. The procedure is safe and is preferred over retrogasserian glycerol injection as it allows for precise lesioning of the ganglion with less risk of aseptic meningitis and subarachnoid hemorrhage. Adverse events include facial dysesthesias, anesthesia dolorosa, corneal sensory loss, and keratitis.

Retrogasserian glycerol injection is percutaneous denervation of the trigeminal roots. Initial response rates are similar to those seen with radiofrequency rhizotomy, but there is a higher recurrence rate with glycerol injection [44]. Advantages of this procedure over radiofrequency trigeminal rhizotomy include a lower incidence of corneal anesthesia and keratitis, and the fact that it is less technically complicated and less expensive than radiofrequency. Disadvantages include lower precision and a higher recurrence rate, and need for repeat injections than is seen with radiofrequency trigeminal rhizotomy [41].

Extracranial peripheral denervation includes denervating the supraorbital nerve at the supraorbital notch in patients with pain predominantly around the eye or at the infraorbital notch if the pain also involves the maxillary region. Denervation with alcohol or nerve avulsion evokes pain relief lasting for 6–30 months. There is no risk of corneal denervation or keratitis associated with this procedure [41].

The trigeminal nerve root can be sectioned at the root entry zone via a suboccipital craniotomy [45, 46]. Studies suggest that better benefits are attained with complete compared to incomplete lesioning of the nerve root.

Gamma-knife stereotactic radiosurgery is a minimally invasive procedure designed to precisely lesion the trigeminal nerve root entry zone [47, 48]. Adverse effects include paresthesias, hypoesthesia, and deafferentation pain. The beneficial effects may be delayed for several weeks.

Microvascular decompression is a surgical procedure that aims to separate the vascular loops compressing the trigeminal nerve root. It may be combined with sectioning and/or decompression of the nervus intermedius [49]. The role of microvascular decompression in the management of refractory cluster headache is problematic.

Peripheral neuromodulation

Since 1999, greater occipital nerve stimulation has been used as a treatment for refractory primary headache disorders, especially chronic migraine and occipital neuralgia. A few studies of implantation of a suboccipital nerve stimulator on the side ipsilateral to the cluster headache have reported improvement [50, 51]. Disabling paresthesias or local infection required the removal of the stimulator. The benefit of the stimulator may take several weeks to become apparent, and the intensity of attacks begins to decrease before the frequency. Patients may still have autonomic symptoms in the absence of pain after successful implantation [52].

One small study of vagus nerve stimulation in two patients with CCH noted an improvement in headache and in disability [53]. The efficacy of the device is doubtful.

Sphenopalatine ganglion stimulation

A small study of patients with refractory CCH evaluated the efficacy of sphenopalatine ganglion stimulation. Complete resolution was seen in 11 attacks, partial resolution (>50% pain reduction) in three patients, and minimal to no relief in nine patients. In cases of complete or partial response, pain relief occurred within 1–3 minutes of stimulation [54].

Hypothalamic deep brain stimulation

The ipsilateral posterior inferior hypothalamus plays an important role in the generation of cluster headaches, and hypothalamic deep brain stimulation has thus been investigated as a therapy for refractory cluster headache. Several studies have shown a positive response [55, 56, 57, 58, 59, 60, 61, 62]. The most common adverse event was transient diplopia. One patient developed a fatal intracranial hemorrhage several hours after surgery, and one patient had a small asymptomatic hemorrhage within the third ventricle. This procedure should be reserved for refractory cases that have failed medical management and have not responded to peripheral neuromodulation.

Paroxysmal hemicrania

The treatment of paroxysmal hemicrania is aimed at preventive therapy, as individual attacks are too brief to allow for effective acute treatment. The importance of making an accurate diagnosis cannot be overstated, as paroxysmal hemicrania is typically exquisitely responsive to indomethacin. Treatment becomes more complicated if the patient is either unresponsive to or is unable to tolerate indomethacin as no other therapy is consistently as effective.

Indomethacin

Indomethacin is the treatment of choice for paroxysmal hemicrania. Complete resolution can be expected within 1–2 days of reaching an effective dose. The vast majority of patients respond within 8–24 hours to a dose of 75–150 mg daily. The response to intramuscular indomethacin is even more robust, but this formulation is not available in the USA [63, 64, 65]. Given the risk of peptic ulcers associated with long-term indomethacin therapy, patients should also be given prophylaxis to protect the stomach. The suppository formulation can be utilized to reduce gastric exposure.

Maintenance doses usually fall in the range of 25–100 mg daily, but may be as low as 12.5 mg daily and as high as 300 mg daily. If higher doses are needed, a secondary cause should be sought [66]. The required dose may fluctuate over time [67, 68]. For patients with episodic paroxysmal hemicrania, the dose should be tapered off after the expected duration of a bout.

Other nonsteroidal anti-inflammatory drugs and cyclooxygenase-2 inhibitors

Nearly all other nonsteroidal anti-inflammatory drugs have been tried, with limited success. Isolated case reports have demonstrated efficacy with the use of aspirin, ketoprofen, ibuprofen, naproxen, and piroxicam B–cyclodextrin [69, 70, 71, 72]. There have been case reports of success with rofecoxib and celecoxib [73, 74, 75]. None of these medications has been as consistently effective as indomethacin.

Other medications

Isolated case reports of successful treatment with calcium channel antagonists (verapamil, flunarizine, and nicardipine), acetazolamide, prednisone, ergotamines, lithium, sumatriptan, carbamazepine, and topiramate exist, but the response is inconsistent. There is one case report of successful treatment with botulinum toxin A injected into the ipsilateral temporalis muscle [76, 77, 78, 79, 80, 81, 82, 83, 84].

Local blockades and invasive surgical procedures

Rare cases of a positive response to blockade with lidocaine or bupivacaine in combination with methylprednisolone have been reported [85, 86, 87, 88], and one patient had stellate ganglionectomy that rendered him completely pain-free. With the exception of the latter single case report, surgical procedures are ineffective.

Short-lasting unilateral neuralgiform headache with conjunctival injection and tearing

With individual attacks lasting on average between 2 and 240 seconds, acute therapy is untenable. Short-term prevention in a hospital setting is indicated if attacks are of sufficient severity to render the patient disabled. Short-term prevention strives to rapidly suppress attacks during the interval of time required for the longer acting maintenance prophylactic agents to take effect.

Short-term prevention

Lidocaine

Intravenous lidocaine (1.3–3.3 mg/kg per hour) has been extremely effective in suppressing headache attacks in short-lasting unilateral neuralgiform headache with conjunctival injection and tearing (SUNCT) [89, 90, 91]. The longest pain-free period was 3 weeks in a patient with chronic SUNCT, 12 weeks in a patient with chronic short-lasting unilateral neuralgiform headache with cranial autonomic features (SUNA), and 6 months in a patient with episodic SUNCT [92]. Lidocaine administered intranasally was ineffective, and lidocaine mouthwash resulted in a possible improvement in two of five patients [89].

Long-term prevention

Lamotrigine

As one might expect in the treatment of rare diseases, only small open-label studies and case reports are available. Except for some antiepileptic drugs, most therapies have been found to be ineffective. As usual, single cases of apparent success are reported.

Lamotrigine is the treatment of choice in the management of SUNCT and SUNA syndromes. Results ranged from highly effective to nil [93, 94, 95, 96, 97, 98, 99]. The dose ranged from 100 mg to 400 mg daily. Stevens–Johnson syndrome is a potentially serious adverse effect.

Topiramate

The response to topiramate was variable in a few cases. The dose ranged from 50 mg to 300 mg daily [89, 92, 100, 101]. One study reported a good response in half of patients with SUNCT, but the response in SUNA was less obvious [91].

Gabapentin

The effect of gabapentin has been studied in a small number of cases [89, 102, 103, 104, 105].

Doses ranged from 800 mg to 2700 mg daily. In one open-label trial, gabapentin was effective in 45% of SUNCT cases and 60% of SUNA cases.

Carbemazapine

There was no response of SUNCT to carbamazepine monotherapy [90, 103, 106, 107] but some patients reported a good response when carbamazepine was administered in conjunction with other agents such as naloxone, verapamil, lithium, or steroids [92, 108, 109, 110].

Other drugs

Numerous other drugs have been tried in open-label studies and have been found to be ineffective with the exception of isolated case reports [89, 108, 109, 111].

Surgical procedures

Local nerve blockades

Local blockade of multiple pericranial nerves have been attempted and are generally regarded as ineffective [89, 98, 112]. A few patients appeared to respond to greater occipital nerve blocks with lidocaine and methylprednisolone.

Invasive surgical procedures involving the trigeminal nerve

Most of the procedures utilized for cluster headache have been tried for the treatment of SUNCT without consistent success [106, 113, 114, 115, 116, 117]. One patient with intractable chronic SUNCT, averaging 77 attacks daily, was successfully treated with ipsilateral posterior inferior hypothalamic deep brain stimulation [118].

References

1. Ekbom K. The sumatriptan cluster headache study group. Treatment of acute cluster headache with sumatriptan. *New Eng J Med* 1991;**325**(5):322–6.
2. Gobel H, Lindner V, Heinze A, Ribbat M, Deuschl G. Acute therapy for cluster headache with sumatriptan: findings of a one-year long-term study. *Neurology* 1998;**51**(3):908–11.
3. Ekbom K, Krabbe A, Micieli G, et al. Cluster headache attacks treated for up to three months with subcutaneous sumatriptan (6mg). *Cephalalgia* 1995;**15**:230–6.
4. Van Vliet JA, Bahra A, Martin V, et al. Intranasal sumatriptan in cluster headache: randomized placebo-controlled double-blind study. *Neurology* 2003;**60**:630–3.
5. Hardebo JE, Dahlof C. Sumatriptan nasal spray (20mg/dose) in the acute treatment of cluster headache. *Cephalalgia* 1998;**18**: 487–9.
6. Kudrow L. Response of cluster headache attacks to oxygen inhalation. *Headache* 1981;**21**:1–4.
7. Fogan L. Treatment of cluster headache. A double-blind comparison of oxygen vs. air inhalation. *Arch Neurol* 1985;**42**:362–3.
8. Cohen AS, Burns B, Goadsby PJ. High-flow oxygen for treatment of cluster headache: a randomized trial. *JAMA* 2009;**302**(22): 2451–7.
9. Rozen TF. High oxygen flow rates for cluster headache. *Neurology* 2004;**63**:593.
10. Dodick DW, Rozen TD, Goadsby PJ, Silberstein SD. Cluster headache. *Cephalalgia* 2000;**20**:787–803.
11. Anderson PG, Jesperson LT. Dihydroergotamine nasal spray in the treatment of attacks of cluster headache. *Cephalalgia* 1996;**6**:51–4.
12. Bahra A, Becker WJ, Blau JN. Efficacy of oral zolmitriptan in acute treatment of cluster headache. *Cephalalgia* 1999;**19**:457.
13. Mathew NT, Kailasam J, Seifer T, Bouton T. Zolmitriptan (Zomig) nasal spray in cluster headache attacks; a single-blind observation—a preliminary report. *Headache* 2004; **44**:483.
14. Cittadini E, May A, Straube A, Evers S, Bussone G, Goadsby PJ. Effectiveness of intranasal zolmitriptan in acute cluster headache: a randomized, placebo-controlled, double-blind crossover study. *Arch Neurol* 2006;**63**:1537–42.
15. Robbins L. Intranasal lidocaine for cluster headache. *Headache* 1995;**35**:83–4.
16. Kudrow L. *Cluster Headache: Mechanisms and Management*. Oxford: New York: Oxford University Press; 1980.
17. Anthony M, Daher BN. Mechanism of action of steroids in cluster headache. In Clifford RF (ed.), *New Advances in Headache Research, 2*. London: Smith Gordon; 1992: pp. 271–4.

18. Magnoux E, Zlotnik G. Outpatient intravenous dihydroergotamine for refractory cluster headache. *Headache* 2004;**44**: 249–55.

19. Peres MFP, Stiles MA, Siow HC, Rozen TD, Young WB, Silberstein SD. Greater occipital nerve blockade for cluster headache. *Cephalalgia* 2002;**22**:520–2.

20. Afridi SK, Shields KG, Bhola R, Goadsby PJ. Greater occipital nerve injection in primary headache syndromes – prolonged effects from a single injection. *Pain* 2006;**122**: 126–9.

21. Ambrosini A, Vandenheede M, Rossi P, Aloj F, Sauli E, Buzzi MG. Suboccipital (GON) injection with long-acting steroids in cluster headache: a double-blind placebo-controlled study. *Cephalalgia* 2003;**23**:734.

22. Gabaj IJ Spierings EHL. Prophylactic treatment of cluster headache with verapamil. *Headache* 1989;**29**:167–8.

23. Leone M, D'Amico D, Allanasio A, et al. Verapamil is an effective prophylactic for cluster headache: results of a double-blind multicenter study versus placebo. In Olesen J, Goadsby PJ (eds.), *Cluster Headache and Related Conditions*. Oxford: Oxford University Press;1999: pp. 296–9.

24. Gobel H, Holzgreve H, Heinze A, Deuschl G, Engel C, Kuhn K. Retarded verapamil for cluster headache prophylaxis. *Cephalalgia* 1999;**19**:458–9.

25. Hering R, Kuritzky A. Sodium valproate in the treatment of cluster headache: an open trial. *Cephalalgia* 1989;**9**:195–8.

26. Wheeler S. Significance of migrainous features in cluster headache: divalproex responsiveness. *Headache* 1998;**38**:547–51.

27. El Amrani M, Massiou H, Bousser MG. A negative trial of sodium valproate in cluster headache: methodological issues. *Cephalalgia* 2002;**22**:205–8.

28. Wheeler S, Carrazana EJ. Topiramate-treated cluster headache. *Neurology* 1999; **53**:234–6.

29. Forderrenther S, Mayer M, Straube A. Treatment of cluster headache with topiramate: effects and side-effects in five patients. *Cephalalgia* 2002;**22**:186–9.

30. Lainez MJA, Pascual J, Pascual AM, et al. Topiramate in the prophylactic treatment of cluster headache. *Headache* 2003;**43**: 784–9.

31. Leone M, Dodick D, Rigamonti A, et al. Topiramate in cluster headache prophylaxis: an open trial. *Cephalalgia* 2003;**23**: 1001–2.

32. Ekbom K. Lithium for cluster headache: review of the literature and preliminary results of long-term treatment. *Headache* 1981;**21**(4):132–9.

33. Manzoni GC, Bono G, Lanfranchi M, et al. Lithium carbonate in cluster headache: assessment of its short and long-term therapeutic efficacy. *Cephalalgia* 1983;**3**: 109–14.

34. Bussone G, Leone M, Peccarisi C. Double-blind comparison of lithium and verapamil in cluster headache prophylaxis. *Headache* 1990;**30**:411–7.

35. Leandri M, Luzzani M, Cruccu G, Gottlieb A. Drug-resistant cluster headache responding to gabapentin: a pilot study. *Cephalalgia* 2001;**21**:744–6.

36. Schuh-Hofer S, Israel H, Need L, Reuter U, Arnold G. The use of gabapentin in chronic cluster patients refractory to first-line treatment. *Eur J Neurol* 2007;**14**(6):694–6.

37. Leone M, Lucini V, D'Amico D, et al. Twenty-four hour melatonin and cortisol plasma levels in relation to timing of cluster headache. *Cephalalgia* 1995;**15**:224–9.

38. Leone M, D'Amico D, Moschiano F, et al. Melatonin versus placebo in the prophylaxis of cluster headache" a double-blind pilot study with parallel groups. *Cephalalgia* 1996;**16**:494–6.

39. Peres MF, Rozen TD. Melatonin in preventive treatment of chronic cluster headache. *Cephalalgia* 2001;**21**:993–5.

40. Pringsheim T, Magnou E, Dobson CF, Jamel E, Aube M. Melatonin as adjunctive therapy in the prophylaxis of cluster headache: a pilot study. *Headache* 2002;**42**(8): 787–92.

41. Rozen TD. Interventional treatment for cluster headache: a review of the options. *Curr Pain Head Rep* 2002;**6**:57–64.

42. Mathew NT, Hurt W. Percutaneous radiofrequency trigeminal gangliorhizolysis in intractable cluster headache. *Headache* 1988; **28**:328–31.

43. Taha JM, Tew JM. Long-term results of radiofrequency rhizotomy in the treatment of cluster headache. *Headache* 1995;**35**:193–6.

44. Pieper DR, Dickerson J. Hassenbusch SJ. Percutaneous retrogasserian glycerol rhizolysis for treatment of chronic intractable cluster headaches: long-term results. *Neurosurgery* 2000;**46**:363–8.

45. Kirkpatrick PJ, O'Brien MD, MacCabe JJ. Trigeminal nerve section for chronic migrainous neuralgia. *Br J Neurosurg* 1993; **7**:483–90.

46. Jarrar RG, Black DF, Dodick DW, Davis DH. Outcome of trigeminal nerve section in the treatment of cluster headache. *Neurology* 2003;**60**:1360–2.

47. Ford RG, Ford KT, Swaid S, Young P, Jennelle R. Gamma knife treatment of refractory cluster headache. *Headache* 1998;**38**:3–9.

48. Donnet A, Valade D, Regis J. Gamma knife treatment for refractory cluster headache: prospective open trial. *J Neurol Neurosurg Psychiatry* 2005;**76**:218–21.

49. Lovely TJ, Kotsiakis X, Jannetta PJ. The surgical management of chronic cluster headache. *Headache* 1998;**38**:590–4.

50. Magis D, Allena M, Bolla M, De Pasqua V, Remacle J-M, Schoenen J. Occipital nerve stimulation for drug-resistant chronic cluster headache. *Lancet Neurol* 2007;**6**: 314–21.

51. Burns B, Watkins L, Goadsby PJ. Treatment of medically intractable cluster headache by occipital nerve stimulation: long-term follow-up of eight patients. *Lancet.* 2007;**369**: 1099–106.

52. Schwedt T, Dodick D, Trentman T, Zimmerman R. Occipital nerve stimulation for chronic cluster headache and hemicrania continua: pain relief and persistence of autonomic features. *Cephalalgia* 2006;**26**: 1025–7.

53. Mauskop A. VNS relieves chronic refractory migraine and cluster headache. *Cephalalgia* 2005;**25**(2):82–6.

54. Ansarinia M, Rezai A, Tepper SJ, et al. Electrical stimulation of sphenopalatine ganglion for acute treatment of cluster headaches. *Headache* 2010;**50**:1164–74.

55. Leone M, Proletti Cecchini A, Franzini A, et al. Lessons from 8 years experience of

56. Leone M, Franzini A, Broggi G, Bussone G. Hypothalamic stimulation for intractable cluster headache: long-term experience. *Neurology* 2006;**67**:150–2.

57. Schoenen J, Di Clemente L, Vandenheede M, et al. Hypothalamic stimulation in chronic cluster headache: a pilot study of efficacy and mode of action. *Brain* 2005;**128**:940–7.

58. Starr PA, Barbaro NM, Raskin NH, Ostrem JL. Chronic stimulation of the posterior hypothalamic region for cluster headache: technique and 1-year results in four patients. *J Neurosurg* 2007;**106**:999–1005.

59. Bartsch T, Pinsker MO, Rasche D, et al. Hypothalamic deep brain stimulation for cluster headache—experience from a new multicase series. *Cephalalgia* 2008;**28**: 285–95.

60. Leone M, Franzini A, Bussone G. Stereotactic stimulation of posterior hypothalamic gray matter for intractable cluster headache. *N Engl J Med* 2001;**345**:1428–9.

61. Leone M, Franzini A, Broggi G, May A, Bussone G. Long-term follow up of bilateral hypothalamic stimulation for intractable cluster headache. *Brain* 2004;**127**: 2259–64.

62. Franzini A, Ferroli P, Leone M, Bussone G, Broggi G. Hypothalamic deep brain stimulation for the treatment of chronic cluster headache: a series report. *Neuromodulation* 2004;**1**:1–8.

63. Sjaastad O. Chronic paroxysmal hemicrania. In Vinken P, Bruyn G, Klawans H, et al. (eds.), *Handbook of Clinical Neurology*, Vol. 48. Amsterdam: Elsevier; 1986: pp. 257–66

64. Pareja J, Sjaastad O. Chronic paroxysmal hemicrania and hemicrania continua. Interval between indomethacin administration and response. *Headache* 1996;**36**: 20–3.

65. Antonaci F, Pareja JA, Caminero AB, Sjaastad O. Chronic paroxysmal hemicrania and hemicrania continua. Parenteral indomethacin: the "indotest." *Headache* 1998;**38**: 122–8.

66. Sjaastad O, Stovner LJ, Stolt-Nielsen A, et al. CPH and hemicrania continua: require-

ments of high indomethacin dosages—an ominous sign? *Headache* 1995;**35**:363–7.

67. Pareja JA, Caminero AB, Franco E, et al. Dose, efficacy and tolerability of long-term indomethacin treatment of chronic paroxysmal hemicrania and hemicrania continua. *Cephalalgia* 2001;**21**:906–10.

68. Antonaci F, Sjaastad O. Chronic paroxysmal hemicrania (CPH): a review of the clinical manifestations. *Headache* 1989;**29**:648–56.

69. Kudrow DB, Kudrow L. Successful aspirin prophylaxis in a child with chronic paroxysmal hemicrania. *Headache* 1989;**29**:280–1.

70. Evers S, Husstedt IW. Alternatives in drug treatment of chronic paroxysmal hemicrania. *Headache* 1996;**36**:429–32.

71. Durko A, Klimek A. Naproxen in the treatment of chronic paroxysmal hemicrania. *Cephalalgia* 1987;**7**:361–2.

72. Sjaastad O, Antonaci F. A piroxicam derivative partly effective in chronic paroxysmal hemicrania and hemicrania continua. *Headache* 1995;**35**:49–50.

73. Lisotto C, Maggioni F, Mainardi F. Rofecoxib for the treatment of chronic paroxysmal hemicrania. *Cephalalgia* 2003;**23**:318–20.

74. Siow H. Seasonal episodic paroxysmal hemicrania responding to cyclooxygenase-2 inhibitors. *Cephalalgia* 2004;**24**:414–5.

75. Mathew NT, Kailasam J, Fischer A. Responsiveness to celecoxib in chronic paroxysmal hemicrania. *Neurology* 2000;**55**:316.

76. Shabbir N, McAbee G. Adolescent chronic paroxysmal hemicrania responsive to verapamil monotherapy. *Headache* 1994;**34**:209–10.

77. de Almeida DB, Cunali PA, Santos HL, et al. Chronic paroxysmal hemicrania in early childhood: case report. *Cephalalgia* 2004;**24**:608–9.

78. Zidverc-Trajkovic J, Pavlovic A, Mijajlovic M, et al. Cluster headache and paroxysmal hemicrania: differential diagnosis. *Cephalalgia* 2005;**25**:244–8.

79. Coria F, Claveria LE, Jimenez-Jimenez FJ, de Seijas EV. Episodic paroxysmal hemicrania responsive to calcium channel blockers. *J Neurol Neurosurg Psychiatr* 1992;**55**:166.

80. Warner JS, Wamil AW, McLean MJ. Acetazolamide for the treatment of chronic paroxysmal hemicrania. *Headache* 1994;**34**:597–9.

81. Hannerz J, Jogestrand T. Intracranial hypertension and sumatriptan efficacy in a case of chronic paroxysmal hemicrania which became bilateral. (The mechanism of indomethacin in CPH). *Headache* 1993;**33**:320–3.

82. Pascual J, Quijano J. A case of chronic paroxysmal hemicrania responding to subcutaneous sumatriptan. *J Neurol Neurosurg Psychiatry* 1998;**65**:407.

83. Cohen AS, Goadsby PJ. Paroxysmal hemicrania responding to topiramate. *J Neurol Neurosurg Psychiatry* 2007;**78**:96–7.

84. Gobel H, Heinze A, Heinze-Kuhn K. Botulinum toxin A in the treatment of chronic paroxysmal hemicrania—a case report. *Cephalalgia* 2001;**21**:506.

85. Antonaci F, Pareja JA, Caminero AB, et al. Chronic paroxysmal hemicrania and hemicrania continua: blockade of pericranial nerves. *Funct Neurol* 1997;**12**:11–5.

86. Rossi P, Di Lorenzo G, Faroni J, et al. Seasonal, extratrigeminal, episodic paroxysmal hemicrania successfully treated with single suboccipital steroid injection. *Eur J Neurol* 2005;**12**:903–6.

87. Afridi SK, Shields KG, Bhola R, et al. Greater occipital nerve injection in primary headache syndromes—prolonged effects from a single injection. *Pain* 2006;**122**:126–9.

88. Antonaci F, Sjaastad O. Chronic paroxysmal hemicrania: a review of the clinical manifestations. *Headache* 1989;**29**:648–56.

89. Pareja JA, Kruszewski P, Sjaastad O. SUNCT syndrome: trials of drugs and anesthetic blockades. *Headache* 1995;**35**:138–42.

90. Matharu MS, Cohen AS, Goadsby PJ. SUNCT syndrome responsive to intravenous lidocaine. *Cephalalgia* 2004;**24**:985–92.

91. Cohen AS, Matharu MS, Goadsby PJ. Suggested guidelines for treating SUNCT and SUNA. *Cephalalgia* 2005;**25**:1200.

92. Matharu MS, Boes CJ, Goadsby PJ. SUNCT syndrome: prolonged attacks, refractoriness and response to topiramate. *Neurology* 2002;**58**:1307.

93. D'Andrea G, Granella F, Ghiotto N, Nappi G. Lamotrigine in the treatment of SUNCT syndrome. *Neurology* 2001;**57**:1723–5.

94. Gutierrez-Garcia JM. SUNCT syndrome responsive to lamotrigine. *Headache* 2002; **42**:823–5.

95. Chakravarty A, Mukherjee A. SUNCT syndrome responsive to lamotrigine: documentation of the first Indian case. *Cephalalgia* 2003;**23**:474–5.

96. Leone M, Rigamonte A, Usai S, et al. Two new SUNCT cases responsive to lamotrigine. *Cephalalgia* 2000;**20**:845–7.

97. D'Andrea G, Granella F, Cadaldini M. Possible usefulness of lamotrigine in the treatment of SUNCT syndrome. *Neurology* 1999;**53**:1609.

98. Piovesan EJ, Siow C, Kowacs PA, Werneck LC. Influence of lamotrigine in the treatment of SUNCT syndrome: one patient follow-up for two years. *Arq Neuropsiquiatr* 2003;**61**:691–4.

99. Malik K, Rizvi S, Vaillancourt PD. The SUNCT syndrome: successfully treated with lamotrigine. *Pain Med* 2002;**3**:167–8.

100. Rossi P, Cesarino F, Faroni J, et al. SUNCT syndrome successfully treated with topiramate: case reports. *Cephalalgia* 2003;**23**: 474–5.

101. Kuhn J, Vosskaemper M, Bewermeyer H. SUNCT syndrome: a possible bilateral case responding to topiramate. *Neurology* 2005; **64**:2159.

102. Matharu MS, Cohen AS, Boes CA, et al. Short-lasting unilateral neuralgiform headache with conjunctival injection and tearing syndrome: a review. *Curr Pain Headache Rep* 2003;**7**:308–18.

103. Graff-Radford SB. SUNCT syndrome responsive to gabapentin. *Cephalalgia* 2000; **20**:515–7.

104. Hunt CH, Dodick DW, Bosch EP. SUNCT syndrome responsive to gabapentin. *Neurology* 2002;**42**:525–6.

105. Porta-Etessam J, Benito-Leon J, Martinez-Salio A, et al. Gabapentin in the treatment of SUNCT syndrome. *Headache* 2002;**42**: 523–4.

106. Black DF, Dodick DW. Two cases of medically and surgically intractable SUNCT: a reason for caution and an argument for a central mechanism. *Cephalalgia* 2002;**22**: 201–4.

107. Goadsby PJ, Lipton RB. A review of paroxysmal hemicranias, SUNCT syndrome and other short lasting headaches with autonomic feature, including new cases. *Brain* 1997;**120**:193–209.

108. Montes E, Alberca R, Lozano P, et al. Status-like SUNCT in two young women. *Headache* 2001;**41**:826–9.

109. Sabatowski R, Huber M, Meuser T, et al. SUNCT syndrome: a treatment option with local opioid blockade of the superior cervical ganglion? A case report. *Cephalalgia* 2001;**21**:154–6.

110. Raimondi E, Gardella L. SUNCT syndrome. Two cases in Argentina. *Headache* 1998;**38**: 369–71.

111. Hannerz J, Greitz D, Hansson P, et al. SUNCT may be another manifestation of orbital venous vasculitis. *Headache* 1992;**32**:384–9.

112. Hannerz J, Linderoth B. Neurosurgical treatment of short-lasting, unilateral, neuralgiform hemicrania with conjunctival injection and tearing. *Br J Neurosurg* 2002;**16**:55–8.

113. Koseoglu E, Karaman Y, Kucuk S, et al. SUNCT syndrome associated with compression of trigeminal nerve. *Cephalalgia* 2005;**25**:473–5.

114. Sprenger T, Valet M, Platzer S, et al. SUNCT: bilateral hypothalamic activation during headache attacks and resolving of symptoms after trigeminal decompression. *Pain* 2005;**113**:422–6.

115. Matharu MS, Goadsby PJ. Persistence of attacks of cluster headache after trigeminal nerve root section. *Brain* 2002;**125**:976–84.

116. Gardella L, Viruega A, Rojas H, Nagel J. A case of a patient with SUNCT syndrome treated with Jannetta procedure. *Cephalalgia* 2001;**21**:996–9.

117. Lenaerts M, Diederich N, Phuce K. A patient with SUNCT cured by the Jannetta procedure. *Cephalalgia* 1997;**17**:461.

118. Leone M, Franzini A, D'Andrea G, Broggi G, Casucci G, Bussone G. Deep brain stimulation to relieve drug-resistant SUNCT. *Ann Neurol* 2005;**57**:924–7.

Part V

Other Headache Disorders

New Daily Persistent Headache

Matthew S. Robbins

Albert Einstein College of Medicine, Bronx, NY, USA

Introduction

Chronic daily headache (CDH) of long duration is a heterogeneous syndrome, encompassing four primary headache disorders that cause head pain on 15 or more days per month over at least 3 months, with untreated pain lasting at least 4 hours on each day of headache [1]. CDH has four subtypes: chronic migraine (CM), chronic tension-type headache (CTTH), hemicrania continua (HC), and new daily persistent headache (NDPH) [2]. CM, CTTH, and HC are each covered separately within this volume.

NDPH distinguishes itself from the other forms of CDH based on its defining feature of continuous headache since its onset, lacking the gradual evolution from pre-existing episodic headache that defines CM and CTTH (Figure 18.1). Here we review the available literature on this unusual disorder, highlighting its diagnosis, potential initiating features, clinical features, epidemiology, prognosis, and management.

Making the diagnosis

NDPH is defined as the acute onset of a constant and continuous or near-continuous headache without any identifiable cause. A patient presenting with the acute onset of a daily headache at any age warrants an exhaustive search for an underlying cause and 3 months to elapse before NDPH can be diagnosed. The treating physician should probe for all of the usual "red flags," as outlined earlier in this volume. All patients should undergo a detailed history, physical examination, neurologic examination (including fundoscopy), and a neuroimaging study. Serologic tests and a lumbar puncture for opening pressure and cerebrospinal fluid examination should also be performed in selected patients where systemic disease or derangements of intracranial pressure are suspected.

> ### ✋ CAUTION!
>
> When considering the diagnosis of NDPH, the possibility of spontaneous intracranial hypotension from a spinal cerebrospinal fluid leak should always be entertained. This disorder usually provokes a daily headache with orthostatic features, but in some patients the positional component is absent. In these patients, a "second half of the day" pattern can be observed, where the patient awakens after a night in recumbency headache-free, and as the day progresses a worsening headache develops while the patient is upright [3].

Headache, First Edition. Edited by Matthew S. Robbins, Brian M. Grosberg, and Richard B. Lipton.
© 2013 John Wiley & Sons, Ltd. Published 2013 by John Wiley & Sons, Ltd.

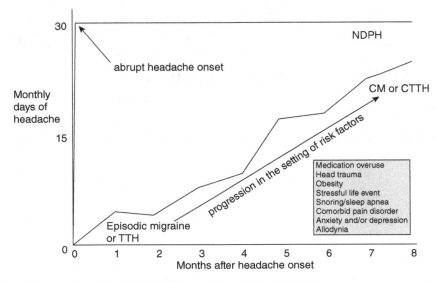

Figure 18.1. Temporal profile of NDPH compared to CM and CTTH.

The diagnostic criteria for NDPH have been disputed, largely based on controversy regarding the features associated with the daily headache. The second edition of the International Classification of Headache Disorders (ICHD-2) states that when a new-onset headache fulfilling the criteria of CTTH starts abruptly or within 3 days of onset and without a history of escalating episodic tension-type headache (ETTH), the diagnosis of NDPH should be made (Table 18.1) [2]. However, not all investigators agree with the ICHD-2, and other criteria have been used in clinical studies. The Silberstein–Lipton criteria for NDPH do not exclude patients with migraine features, but like other forms of CDH, patients must have headache on 15 or more days per month over at least 3 months, although not necessarily daily or continuous pain [4]. The most appropriate criteria have been used in two large series of NDPH, where only criteria A, B, and E of the ICHD-2 are required for the diagnosis (Table 18.1) [5, 6]. The essence of these modified ICHD-2 criteria is that NDPH is a CDH of acute onset featuring continuous and daily pain without restriction on the pain characteristics or associated features.

In the largest series of NDPH patients reported, only 43.7% would have fulfilled the ICHD-2 criteria [6]. When separated into groups with

Table 18.1. ICHD-2 criteria for NDPH [2]

A. Headache for more than 3 months fulfilling criteria B–D
B. Headache is daily and unremitting from onset or less than 3 days from onset
C. At least 2 of the following pain characteristics:
   1. Bilateral location
   2. Pressing/tightening (nonpulsating) quality
   3. Mild or moderate intensity
   4. Not aggravated by routine physical activity such as walking or climbing stairs
D. Both of the following:
   1. No more than one of photophobia, phonophobia, or mild nausea
   2. Neither moderate or severe nausea or vomiting
E. Not attributed to another disorder

The recently used revised criteria for NDPH [5, 6] do not require criterion C or D to be fulfilled.

migraine features (not fulfilling ICHD-2) and without migraine features (fulfilling ICHD-2), they were very similar clinically, although the group with features of migraine was younger, included more women, and was associated with a higher rate of depression, which could suggest an underlying biologic link to migraine. The two groups had no differences in their long-term prognosis.

Onset of NDPH and clues to its underlying pathophysiology

As NDPH is characterized by the acuity of its onset, elucidating precipitating factors may give clues to its underlying pathophysiology, which remains unknown. A heterogeneous set of inciting factors have been reported. Many patients with NDPH report an antecedent febrile illness, which often has upper respiratory symptoms. In children, almost half of all NDPH patients report onset of the headache during an infection [7], whereas in adults anywhere from 14% [6] to 30% [8] of patients report this trigger. In one series, 84% of NDPH patients compared with 25% of controls had evidence of active Epstein–Barr virus infection [9]. Other infectious triggers have also been reported, including herpes simplex virus and cytomegalovirus [10]. Patients with treatment-refractory NDPH and CM may have high cerebrospinal fluid levels of tumor necrosis factor-alpha, a pro-inflammatory cytokine, although patients reporting an infectious trigger do not necessarily have higher levels of this [11]. Perhaps related to an infectious etiology in some patients with NDPH could be the seasonal variation noticed in its onset. In the largest series, NDPH had a biannual peak, with an onset most often occurring in the months of September and March [6].

Aside from infections, other inciting factors have been reported, including stressful life events [6, 8], which can also provoke transition to other forms of CDH in episodic headache sufferers [12]. Other factors reported include extracranial surgery [7, 8, 10], athletic activity [11], childbirth [11], menarche [6], human papillomavirus vaccination [6], and tapering of selective serotonin reuptake inhibitors used for depression [6]. Other hypothesized clues to the etiology of NDPH include a higher rate of hypothyroidism [13], cervical spine joint hypermobility [14], and defective internal jugular venous drainage [15], all studied in small series of patients. It is likely that NDPH is not a single entity but a heterogeneous syndrome encompassing unrecognized secondary headache disorders, as well as the acute onset of a continuous primary headache disorder resembling migraine or CTTH.

Clinical features

NDPH shares some similarities to the other forms of CDH (Table 18.2). Although some of the clinical features of NDPH are variable, the most striking feature of the disorder is its abrupt onset that is almost always memorable. Patients usually recall the exact day or moment of onset. In one series, 42% of patients recalled the exact day of onset, while an additional 41% recalled at least the month and the year of onset [6]. In other series, recall of the precise day of onset was as high as 82% [8]. The ability to recall the precise date of onset or the presence of an inciting factor does not seem to impart a different long-term prognosis [6].

The quality of NDPH pain is variable, and is most commonly pulsating or dull [6, 8]. Most patients have bilateral head pain, but unilateral pain may occur occasionally [6, 8]. The pain is often aggravated by physical activity and usually continuous, [6, 8, 16], with the baseline level of pain most often being moderate [6]. When Vanast first described the disorder in 1986, many of his patients had features of migraine [16]. In retrospective studies at tertiary headache centers using more inclusive diagnostic criteria, migraine features are found to be common. In one large series, nausea was the most common associated symptom (68%), followed by photophobia (66%) and phonophobia (61%) [8]. Nausea may be less common in adolescents with NDPH [5], and vomiting is rare [6, 8]. Aura may occur in patients with NDPH, which is usually visual [6, 8], although one patient has had an olfactory aura [17]. A minority of patients may have unilateral or bilateral cranial autonomic symptoms associated with exacerbations of pain, such as lacrimation, ptosis, miosis, and nasal discharge. Bilateral facial flushing, lasting minutes, with painful headache exacerbations may also occur [6]. In one series, cutaneous allodynia was found in a quarter of NDPH patients [6], far less common than the two-thirds of patients with migraine who have this phenomenon, which is thought to be a clinical marker of central sensitization [18].

Patients with NDPH may have a pre-existing history of episodic headaches, most often ETTH or episodic migraine [6, 8]. Anywhere from one-third [8] to one-half [6] of patients with

Table 18.2. Comparison of the clinical features of NDPH, CM, CTTH, and HC

Feature	NDPH	CM	CTTH	HC
Onset	Sudden	Gradual, evolving from episodic migraine	Gradual, evolving from ETTH	Sudden or gradual
Pre-existing headache	Occasional episodic migraine or ETTH	Episodic migraine	ETTH	Occasional episodic migraine or ETTH
Headache frequency	Daily and continuous, for ≥3 months	≥15 days per month, sometimes daily and continuous, for ≥3 months	≥15 days per month, sometimes daily and continuous, for ≥3 months	Daily and continuous, for ≥3 months
Pain character	Pulsating or dull	Pulsating or dull	Dull	Pulsating or dull
Pain location	Bilateral	Unilateral or bilateral	Bilateral	Strictly unilateral
Photophobia and phonophobia	Common	Common	Uncommon	Occasionally with exacerbations; photophobia often unilateral
Nausea	Common	Common	Uncommon, mild if present	Occasionally with exacerbations
Vomiting	Uncommon but occasional	Common	Rare	Occasionally with exacerbations
Aura	Uncommon but occasional	Common	Rare	Uncommon but occasional
Aggravation by physical activity	Common	Common	Uncommon	Occasional
Autonomic symptoms	Occasional	Occasional	Rare	Unilateral and prominent
Allodynia	Occasional	Common	Occasional	Occasional

NDPH report a family history of headache. Pre-existing and coexisting depression and anxiety are also fairly common [6, 19]. One small series has described panic disorder occurring *de novo* with onset of NDPH [20].

Epidemiology and prognosis

Only two population studies have been performed to capture the epidemiology of NDPH. The first was performed in Spain and used the less restrictive Silberstein–Lipton criteria, documenting a 1-year population prevalence of 0.1% [21]. This prevalence was far less common than that of CTTH (2.2%) and transformed migraine (2.4%). A more recent study undertaken in Norway used the more restrictive ICHD-2 criteria [2], documenting an NDPH prevalence of 0.03%, compared to a CTTH prevalence of 1.3% [22].

Clinic-based studies in tertiary care suggest that, in this setting, CM is the most common form of CDH, but NDPH is more common than CTTH in both adolescents and adults [23, 24]. One small study of CDH from a pediatric headache center found that NDPH may actually be more common in that setting than CM [24]. Patients with less severe, albeit frequent, headache such as CTTH sufferers are less likely to present to a headache center, and these studies may simply reflect a referral bias. Therefore, in the population NDPH is relatively uncommon, but in tertiary care NDPH presents more commonly to the practitioner than does CTTH, although less commonly than CM.

★ TIPS AND TRICKS

Most patients with NDPH who seek treatment at headache centers or other tertiary care facilities have not previously been diagnosed and are felt to have other forms of CDH, such as CM or CTTH. Many patients are erroneously diagnosed with "sinus headache," as they often have an antecedent upper respiratory infection at the time of headache onset, and often have ongoing unilateral or bilateral cranial autonomic symptoms such as lacrimation or rhinorrhea during painful exacerbations. The ICHD-2 does not consider chronic sinusitis as a cause of headache unless it relapses into an acute phase.

Like CM and CTTH, NDPH occurs more commonly in women, with female:male ratios ranging from 1.4:1 to 2.6:1 [5, 6, 8, 16]. However, one study of NDPH patients in Japan demonstrated a slight male predominance (57%) [25]. NDPH occurs in a wide age range, from young children to septuagenarians. The onset occurs most commonly in women in their third decade, although in men the peak onset has been demonstrated to occur in either the third or fifth decade [6, 8].

Patients from North America, Europe, and Asia have been identified with NDPH, including white, African-American, Hispanic, and Asian individuals [5, 6, 8, 10, 16, 22, 25, 26], but no racial predilection has been elucidated.

Although the long-term prognosis of both CM and CTTH are favorable [27, 28], the prognosis of NDPH is less certain. The initial description of this disorder by Vanast described freedom from headache in 86% of men and 73% of women within 2 years of onset [16]. Subsequent case series have shown the disorder to be more refractory to treatment and often with a poor prognosis [6, 8, 25]. The prognosis of NDPH can be divided into three subforms: persisting, remitting, and relapsing–remitting [6]. Most patients in tertiary care have the persisting subform, and over half of these patients have daily headache that persist for at least 2 years [6]. These patients are more likely to be white, have comorbid anxiety or depression, and have an onset of NDPH at a younger age [6].

Most patients with NDPH that remit do so within 2 years of onset [6]. Patients who have the relapsing–remitting subform, where periods of continuous headache are interspersed with pain-free weeks or months, usually have their first remission within 2 years as well [6]. In reality, many patients with a self-limited remitting form of NDPH do not perhaps reach tertiary care centers or neurologists, or even come to medical attention at all.

Treatment

As the natural history of NDPH is so variable, the impact of prophylactic treatment is uncertain. The literature on therapies specifically aimed at addressing NDPH is scarce. In the largest case series, 10 of the 11 patients whose NDPH remitted did so while on preventive medications, most frequently nortriptyline and topiramate [6].

Other prophylactic therapies that have been reported to be beneficial specifically for NDPH in either short case reports or small case series include clonazepam [29], botulinum toxin A [30], and mexiletene [31].

⌘ SCIENCE REVISITED

A preliminary report has suggested open-label success with the antibiotic doxycycline based on its inhibition of tumor necrosis factor-alpha in four NDPH patients with elevated cerebrospinal fluid levels of this inflammatory cytokine [32]. This is a novel area of therapy, but the full details of the study have not been published, and its efficacy needs to be further explored in controlled studies.

For acute treatments, symptomatic therapy with triptans seems reasonable. Around one-third of patients with NDPH find triptans at least partially beneficial, even if patients lack features of migraine [6]. The triptan-responder group includes patients who have more of a CTTH headache phenotype, distinguishing NDPH from actual pure TTH, where patients do not benefit from triptan therapy [33]. Intravenous methylprednisolone has recently been reported to cause partial or complete remission in a small open-label series of nine NDPH patients who reported an infectious trigger [34]. Intravenous haloperidol [35] and intravenous magnesium [11] have also been reported to demonstrate some efficacy. Over half of patients treated with peripheral nerve blocks using bupivacaine in the largest series found them at least temporarily effective [6].

As there are no guidelines or randomized trials to guide the management of NDPH, it is perhaps best treated similarly to the manifesting headache phenotype, mainly CM or CTTH [36]. Medication overuse also must be addressed, as it may develop in up to half of all adult patients with NDPH [6]. Medication overuse is much less common in adolescents with NDPH [5].

Conclusion

NDPH is an uncommon syndrome in the population characterized by the abrupt onset of CDH without any identifiable underlying cause. Although the pathophysiology is unknown, a number of inciting factors have been identified, and it likely encompasses a heterogeneous set of unrecognized or undiagnosed secondary headache disorders as well as the acute onset of a chronic primary headache disorder such as CM or CTTH. The headache phenotype more often resembles CM, but can be similar to CTTH as well. The prognosis is uncertain, and while the majority of patients have a protracted course of continuous pain, a sizeable number of patients do improve. No blinded studies exist for NDPH therapy, but many patients respond to therapies aimed at CM and CTTH.

References

1. Silberstein S, Lipton R, Sliwinski M. Classification of daily and near-daily headaches: field trial of revised IHS criteria. *Neurology* 1996;**47**(4):871–5.
2. The International Classification of Headache Disorders: 2nd edition. *Cephalalgia* 2004; **24**(Suppl. 1):9–160.
3. Mokri B. Spontaneous low cerebrospinal pressure/volume headaches. *Curr Neurol Neurosci Rep* 2004;**4**(2):117–24.
4. Siberstein SD, Lipton RB, Solomon S, Mathew NT. Classification of daily and near-daily headaches: proposed revisions to the IHS criteria. *Headache* 1994;**34**(1):1–7.
5. Kung E, Tepper SJ, Rapoport AM, Sheftell FD, Bigal ME. New daily persistent headache in the paediatric population. *Cephalalgia* 2009;**29**(1):17–22.
6. Robbins M, Grosberg B, Napchan U, Crystal S, Lipton R. Clinical and prognostic subforms of new daily-persistent headache. *Neurology* 2010;**74**(17):1358–64.
7. Mack K. What incites new daily persistent headache in children? *Pediatr Neurol* 2004;**31**(2):122–5.
8. Li D, Rozen TD. The clinical characteristics of new daily persistent headache. *Cephalalgia* 2002;**22**(1):66–9.
9. Diaz-Mitoma F, Vanast WJ, Tyrrell DL. Increased frequency of Epstein–Barr virus excretion in patients with new daily persistent headaches. *Lancet* 1987;**1**:411–5.
10. Meineri P, Torre E, Rota E, Grasso E. New daily persistent headache: clinical and serological

characteristics in a retrospective study. *Neurol Sci* 2004;**25**(Suppl. 3):S281–2.

11. Rozen T, Swidan SZ. Elevation of CSF tumor necrosis factor alpha levels in new daily persistent headache and treatment refractory chronic migraine. *Headache* 2007;**47**(7): 1050–5.

12. Scher A, Stewart W, Buse D, Krantz D, Lipton R. Major life changes before and after the onset of chronic daily headache: a population-based study. *Cephalalgia* 2008;**28**(8):868–76.

13. Bigal ME, Sheftell FD, Rapoport AM, Tepper SJ, Lipton RB. Chronic daily headache: identification of factors associated with induction and transformation. *Headache* 2002;**42**(7): 575–81.

14. Rozen T, Roth J, Denenberg N. Cervical spine joint hypermobility: a possible predisposing factor for new daily persistent headache. *Cephalalgia* 2006;**26**(10):1182–5.

15. Donnet A, Levrier O. A consecutive series of ten cases of new daily persistent headache: clinical presentation and morphology of the venous system. *Neurology* 2009;**72**(Suppl. 3):A419.

16. Vanast WJ. New daily persistent headaches: definition of a benign syndrome. *Headache* 1986;**26**:318.

17. Grosberg BM, Tarshish S, Robbins MS. Olfactory hallucinations in primary headache disorders: 8 new cases and a review of the literature. *Cephalalgia* 2009;**29**(Suppl. 1):161.

18. Bigal ME, Ashina S, Burstein R, et al. Prevalence and characteristics of allodynia in headache sufferers: a population study. *Neurology* 2008;**70**(17):1525–33.

19. Robbins MS. New daily-persistent headache and anxiety. *Cephalalgia* 2011;**31**(7):875–6.

20. Peres MF, Lucchetti G, Mercante JP, Young WB. New daily persistent headache and panic disorder. *Cephalalgia* 2011;**31**(2): 250–3.

21. Castillo J, Muñoz P, Guitera V, Pascual J. Kaplan Award 1998. Epidemiology of chronic daily headache in the general population. *Headache* 1999;**39**(3):190–6.

22. Grande R, Aaseth K, Lundqvist C, Russell M. Prevalence of new daily persistent headache in the general population. The Akershus study of chronic headache. *Cephalalgia* 2009;**29**(11):1149–55.

23. Bigal ME, Lipton RB, Tepper SJ, Rapoport AM, Sheftell FD. Primary chronic daily headache and its subtypes in adolescents and adults. *Neurology* 2004;**63**(5):843–7.

24. Gladstein J, Holden EW. Chronic daily headache in children and adolescents: a 2-year prospective study. *Headache* 1996;**36**(6): 349–51.

25. Takase Y, Nakano M, Tatsumi C, Matsuyama T. Clinical features, effectiveness of drug-based treatment, and prognosis of new daily persistent headache (NDPH): 30 cases in Japan. *Cephalalgia* 2004;**24**(11):955–9.

26. Siow C. New daily persistent headache (NDPH)—a Singaporean perspective. *Headache* 2006;**46**(5):896–7.

27. Bigal M, Lipton R. The prognosis of migraine. *Curr Opin Neurol* 2008;**21**(3):301–8.

28. Lyngberg AC, Rasmussen BK, Jorgensen T, Jensen R. Prognosis of migraine and tension-type headache: a population-based follow-up study. *Neurology* 2005;**65**(4):580–5.

29. Tarshish SC, Robbins MS, Napchan U, Buse DC, Grosberg BM. Prophylaxis of new daily persistent headache (NDPH): response to clonazepam in four patients. *Cephalalgia* 2009;**29** (Suppl. 1):49.

30. Spears RC. Efficacy of botulinum toxin type A in new daily persistent headache. *J Headache Pain* 2008;**9**(6):405–6.

31. Marmura MJ, Passero FC, Jr., Young WB. Mexiletine for refractory chronic daily headache: a report of nine cases. *Headache* 2008; **48**(10):1506–10.

32. Rozen TD. Doxycycline for treatment resistent new daily persistent headache. *Neurology* 2008;**70** (Suppl. 1):A348.

33. Brennum J, Brinck T, Schriver L. Sumatriptan has no clinically relevant effect in the treatment of episodic tension-type headache. *Eur J Neurol* 1996;**3**:23–6.

34. Prakash S, Shah ND. Post-infectious new daily persistent headache may respond to intravenous methylprednisolone. *J Headache Pain* 2010;**11**(1):59–66.

35. Loftus BD. Intravenous haloperidol therapy for new daily persistent headache. *Cephalalgia* 2009;**29**(Suppl. 1):49–50.

36. Goadsby PJ, Boes C. New daily persistent headache. *J Neurol Neurosurg Psychiatry* 2002;**72**(Suppl. 2):ii6–9.

Hemicrania Continua

Uri Napchan

Middletown Medical, Middletown, NY, USA

Introduction

The first case series of a headache syndrome characterized by a background unilateral headache with superimposed exacerbation associated with autonomic features was described by Medina and Diamond in 1981 [1]. Of the 54 patients described, 83% responded and 50% achieved complete control with the nonsteroidal anti-inflammatory drug (NSAID) indomethacin. Three years later, the term "hemicrania continua" was coined by Sjaastad and Spierings [2] to describe two patients with phenotypically similar headaches. Following these early reports, a flurry of case reports and series were published, confirming that such a headache syndrome responsive to indomethacin existed in different settings and populations [3, 4, 5, 6, 7, 8, 9, 10].

Classification and diagnosis

It was not until 2004, with the publication of the second edition of the International Classification of Headache Disorders (ICHD-2), that hemicrania continua was formally included in the classification criteria [11]. Hemicrania continua was classified under the "Other primary headaches" section. Diagnostic criteria (Table 19.1) include a side-locked headache lasting longer than 3 months, of at least moderate intensity, that is daily and continuous, with either conjunctival injection/lacrimation or nasal congestion/rhinorrhea. The diagnostic criteria also require a complete response to indomethacin.

A point of contention exists as some individuals may fit the diagnostic criteria except for a positive response to indomethacin [12, 13]. A recently published study of 192 patients with putative hemicrania continua retrospectively attempted to compare indomethacin responders to nonresponders [14]. The authors were not able to find a statistically significant difference between the two groups. In clinical practice, some individuals will not respond to indomethacin, while others may not be able to take indomethacin due to a contraindication or intolerability. In addition, some will improve with other treatment. In these cases, the individual patient will be left in an island of diagnostic uncertainty, without fulfilling the diagnostic criteria for hemicrania continua, although they will have headaches that are phenotypically identical to hemicrania continua.

Hemicrania continua may also be associated with symptoms not listed in the ICHD-2 criteria.

Headache, First Edition. Edited by Matthew S. Robbins, Brian M. Grosberg, and Richard B. Lipton.
© 2013 John Wiley & Sons, Ltd. Published 2013 by John Wiley & Sons, Ltd.

Table 19.1. ICHD-2 diagnostic criteria for hemicrania continua

A. Headache for >3 months fulfilling criteria B–D
B. All of the following characteristics:
   1. Unilateral pain without side-shift
   2. Daily and continuous, without pain-free periods
   3. Moderate intensity, but with exacerbations of severe pain
C. At least one of the following autonomic features occurs during exacerbations and ipsilateral to the side of pain:
   1. Conjunctival injection and/or lacrimation
   2. Nasal congestion and/or rhinorrhea
   3. Ptosis and/or miosis
D. Complete response to therapeutic doses of indomethacin
E. Not attributed to another disorder

For example, other autonomic features besides conjunctival injection, lacrimation, nasal congestion, or rhinorrhea may include eyelid edema, forehead and facial swelling, and a sensation of aural fullness or swelling [3]. The primary essence of hemicrania continua is the unilaterality of the pain. However, a case of bilateral pain has been reported [15]. There have also been reports of hemicrania continua with side-shifting [16, 17, 18, 19, 20, 21]. As with other primary headache disorders, there have also been cases of auras associated with hemicrania continua, [17, 22] as well as a pure menstrual form [23].

> ★ **TIPS AND TRICKS**
>
> One underrecognized symptom seen in hemicrania continua patients is the sensation of an ocular foreign body ipsilateral to the pain and cranial autonomic symptoms. It is seen in a sizeable minority of hemicrania continua patients, and is often described as having the feeling of an eyelash or sand in the eye, or a gritty sensation.

The natural history of hemicrania continua can be divided into a continuous or a remitting form. In the continuous form, the headache is continuous, without a meaningful break from the pain, and can last for years. In the remitting form, there are distinct headache phases lasting weeks to months, with pain-free periods in between [24, 25, 26]. The remitting form may evolve from the continuous form [27], or the opposite may also occur where a transition occurs from a remitting form to a continuous phase [28].

There have been over 100 case reports of hemicrania continua reported in the literature, but the true prevalence in the population is currently unknown. Hemicrania continua may be more common than previously thought, as relatively large case series continue to be reported from different centers [3, 29]. In one clinic-based study, hemicrania continua represented 0.8% of chronic daily headaches in adults [30].

For classification purposes, hemicrania continua may be grouped alongside the trigeminal autonomic cephalalgias (TACs; cluster headache, paroxysmal hemicrania, and short-lasting unilateral neuralgiform headache attacks with conjunctival injection and tearing) due to the common presence of cranial autonomic symptoms ipsilateral to the head pain that are seen in both [31, 32]. Some, however, prefer to classify hemicrania continua with the other chronic daily headaches of long duration—chronic migraine, new daily persistent headache, and chronic tension-type headache [33].

Clinical features

The evaluation of patients with hemicrania continua requires a detailed history and physical examination. Hemicrania continua may sometimes be mistaken for another primary headache disorder. For example, patients with hemicrania continua may be misdiagnosed with migraine when the clinician or patient fails to identify the constant baseline pain and focus only on the more severe exacerbations. Another important factor that may lead to a mistaken diagnosis of migraine instead of hemicrania continua is the very common migrainous features that are seen in hemicrania continua, such as photophobia, phonophobia, nausea, vomiting, and sensitivity to motion [3]. An astute clinician must also realize that migraine may also be associated with autonomic features (i.e. ptosis, lacrimation, and conjunctival injection) [34, 35] and be strictly side-locked [36]. One important pearl that is helpful in differentiating hemicrania continua from migraine in cases where phenotypic overlap occurs is that photophobia and phonophobia occur more often unilaterally in individuals with hemicrania continua compared to those with migraine [37].

Clinicians must also distinguish hemicrania continua from the TACs such as cluster headache, paroxysmal hemicrania, and short-lasting unilateral neuralgiform headache attacks with conjunctival injection and tearing, as they are a group of primary headache disorders associated with prominent cranial autonomic features. The TACs, however, lack the interictal pain of hemicrania continua, and the pain is short-lasting, whereas the painful exacerbations of hemicrania continua usually last for hours. Cervicogenic headache and occipital neuralgia are also in the differential diagnosis, as both can be side-locked; however, they are easily dismissed due to the lack of autonomic features. Infrequently, new daily persistent headache and chronic tension-type headache may also be side-locked; however, they lack the autonomic features found in hemicrania continua.

Pathophysiology and secondary causes

Hemicrania continua has been associated with other primary headache and pain disorders, suggesting a common pathophysiologic origin. For example, cases have been described of hemicrania continua in individuals with other trigeminal autonomic cephalalgias [38, 39]. An association with temporomandibular dysfunction has also been reported [40, 41]. Other case reports have described patients who developed hemicrania continua evolving from cluster headache [42, 43], Raeder syndrome [44], paroxysmal hemicrania [45], migraine [46], familial hemiplegic migraine [47], and cervicogenic headache [48, 49].

The cause of hemicrania continua remains unknown, much like the other primary headache disorders. However, one study found activation of the dorsal pons using positron-emission tomography [50], while another found activation of the contralateral posterior hypothalamus and ipsilateral dorsal rostral pons [51].

Table 19.2. Secondary causes of hemicrania continua

Tumor
Metastatic lung cancer
Nonmetastatic lung cancer
Pituitary tumor
Osteoid osteoma of the ethmoid sinus
Sphenoid bone tumor
Infection
Leprosy
Vascular
Ipsilateral brainstem stroke
Internal carotid artery dissection
Unruptured saccular aneurysm
Other
Surgery: post tubal ligation under spinal anesthesia
Pineal cyst
Head trauma
Postpartum

A workup for secondary causes may be warranted as several cases of secondary hemicrania continua have been published (Table 19.2). For example, cases of hemicrania continua associated with metastatic lung cancer [52], nonmetastatic lung cancer [53, 54], pituitary tumor [55, 56, 57], osteoid osteoma of the ethmoid sinus [58], surgery [59], leprosy [60], ipsilateral brainstem lesion [61], internal carotid artery dissection [62, 63], unruptured saccular aneurysm [64], pineal cyst [65], and sphenoid bone tumor [66] have been reported. Hemicrania continua headaches have also been seen in individuals following head trauma [67, 68] and postpartum [69].

Although early reports indicated a potential underlying symptomatic cause when very high doses of indomethacin were required for hemicrania continua [70], a recent large review seems to have dispelled this notion [59].

Treatment

A positive response to indomethacin is a requirement in order to meet the ICHD-2 criteria for hemicrania continua and remains the definitive treatment of choice. The "Indotest" is a useful tool in an office setting to help diagnose hemicrania continua. This test involves injecting 50 mg of indomethacin intramuscularly (not available in the USA) and observing for a response. The time to complete pain relief is 73 ± 66 minutes (standard deviation) with pain relief lasting on average for 13 hours [71].

> ⭐ **TIPS AND TRICKS**
>
> Some patients with chronic daily headaches not fulfilling the complete criteria for hemicrania continua may also respond to indomethacin. For example, patients with side-locked headaches without autonomic features and patients with bilateral daily headaches with autonomic features may also respond to indomethacin.

In the USA, indomethacin is commercially available in an oral instant-release form at 25 mg and 50 mg, and a 75 mg extended-release form. Indomethacin is also available as a suppository (50 mg) and in an oral suspension. A "black box" warning exists for indomethacin as well as all other NSAIDs due to the cardiovascular and gastrointestinal risks. Prophylaxis with proton pump inhibitors, H2-receptor blockers, or sucralfate is recommended while using indomethacin, although no clinical data exists to support this recommendation.

A typical oral indomethacin trial consists of taking 25 mg three times a day for up to 3–5 days. If there is no or only a partial benefit, the dose may be increased to 50 mg three times a day for 3–5 days. If there is again no or only a partial benefit, a trial of 75 mg three times a day is warranted for at least a week. Patients usually experience a significant relief early on, and the response is almost never in doubt. However, recent case reports suggest that some may respond only after months of treatment [72]. The effective dose of indomethacin varies, ranging from 25 mg every 2 days to 300 mg a day [73]. The clinician and patient must decide on the duration of indomethacin treatment once an effective dose has been found. Some patients may be able to decrease the indomethacin dose over time [74], and Rozen has suggested that indomethacin may be acting as a disease-modifying agent [75].

> ⭐ **TIPS AND TRICKS**
>
> A proper trial to evaluate for a definitive indomethacin response in a patient with suspected hemicrania continua consists of:
>
> - 25 mg three times a day for 3–5 days
> - 50 mg three times a day for 3–5 days
> - 75 mg three times a day for 7 days.
>
> The use of a proton pump inhibitor, H2-receptor antagonist, or sucralfate is recommended for gastrointestinal prophylaxis during the trial or duration of therapy.

Although indomethacin remains the most potent treatment option, long-term use may not be viable for some due to intolerance and side effects. Patients with hemicrania continua often respond to other NSAIDs, including other cyclooxygenase-2 (COX-2) inhibitors [76, 77, 78] and piroxicam [79, 80]. Other treatment options include occipital nerve blocks [81], trochlear injection [82], botulinum toxin [83], gabapentin [84, 85], intravenous methylprednisolone [86], occipital nerve stimulation [87, 88, 89], topiramate [16, 90, 91, 92], valproic acid [42], melatonin [93, 94], and verapamil [95, 96] (Table 19.3).

Table 19.3. Reported beneficial therapies for hemicrania continua aside from indomethacin

NSAIDs
Piroxicam
Naproxen
Celecoxib
Other medications
Gabapentin
Methylprednisolone
Topiramate
Valproic acid
Melatonin
Verapamil
Interventional
Occipital nerve blocks
Botulinum toxin
Trochlear injections
Occipital nerve stimulation

CAUTION!

A black box warning exists for indomethacin. Discuss with patients the increased risk of serious cardiovascular and gastrointestinal events associated with the use of indomethacin.

In clinical practice, indomethacin is given at the lowest possible dose. Once the patient is clinically stable, the clinician may attempt to decrease the indomethacin dose. Another alternative is to add another agent, such as the aforementioned drugs used for migraine prophylaxis, to take alongside indomethacin. Once the appropriate dose (generally that used for migraine prophylaxis) is reached, one may attempt to taper the indomethacin. If successful, the additional medication may produce an "indomethacin-sparing effect" where either the patient is completely weaned off the indomethacin, or the dose required is minimal.

SCIENCE REVISITED

The reason for the particular efficacy of indomethacin in treating hemicrania continua is not known. Indomethacin is a potent COX-1 and COX-2 inhibitor, may decrease cerebral blood flow, and may reduce intracranial pressure. It may also inhibit the synthesis of nitric oxide.

Conclusion

Hemicrania continua is an idiopathic unique disorder that should never be missed by the clinician because of its typical definitive treatment with indomethacin.

References

1. Medina JL, Diamond S. Cluster headache variant. Spectrum of a new headache syndrome. *Arch Neurol* 1981;**38**(11):705–9.
2. Sjaastad O, Spierings EL. "Hemicrania continua": another headache absolutely responsive to indomethacin. *Cephalalgia* 1984;**4**(1): 65–70.
3. Cittadini E, Goadsby PJ. Hemicrania continua: a clinical study of 39 patients with diagnostic implications. *Brain* 2010;**133**(Pt 7):1973–86.
4. Bigal ME, Tepper SJ, Sheftell FD, Rapoport AM. Hemicrania continua: a report of ten new cases. *Arq Neuropsiquiatr* 2002;**60**(3-B): 695–8.
5. Newman LC, Lipton RB, Solomon S. Hemicrania continua: ten new cases and a review of the literature. *Neurology* 1994;**44**(11): 2111–4.
6. Pareja JA, Palomo T, Gorriti MA, et al. Hemicrania continua. The first Spanish case: a case report. *Cephalalgia* 1990;**10**(3):143–5.
7. Iordanidis T, Sjaastad O. Hemicrania continua: a case report. *Cephalalgia* 1989;**9**(4): 301–3.
8. Sjaastad O, Tjørstad K. "Hemicrania continua": a third Norwegian case. *Cephalalgia* 1987;**7**(3):175–7.
9. Zukerman E, Hannuch SN, Carvalho DdeS, Fragoso YD, Jenger KA. "Hemicrania continua": a case report. *Cephalalgia* 1987;**7**(3): 171–3.
10. Wheeler SD. Hemicrania continua in African Americans. *J Natl Med Assoc* 2002;**94**(10): 901–7.
11. Headache Classification Committee (2004). The International Headache Classification of Headache Disorders, 2nd edition. *Cephalalgia* **24**:1–160.
12. Prakash S, Shah ND, Marmura MJ. Hemicrania continua unresponsive to indomethacin do exist. *Cephalalgia* 2010;**30**(1):123–5.
13. Kuritzky A. Indomethacin-resistant hemicrania continua. *Cephalalgia* 1992;**12**(1):57–9.
14. Marmura MJ, Silberstein SD, Gupta M. Hemicrania continua: who responds to indomethacin? *Cephalalgia* 2009;**29**(3): 300–7.
15. Pasquier F, Leys D, Petit H. "Hemicrania continua": the first bilateral case? *Cephalalgia* 1987;**7**(3):169–70.
16. Matharu MS, Bradbury P, Swash M. Hemicrania continua: side alternation and response to topiramate. *Cephalalgia.* 2006; **26**(3):341–4.
17. Peres MF, Masruha MR, Young WB. Side-shifting hemicrania continua with aura (migraine with aura with autonomic symptoms responsive to indomethacin?). *Cephalalgia* 2006;**26**(8):917–9.

18. Newman LC, Spears RC, Lay CL. Hemicrania continua: a third case in which attacks alternate sides. *Headache* 2004;**44**(8): 821–3.

19. Marano E, Giampiero V, Gennaro DR, di Stasio E, Bonusa S, Sorge F. "Hemicrania continua": a possible case with alternating sides. *Cephalalgia* 1994;**14**(4):307–8.

20. Sjaastad O, Vincent M, Stovner LJ. Side alternation of pain in hemicrania continua. *Headache* 1993;**33**(1):43–5.

21. Newman LC, Lipton RB, Russell M, Solomon S. Hemicrania continua: attacks may alternate sides. *Headache* 1992;**32**(5):237–8.

22. Peres MF, Siow HC, Rozen TD. Hemicrania continua with aura. *Cephalalgia* 2002;**22**(3): 246–8.

23. Prakash S, Shah ND. Pure menstrual hemicrania continua: does it exist? A case report. *Cephalalgia* 2010;**30**(5):631–3.

24. Newman LC, Lipton RB, Solomon S. Hemicrania continua: ten new cases and a review of the literature. *Neurology* 1994;**44**:2111–4.

25. Sjaastad O, Tjorstad K. "Hemicrania continua": a third Norwegian case. *Cephalalgia* 1987;**7**:175–7.

26. Peres MF, Stiles MA, Oshinsky M, Rozen TD. Remitting form of hemicrania continua with seasonal pattern. *Headache* 2001;**41**(6): 592–4.

27. Pareja JA. Hemicrania continua: remitting stage evolved from the chronic form. *Headache* 1995;**35**(3):161–2.

28. Sjaastad O, Antonaci F. Chronic paroxysmal hemicrania (CPH) and hemicrania continua: transition from one stage to another. *Headache* 1993;**33**(10):551–4.

29. Peres MF, Silberstein SD, Nahmias S, et al. Hemicrania continua is not that rare. *Neurology* 2001;**57**(6):948–51.

30. Bigal ME, Lipton RB, Tepper SJ, Rapoport AM, Sheftell FD. Primary chronic daily headache and its subtypes in adolescents and adults. *Neurology* 2004;**63**(5):843–7.

31. Goadsby PJ, Lipton RB. A review of paroxysmal hemicranias, SUNCT syndrome and other short-lasting headaches with autonomic feature, including new cases. *Brain* 1997;**120**(Pt 1):193–209.

32. Goadsby PJ, Cittadini E, Cohen AS. Trigeminal autonomic cephalalgias: paroxysmal hemicrania, SUNCT/SUNA, and hemicrania continua. *Semin Neurol* 2010;**30**(2): 186–91.

33. Silberstein SD, Lipton RB, Solomon S, Mathew NT. Classification of daily and near-daily headaches: proposed revisions to the IHS criteria. *Headache* 1994;**34**(1):1–7.

34. Lai TH, Fuh JL, Wang SJ. Cranial autonomic symptoms in migraine: characteristics and comparison with cluster headache. *J Neurol Neurosurg Psychiatry* 2009;**80**(10): 1116–9.

35. Gupta R, Bhatia MS. A report of cranial autonomic symptoms in migraineurs. *Cephalalgia* 2007;**27**(1):22–8.

36. Selby G, Lance JW. Observation on 500 cases of migraine and allied vascular headaches. *J Neurol Neurosurg Psychiatry* 1960;**23**: 23–32.

37. Irimia P, Cittadini E, Paemeleire K, Cohen AS, Goadsby PJ. Unilateral photophobia or phonophobia in migraine compared with trigeminal autonomic cephalalgias. *Cephalalgia* 2008;**28**(6):626–30.

38. Cosentino G, Fierro B, Puma AR, Talamanca S, Brighina F. Different forms of trigeminal autonomic cephalalgias in the same patient: description of a case. *J Headache Pain* 2010;**11**(3):281–4.

39. Robbins MS, Grosberg BM, Lipton RB. Coexisting trigeminal autonomic cephalalgias and hemicrania continua. *Headache* 2010; **50**(3):489–96.

40. Fragoso YD, Carvalho Alves HH, Garcia SO. Association of hemicrania continua and temporomandibular dysfunction: the role of each team player. *Headache* 2009;**49**(10): 1547–8.

41. Taub D, Stiles A, Tucke AG. Hemicrania continua presenting as temporomandibular joint pain. *Oral Surg Oral Med Oral Pathol Oral Radiol Endod* 2008;**105**(2):e35–7.

42. Lambru G, Castellini P, Bini A, Evangelista A, Manzoni GC, Torelli P. Hemicrania continua evolving from cluster headache responsive to valproic acid. *Headache* 2008;**48**(9): 1374–6.

43. Lisotto C, Mainardi F, Maggioni F, Zanchin G. Hemicrania continua with contralateral episodic cluster headache: a case report. *Cephalalgia* 2003;**23**:929–30.

44. Koutsis G, Andreadou E, Matsi S, Evangelo-poulos ME, Sfagos C. Benign Raeder syndrome evolving into indomethacin-responsive hemicranial headache. *Headache* 2008;**48**(10):1534–6.

45. Castellanos-Pinedo F, Zurdo M, Martínez-Acebes E. Hemicrania continua evolving from episodic paroxysmal hemicrania. *Cephalalgia* 2006;**26**(9):1143–5.

46. Palmieri A, Mainardi F, Maggioni F, Dainese F, Zanchin G. Hemicrania continua evolving from migraine with aura: clinical evidence of a possible correlation between two forms of primary headache. *Cephalalgia* 2004; **24**(11):1007–8.

47. Evers S, Bahra A, Goadsby PJ. Coincidence of familial hemiplegic migraine and hemicrania continua? A case report. *Cephalalgia* 1999; **19**(5):533–5.

48. Sjaastad O, Joubert J, Elsås T, Bovim G, Vincent M. Hemicrania continua and cervi-cogenic headache. Separate headaches or two faces of the same headache? *Funct Neurol* 1993;**8**(2):79–83.

49. Rothbart P. Unilateral headache with features of hemicrania continua and cervicogenic headache—a case report. *Headache* 1992; **32**(9):459–60.

50. Irimia P, Arbizu J, Prieto E, Fernández-Torrón R, Martínez-Vila E. Activation of the brainstem but not of the hypothalamus in hemicrania continua without autonomic symptoms. *Cephalalgia* 2009;**29**(9):974–9.

51. Matharu MS, Cohen AS, McGonigle DJ, Ward N, Frackowiak RS, Goadsby PJ. Posterior hypothalamic and brainstem activation in hemicrania continua. *Headache* 2004;**44**(8): 747–61.

52. Robbins MS, Grosberg BM. Hemicrania continua-like headache from metastatic lung cancer. *Headache* 2010;**50**(6):1055–6.

53. Evans RW. Hemicrania continua-like head-ache due to nonmetastatic lung cancer—a vagal cephalalgia. *Headache* 2007;**47**(9): 1349–51.

54. Eross EJ, Swanson JW, Dodick DW. Hemicra-nia continua: an indomethacin-responsive case with an underlying malignant etiology. *Headache* 2002;**42**(6):527–9.

55. Wang SJ, Hung CW, Fuh JL, Lirng JF, Hwu CM. Cranial autonomic symptoms in patients

with pituitary adenoma presenting with headaches. *Acta Neurol Taiwan* 2009; **18**(2):104–12.

56. Levy MJ, Matharu MS, Meeran K, Powell M, Goadsby PJ. The clinical characteristics of headache in patients with pituitary tumours. *Brain* 2005;**128**(Pt 8):1921–30.

57. Levy MJ, Matharu MS, Goadsby PJ. Prolac-tinomas, dopamine agonists and headache: two case reports. *Eur J Neurol* 2003;**10**(2): 169–73.

58. Kim K, Yang HS. A possible case of sympto-matic hemicrania continua from an osteoid osteoma of the ethmoid sinus. *Cephalalgia* 2010;**30**:242–8.

59. Prakash S, Shah ND, Soni RK. Secondary hemicrania continua: case reports and a lit-erature review. *J Neurol Sci* 2009;**280**(1–2): 29–34.

60. Prakash S, Dholakia SY. Hemicrania continua-like headache with leprosy: casual or causal association? *Headache* 2008;**48**(7):1132–4.

61. Valença MM, Andrade-Valença LP, da Silva WF, Dodick DW. Hemicrania continua sec-ondary to an ipsilateral brainstem lesion. *Headache* 2007;**47**(3):438–41.

62. Ashkenazi A, Abbas MA, Sharma DK, Silber-stein SD. Hemicrania continua-like head-ache associated with internal carotid artery dissection may respond to indomethacin. *Headache* 2007;**47**(1):127–30.

63. Rogalewski A, Evers S. Symptomatic hemicra-nia continua after internal carotid artery dis-section. *Headache* 2005;**45**(2):167–9.

64. Vikelis M, Xifaras M, Magoufis G, Gekas G, Mitsikostas DD. Headache attributed to unruptured saccular aneurysm, mimicking hemicrania continua. *J Headache Pain* 2005;**6**(3):156–8.

65. Peres MF, Zukerman E, Porto PP, Brandt RA. Headaches and pineal cyst: a (more than) coincidental relationship? *Headache* 2004; **44**(9):929–30.

66. Antonaci F, Sjaastad O. Hemicrania continua: a possible symptomatic case, due to mesen-chymal tumor. *Funct Neurol* 1992;**7**(6): 471–4.

67. Lay CL, Newman LC. Posttraumatic hemicra-nia continua. *Headache* 1999;**39**(4):275–9.

68. Evans RW, Lay CL. Posttraumatic hemicrania continua? *Headache* 2000;**40**(9):761–2.

69. Spitz M, Peres MF. Hemicrania continua postpartum. *Cephalalgia* 2004;**24**(7):603–4.

70. Sjaastad O, Stovner LJ, Stolt-NielsenA, Antonaci F, Fredriksen TA. CPH and hemicrania continua: requirements of high indomethacin dosages – an ominous sign? *Headache* 1995;**35**:363–7.

71. Antonaci F, Pareja JA, Caminero AB, Sjaastad O. Chronic paroxysmal hemicrania and hemicrania continua. Parenteral indomethacin: the "indotest". *Headache* 1998;**38**(2): 122–8.

72. Prakash S, Shah N. Delayed response of indomethacin in patients with hemicrania continua: real or phantom headache? *Cephalalgia* 2010;**30**:375–9.

73. Pareja JA, Antonaci F, Vincent M. The hemicrania continua diagnosis. *Cephalalgia* 2001;**21**:940–6.

74. Pareja JA, Caminero AB, Franco E, Casado JL, Pascual J, Sanchez del Rio M. Dose, efficacy and tolerability of long-term indomethacin treatment for chronic paroxysmal hemicrania and hemicrania continua. *Cephalalgia* 2001;**21**:906–10.

75. Rozen TD. Can indomethacin act as a disease modifying agent in hemicrania continua? A supportive clinical case. *Headache* 2009; **49**(5):759–61.

76. Porta-Etessam J, Cuadrado M, Rodríguez-Gómez O, García-Ptacek S, Valencia C. Are Cox-2 drugs the second line option in indomethacin responsive headaches? *J Headache Pain* 2010;**11**(5):405–7.

77. Peres MF, Silberstein SD. Hemicrania continua responds to cyclooxygenase-2 inhibitors. *Headache* 2002;**42**(6):530–1.

78. Peres MF, Zukerman E. Hemicrania continua responsive to rofecoxib. *Cephalalgia* 2000; **20**(2):130–1.

79. Sjaastad O, Antonaci F. A piroxicam derivative partly effective in chronic paroxysmal hemicrania and hemicrania continua. *Headache* 1995;**35**(9):549–50.

80. Trucco M, Antonaci F, Sandrini G. Hemicrania continua: a case responsive to piroxicam-beta-cyclodextrin. *Headache* 1992;**32**(1): 39–40.

81. Tobin J, Flitman S. Occipital nerve blocks: when and what to inject? *Headache* 2009; **49**(10):1521–33.

82. Cuadrado M, Porta-Etessam J, Pareja J, Matías-Guiu J. Hemicrania continua responsive to trochlear injection of corticosteroids. *Cephalalgia* 2010;**30**(3):373–4.

83. Garza I, Cutrer F. Pain relief and persistence of dysautonomic features in a patient with hemicrania continua responsive to botulinum toxin type A. *Cephalalgia* 2010;**30**(4): 500–3.

84. Spears RC. Is gabapentin an effective treatment choice for hemicrania continua? *J Headache Pain* 2009;**10**(4):271–5.

85. Mariano Da Silva H, Alcantara MC, Bordini CA, Speciali JG. Strictly unilateral headache reminiscent of hemicrania continua resistant to indomethacin but responsive to gabapentin. *Cephalalgia* 2002;**22**(5):409–10.

86. Prakash S, Husain M, Sureka DS, Shah NP, Shah ND. Is there need to search for alternatives to indomethacin for hemicrania continua? Case reports and a review. *J Neurol Sci* 2009;**277**(1–2):187–90.

87. Pascual J. Treatment of hemicrania continua by occipital nerve stimulation with a bion device. *Curr Pain Headache Rep* 2009; **13**(1):3–4.

88. Burns B, Watkins L, Goadsby PJ. Treatment of hemicrania continua by occipital nerve stimulation with a bion device: long-term follow-up of a crossover study. *Lancet Neurol* 2008;**7**(11):1001–12.

89. Schwedt TJ, Dodick DW, Hentz J, Trentman TL, Zimmerman RS. Occipital nerve stimulation for chronic headache—long-term safety and efficacy. *Cephalalgia* 2007;**27**(2):153–7.

90. Prakash S, Husain M, Sureka DS, Shah NP, Shah ND. Is there need to search for alternatives to indomethacin for hemicrania continua? Case reports and a review. *J Neurol Sci* 2009;**277**(1–2):187–90.

91. Camarda C, Camarda R, Monastero R. Chronic paroxysmal hemicrania and hemicrania continua responding to topiramate: two case reports. *Clin Neurol Neurosurg* 2008;**110**(1): 88–91.

92. Brighina F, Palermo A, Cosentino G, Fierro B. Prophylaxis of hemicrania continua: two new cases effectively treated with topiramate. *Headache* 2007;**47**(3):441–3.

93. Rozen TD. Melatonin responsive hemicrania continua. *Headache* 2006;**46**(7):1203–4.

94. Spears RC. Hemicrania continua: a case in which a patient experienced complete relief on melatonin. *Headache* 2006;**46**(3):524–7.

95. Rozen TD. Verapamil-responsive hemicrania continua in a patient with episodic cluster headache. *Cephalalgia* 2006;**26**(3): 351–3.

96. Rajabally YA, Jacob S. Hemicrania continua responsive to verapamil. *Headache* 2005; **45**(8):1082–3.

Unusual Short-duration Primary Headaches

Sarah Vollbracht and Brian M. Grosberg

Albert Einstein College of Medicine, Bronx, NY, USA

Introduction

Although rare, the short-duration primary head-ache disorders described in this chapter are important to recognize because the sufferers tend to be desperate, often misdiagnosed, and mismanaged. Prompt recognition of these head-ache disorders may be confounded by their brevity, unpredictable occurrence, and coexistence with other common primary disorders. Assigning a diagnosis of a short-duration primary headache disorder is predicated on the exclusion of secondary mimics by thorough investigation. Once secondary disorders have been excluded, establishing an accurate diagnosis of one these unusual short-duration primary headaches using the criteria outlined in the second edition of the International Classification of Headache Disorders (ICHD-2) can both guide treatment decisions and allow for patient reassurance. This chapter reviews the epidemiology, clinical features, differential diagnosis, and available treatment options for these unusual short-duration primary headache disorders.

Primary stabbing headache

Primary stabbing headache is a benign headache disorder, with a lifetime prevalence of 1%–2% [1].

The disorder typically affects women and occurs in the middle or later years of life, with a mean age of onset of approximately 47 years [2]. Primary stabbing headache is characterized by sudden, unprovoked, ultrashort (1–10 seconds) paroxysms of severe head pain. The fleeting head pain is moderate to severe in intensity and usually occurs as either a single stab or a series of stabs in the distribution of the first division of the trigeminal nerve [2], although attacks can also occur in extratrigeminal locations [3, 4]. The pain is described as sharp, pricking, or stabbing in quality. Individual attacks last between 1 and 10 seconds, with more than two-thirds of reported attacks lasting 1 second. Attacks are typically unilateral, but may be bilateral, and vary in location between or within an individual attack. The pattern and frequency of attacks is also quite variable, ranging from one attack per year to 50 attacks daily. There are no accompanying symptoms. In more than 50% of cases, primary stabbing headache is associated with other headache disorders, such as migraine, cluster headache, tension-type headache, hemicrania continua, cervicogenic headache, and chronic paroxysmal hemicrania [2, 5, 6, 7, 8]. The diagnostic criteria for primary stabbing headache are outlined in Table 20.1.

Headache, First Edition. Edited by Matthew S. Robbins, Brian M. Grosberg, and Richard B. Lipton.
© 2013 John Wiley & Sons, Ltd. Published 2013 by John Wiley & Sons, Ltd.

Table 20.1. ICHD-2 diagnostic criteria for primary stabbing headache

A. Head pain occurring as a single stab or a series of stabs and fulfilling criteria B–D
B. Exclusively or predominantly felt in the distribution of the first division of the trigeminal nerve (orbit, temple, and parietal area)
C. Stabs last for up to a few seconds and recur with irregular frequency ranging from one to many per day
D. No accompanying symptoms
E. Not attributed to another disorder[a]

[a]History and physical and neurologic examinations do not suggest any of the disorders listed in Groups 5–12, or history and/or physical and/or neurologic examinations do suggest such a disorder but it is ruled out by appropriate investigations, or such a disorder is present but pain does not occur for the first time in close temporal relation to the disorder.

★ TIPS AND TRICKS

The diagnosis of primary stabbing headache can be missed or delayed because of the brevity and unpredictable nature of the attacks, as well as its coexistence with other primary headache disorders. In a patient with a primary headache disorder and a new type of head pain, it is important to consider the possibility of a coexistent primary headache disorder. Making the appropriate diagnosis may influence the treatment and prognosis.

The differential diagnosis of primary stabbing headache includes other recurrent, short-duration primary headache disorders, such as the trigeminal autonomic cephalalgias, particularly short-lasting unilateral neuralgiform headache with conjunctival injection and tearing (SUNCT), cough headache, exertional headache, headache associated with sexual activity, hypnic headache, and trigeminal neuralgia. The absence of associated autonomic features such as lacrimation, ptosis, rhinorrhea, and conjunctival injection excludes the trigeminal autonomic cephalalgias from the diagnosis. Similarly, cough, sexual, exertional, and hypnic headache are excluded by the absence of robust trigger factors such as cough, sex, exercise, and sleep. Trigeminal neuralgia is excluded by the lack of trigger points.

⚠ CAUTION!

When the stabs of pain are strictly localized to one area, organic pathology at this site and in the distribution of the affected cranial nerve must be excluded. The diagnosis of primary stabbing headache is predicated upon the exclusion of secondary causes such as meningiomas, pituitary tumors, temporal arteritis, cerebrovascular disease, cranial and ocular trauma, herpes zoster, and elevated intraocular pressure [2, 6, 9, 10]. Patients should be referred for an ophthalmologic evaluation, an MRI scan of the brain, and laboratory studies, including an erythrocyte sedimentation rate and C-reactive protein level, to help confirm or exclude these secondary disorders.

Patient reassurance is crucial to the successful management of this condition. It is very important to let patients know that the sudden stabs of pain do not automatically imply an ominous underlying condition. Most patients attain complete or partial relief with indomethacin given prophylactically at a dose ranging from 25 mg to 150 mg per day [2, 4, 11, 12, 13]. In patients unable to tolerate indomethacin, success has been reported with melatonin, in doses ranging from 3 mg to 12 mg daily, and gabapentin 400 mg twice daily [14, 15].

Hypnic headache

Hypnic headache is a rare primary headache disorder that primarily affects the elderly, usually beginning after age 50 years, with a mean age at onset of 63 ± 11 years (range 36–83 years) [16]. There has been one case report of hypnic headache occurring in a 9-year-old child, but this is atypical [17]. The prevalence is estimated to be 0.07%–0.1% of all patients evaluated in an outpatient headache clinic, which reflects the relative rarity of this particular headache disorder [16,

Table 20.2. ICHD-2 diagnostic criteria for hypnic headache

A. Dull headache fulfilling criteria B–D
B. Develops only during sleep, and awakens the patient
C. At least two of the following characteristics:
  1. Occurs >15 times per month
  2. Lasts ≥15 minutes after waking
  3. First occurs after age 50 years
D. No autonomic symptoms and no more than one of nausea, photophobia, or phonophobia
E. Not attributed to another disorder[a]

[a]History and physical and neurologic examinations do not suggest any of the disorders listed in Groups 5–12, or history and/or physical and/or neurological examinations do suggest such a disorder but it is ruled out by appropriate investigations, or such a disorder is present but pain does not occur for the first time in close temporal relation to the disorder.

18]. Women are more commonly affected than men, representing approximately 65% of cases. Table 20.2 lists the ICHD-2 criteria for hypnic headache.

☠ CAUTION!

Hypnic headache almost exclusively occurs in patients older than 50 years of age. Any young patient presenting with headaches that awaken them from sleep must be evaluated for potential secondary causes.

Hypnic headache has been referred to as "alarm clock" headache because the attacks predictably occur at approximately the same time each night, usually between 1:00 and 3:00 hours. Rarely, these headaches can occur during a daytime nap [19, 20]. The headaches begin abruptly, typically with dull and throbbing pain of moderate intensity. The pain is most often bilateral, located diffusely or frontotemporally. Less commonly, the pain may be unilateral or bilateral involving the occiput or neck [16, 18, 19, 21, 22].

The duration of an untreated attack of hypnic headache varies from patient to patient. Attacks usually resolve within 1–2 hours (range 15–180 minutes), but longer attacks of up to 10 hours have been reported. The frequency of attacks is high, ranging from one per week to six per night. More than four attacks per week occurred in 70% of patients, and approximately 50% of patients reported daily attacks [16, 20]. Migrainous features such as nausea, photophobia, and phonophobia are rarely associated with an attack. Autonomic features can be present in approximately 8% of sufferers [23].

Secondary causes of hypnic headache must be ruled out before the diagnosis is established. There have been reports of hypnic headache occurring in the setting of a posterior fossa meningioma, pontine infarct, growth hormone-secreting pituitary adenoma, nonfunctioning pituitary macroadenoma, cerebellar hemangioblastoma, intracranial hypotension, and essential hypertension [24, 25, 26, 27, 28, 29]. These cases reinforce the need for neuroimaging in the evaluation of patients presenting with headaches of short duration triggered by sleep.

⚛ SCIENCE REVISITED

The diagnosis and management of hypnic headache must be based upon an understanding of the physiologic mechanisms underlying this disorder. It has been hypothesized that hypnic headache results from a chronobiological disorder, serotonin and melatonin dysregulation, or a disturbance of rapid eye movement (REM) sleep.

The periodicity of this headache, occurring at the same time each night, suggests involvement of the area of the brain responsible for maintaining the circadian rhythm, specifically the suprachiasmatic nucleus. The suprachiasmatic nucleus is connected to the periaqueductal gray matter and dorsal raphe nuclei in the midbrain via serotonergic pathways [30, 31]. Lithium carbonate, the medication most frequently reported to successfully treat this condition, affects serotonin metabolism. By a similar reasoning, dysregulation of melatonin may also be involved. Melatonin is the main product of the pineal gland and is a marker of circadian rhythm. With age, there is a decrease in the activity of the hypothalamic–pineal axis and a subsequent reduction in the nocturnal secretion of melatonin [32]. This decrease may explain the almost exclusive occurrence of this headache in the elderly population.

The fact that hypnic headache occurs exclusively during sleep has led some to postulate that the syndrome is a disorder of REM sleep. REM sleep is associated with decreased levels of serotonin, increases in cerebral blood flow, and a reduction in the activity of the dorsal raphe and locus ceruleus [33]. In most of the patients with hypnic headache who have undergone polysomnographic studies, attacks were associated with REM sleep [16, 34, 35, 36, 37, 38]. Non-REM related attacks, however, have also been reported [39, 40], lending credence to the fact that multiple mechanisms may be involved.

Prompt recognition of this rare, recurrent primary headache disorder is important because there are effective treatments for hypnic headache. The first effective treatment reported for hypnic headache was lithium, initiated at a dose of 300 mg at bedtime with an increase to 600 mg at bedtime within 1 week if needed [20, 37, 41, 42]. Lithium has the greatest efficacy as a prophylactic agent, but is limited by its side effect profile in the elderly. As a result, close monitoring is necessary for the duration of the treatment. Renal and thyroid function should be assessed before initiating therapy, and periodically during treatment. Because lithium has a narrow therapeutic window, serum levels must be monitored to avoid toxicity. Potential side effects include tremor, diarrhea, polydipsia, polyuria, and nephrogenic diabetes insipidus.

Other better-tolerated medications have been reported to be effective. A cup of coffee (caffeine) at bedtime has been effective in many cases and is the most benign prophylactic agent [18, 37, 43].

Additional agents that have been used to treat hypnic headache include flunarizine 5 mg [37, 42, 43], melatonin [36], and indomethacin at a dose of 25–75 mg [18, 37 43, 44]. Of note, indomethacin has been found to be more efficacious in patients with strictly unilateral attacks [45].

Primary thunderclap headache

Primary thunderclap headache (PTCH) is a rare and poorly understood disorder characterized by a severe headache that rapidly reaches peak intensity. Patients often describe this headache as the worst headache of their life. Thunderclap headache should be treated as a neurological emergency, and an expedient and exhaustive investigation must be undertaken to exclude any underlying secondary cause. The pathophysiology of PTCH is poorly understood, and the evidence supporting its existence is inadequate. It has been hypothesized that abnormal activation of the sympathetic nervous system or a direct activation of intracranial pain sensitive structures may play a role [46]. Table 20.3 lists the diagnostic criteria for PTCH.

The pain can involve any region of the head and neck, but is most commonly occipital in location. Associated symptoms may include photophobia, phonophobia, neck stiffness, nausea, and/or vomiting. The typical duration of an attack is several hours, but a low level of head pain may linger for several days to weeks. Repeated attacks may occur within the first 2 weeks or, less commonly, over the following

Table 20.3. ICHD-2 Diagnostic criteria for PTCH

A. Severe head pain fulfilling criteria B and C
B. Both of the following characteristics:
1. Sudden onset, reaching maximum intensity in <1 min
2. Lasting from 1 hour to 10 days
C. Does not recur regularly over subsequent weeks or months[a]
D. Not attributed to another disorder[b]

[a]Headache may recur within the first week after onset.
[b]Normal cerebrospinal fluid (CSF) and normal brain imaging are required.

months to years. The attacks can begin spontaneously while at rest or may be precipitated by exertion, vigorous exercise, bathing in hot water, hyperventilation, or sexual activity. Valsalva-related maneuvers appear to be a provoking factor in up to one-third of patients with PTCH [47]. The majority of patients have a normal neurological examination, although focal deficits have been rarely reported [48].

PTCH is both a diagnosis of inclusion, as certain features must be present, and a diagnosis of exclusion, in that secondary causes must be eliminated. The differential diagnosis of PTCH includes subarachnoid hemorrhage (SAH), intracerebral hemorrhage, cerebral venous sinus thrombosis, arterial dissection, pituitary apoplexy, intracranial hypotension, third ventricular colloid cyst, reversible cerebral vasoconstriction syndrome, intracranial infection, and posterior leukoencephalopathy [46]. Thunderclap headache has also been reported as the presenting symptom of pheochromocytoma, aqueductal stenosis, complicated sinusitis, Vogt–Koyanagi–Harada disease, and acute myocardial infarction [49, 50, 51, 52, 53, 54].

Diagnostic testing should include an emergent noncontrast CT scan of the brain followed by a lumbar puncture to exclude SAH. If the results of these initial studies are normal or inconclusive, further neuroimaging with cerebral MRI, magnetic resonance angiography, and magnetic resonance venography should be performed. If indicated, it is prudent to obtain an MRI of the neck with fat suppression to evaluate the cervical arteries [46]. The ICHD-2 criteria make no mention of the need for angiography. In some patients, magnetic resonance angiography or four-vessel angiography may be necessary to exclude an unruptured intracranial aneurysm or arteriovenous malformation. Some patients with PTCH have angiographic evidence of segmental vasospasm [48, 55, 56, 57]. In these patients, central nervous system vasculitis and reversible cerebral vasoconstriction syndrome should be considered in the differential diagnosis.

Since PTCH is usually a self-limited disorder, treatment may not be necessary. Symptomatic relief has been reported with both oral and intravenous nimodipine. In the absence of vasospasm, a short-term course of oral nimodipine

may be beneficial. If vasospasm is identified, intravenous nimodipine may be warranted to provide symptomatic relief and to reduce the risk of stroke. Recurrent TCH associated with vasospasm leading to stroke has been reported. In these cases, long-term treatment with oral nimodipine may lessen this risk [57, 58, 59, 60].

Primary cough headache

Primary cough headache is an uncommon disorder, with a lifetime prevalence of approximately 1% [61]. This disorder predominantly affects older men, with a mean age of onset of 67 years [62]. The headache is of sudden onset, occurring within seconds of coughing, but may also be precipitated by sneezing, straining, or other Valsalva maneuvers. The pain is usually moderate to severe in intensity and is described as sharp, stabbing, or splitting in quality. It is typically bilateral and maximal in the vertex, frontal, occipital, or temporal regions. The headache typically lasts from 1 second up to 30 minutes, but some sufferers have described a dull ache that can last for several hours afterward [63, 64]. These headaches have no associated neurologic signs or symptoms. Migrainous features such as nausea and vomiting are noticeably absent, and the headache is not associated with autonomic features. The diagnostic criteria for primary cough headache are outlined in Table 20.4.

Table 20.4. ICHD-2 diagnostic criteria for primary cough headache

A. Headache fulfilling criteria B and C
B. Sudden onset, lasting 1 second to 30 min
C. Brought on by and occurring only in association with coughing, straining, and/or a Valsalva maneuver
D. Not attributed to another disorder[a]

[a]History and physical and neurologic examinations do not suggest any of the disorders listed in Groups 5–12, or history and/or physical and/or neurological examinations do suggest such a disorder but it is ruled out by appropriate investigations, or such a disorder is present but pain does not occur for the first time in close temporal relation to the disorder.

Unlike primary cough headache, other headache disorders such as migraine, tension-type headache, cluster headache, and idiopathic intracranial hypertension may be aggravated by coughing, but are not specifically and consistently precipitated by it.

Be on the lookout for these atypical features in the history of a patient with primary cough headache: female, patients who are younger than 40 years of age, attacks lasting longer than 30 minutes, a lack of remission after 2 years, unilateral pain, or associated neurologic symptoms. If a routine MRI of the brain is normal in these cases, further diagnostic testing should be considered.

Although the pathophysiology of primary cough headache is unknown, it has been postulated that these headaches may be the result of a sudden increase in intrathoracic and intra-abdominal pressure causing an increase in intracranial venous pressure. This transient increase in intracranial venous pressure may lead to traction on pain-sensitive structures from downward displacement of the cerebellar tonsils [65]. Hypersensitivity of the pressure receptors of the venous vasculature has also been suggested as a potential mechanism for primary cough headache [66]. In a small series, patients with primary cough headache were found to have reduced volume of the posterior fossa with no other abnormalities [67].

Approximately one-half of all cases of cough headache are due to a secondary cause [68]. Secondary cough headache has been described in patients with posterior fossa lesions, most commonly Chiari type I malformations, but also with posterior fossa brain tumors such as meningiomas and acoustic neuromas. There have also been reports of cough headache associated with vertebrobasilar disease, Paget's disease of the skull, basilar impression, subdural hematoma, carotid artery disease, spontaneous intracranial hypotension, and unruptured intracranial aneurysms [68, 69]. Therefore, all patients who present with a headache that is precipitated by coughing or straining must obtain neuroimaging to exclude secondary causes.

Primary cough headache follows a benign course, with most patients attaining remission within 2 months to 2 years [62, 70]. Treatment with the sustained-release formulation of indomethacin at a dose of 75–150 mg is the treatment of choice for primary cough headache. In patients who do not respond or are unable to tolerate indomethacin, success with naproxen, acetazolamide, methysergide, dihydroergotamine, propranolol, and topiramate has been reported [30, 71, 72]. One small case series demonstrated relief with removal of 40 mL of CSF via lumbar puncture [66]. Regardless of the response to treatment, diagnostic studies must be pursued as secondary cough headache may also respond to medical management.

Primary exertional headache

Primary exertional headache is not an uncommon disorder, with a prevalence of approximately 10% of the general population [73]. Data regarding gender predilection is conflicting; some studies suggest a male predominance, while others report a female predominance [68, 73, 74]. In contrast to primary cough headache, primary exertional headache occurs in a younger patient population, with a mean age of onset of 24 years [68]. As with primary stabbing headache, there is a high comorbidity with migraine; nearly half of all patients with primary exertional headache also have migraine headache [68, 73].

Primary exertional headache is frequently associated with migraine headache, but it is a distinct disorder. Be sure to distinguish between a migraine headache that is aggravated by exertion and a headache that is specifically and reliably triggered by exertion.

Like cough headache, primary exertional headache is sudden in onset and usually bilateral in location. However, unlike cough headache, the quality is often pulsatile and of longer duration (5 minutes to 48 hours). Associated symptoms of nausea, vomiting, photophobia, and phonophobia commonly accompany primary exertional headache [68]. Exertional headache can be precipitated by a variety of physical exercises, including swimming, running, weight-lifting, straining, or bending over [74, 75, 76, 77]. Predisposing factors include heat and humidity, high altitude, hypoglycemia, and ingestion of caffeine and alcoholic beverages [75]. The diagnostic criteria for primary exertional headache are listed in Table 20.5.

Before a diagnosis of primary exertional headache can be made, neuroimaging must be performed to rule out secondary causes. Secondary causes of primary exertional headache include SAH, carotid dissection, Chiari malformation, subdural hematoma, primary or metastatic neoplasm, and platybasia [68].

> ### ✋ CAUTION!
>
> Be on the lookout for "red flags" in the history. Atypical features that are suggestive of a secondary disorder include unilateral location, onset later in life, longer duration (24 hours to weeks), or associated neurological symptoms (such as meningismus).

Table 20.5. ICHD-2 diagnostic criteria for primary exertional headache

A. Pulsating headache fulfilling B and C
B. Lasting 5 min to 48 hours
C. Brought on by and occurring only during physical exertion
D. Not attributed to another disorder[a]

[a]On first occurrence of this headache type, it is mandatory to exclude SAH and arterial dissection.

The pathophysiology of primary exertional headache is unknown. Distension of the venous or arterial blood vessels that occurs following exercise may a play role by releasing vasoactive peptides with subsequent neurogenic inflammation and activation of the trigeminal pain pathways [78].

The first-line therapy of primary exertional headache should include patient reassurance and nonpharmacologic approaches. Warm-up periods before exercise, weight loss, and avoidance of high altitudes, heat, humidity, alcohol, and caffeine may be of benefit if the headaches are infrequent, mild, or slow to build in intensity [79, 80]. If the headaches are severe, frequent, or unpredictable, pharmacotherapy may be given either prophylactically or acutely. Beta-adrenergic blockers have been shown to be beneficial but can interfere with exercise tolerance [81]. Indomethacin taken prophylactically at a dose of 25–250 mg daily or immediately prior to exercise is often the first-line pharmacotherapy. Other nonsteroidal anti-inflammatory medications (such as naproxen) or ergot derivatives taken before exercise may also be of benefit. Life-long treatment is rarely indicated, as the disorder is often self-limited, usually lasting 3–6 months. It is advisable to discontinue the therapy after 6 months of treatment and re-evaluate the patient [68, 82].

Primary headaches associated with sexual activity

Headaches associated with sexual activity are relatively rare, occurring in 0.2%–1.3% of patients evaluated in subspecialty headache clinics [61, 83]. The exact prevalence, however, may be underreported as patients may be reluctant to discuss their sexual experiences [84], and direct questioning is required to elicit this information.

Primary headache associated with sexual activity is more common in men in their fourth decade of life. These headaches are precipitated not only by sexual intercourse, but also by masturbation, nocturnal emissions, and orgasm. Hence, the term primary headache associated with sexual activity came to replace previously used terms such as benign sex headache, benign vascular sexual headache, coital cephalalgia, and benign orgasmic headache [85, 86, 87].

The first edition of the ICHD divided headaches associated with sexual activity into three subtypes: a dull type, an explosive type, and a postural type [88]. The postural subtype, seen in approximately 5% of sufferers, is a post-orgasmic headache that worsens with sitting or standing and is relieved by recumbency. It may be caused by a dural tear that develops spontaneously during sexual activity. This rare subtype has been reassigned in the ICHD-2 to the category of headaches attributed to spontaneous low CSF pressure, and is thus no longer classified as a headache associated with sexual activity. The ICHD-2 classification divides primary headache associated with sexual activity into two subtypes: preorgasmic and orgasmic headaches. The criteria for primary headache associated with sexual activity are listed in Table 20.6.

★ TIPS AND TRICKS

Patients may be hesitant to discuss their sexual experiences with their physician, so direct questioning may be necessary to elicit this information. It is important to make this diagnosis, as the patient and their partner may need reassurance that it is a benign condition and that specific treatments can be offered if the headache interferes with the patient's quality of life.

Table 20.6. ICHD-2 diagnostic criteria for primary headache associated with sexual activity

Preorgasmic headache
A. Dull ache in the head and neck associated with awareness of neck and/or jaw muscle contraction and fulfilling criterion B
B. Occurs during sexual activity and increases with sexual excitement
C. Not attributed to another disorder

Orgasmic headache
A. Sudden severe ("explosive") headache fulfilling criterion B
B. Occurs at orgasm
C. Not attributed to another disorder[a]

[a]On first onset of orgasmic headache, it is mandatory to exclude conditions such as SAH.

Preorgasmic headache is the least common of the two subtypes, occurring in approximately 20% of patients with primary headache associated with sexual activity. Preorgasmic headaches typically begin as a generalized dull ache as sexual excitement begins to escalate. They are bilateral, and many patients describe an awareness of tightness and contraction of the muscles in the neck and jaw. The exact pathophysiology is unknown; some postulate that preorgasmic headache is related to tension-type headache [68, 89, 90].

Orgasmic headache is more common, occurring in approximately 75% of patients with primary headache associated with sexual activity. It has been proposed that orgasmic headache is related to primary exertional headache, caused by brief periods of increased intracranial pressure, while others believe that it is a migraine variant [89, 91]. It has been shown that up to 50% of sufferers have comorbid migraine headaches [89]. These headaches begin suddenly at the moment of orgasm. The pain is severe, often explosive or throbbing in quality and can be frontal, occipital, or generalized. It is not uncommon for this headache to be associated with nausea and vomiting. Headaches typically last anywhere from 1 minutes to 3 hours, but have been reported to last up to 4 days [92].

A diagnosis of primary headache associated with sexual activity cannot be made until secondary causes have been excluded. These include SAH, arterial dissection, posterior fossa masses, obstruction or dysregulation of the CSF, and cervical spine lesions [68, 93]. Once secondary causes have been excluded, the practitioner can reassure the patient that this headache disorder follows a benign and self-limited course.

⚠ CAUTION!

SAH occurs during sexual activity in approximately 10% of cases [83], so it is essential to have a high index of suspicion of any headache that abruptly develops during sexual activity.

Although self-limited, the headaches can be unpredictable and may occur at infrequent intervals throughout the patient's life or in clusters followed by long periods of remission with subsequent recurrence or even complete resolution. As acute therapy is likely to be of little benefit, the goal of therapy should focus on patient reassurance and prevention.

The risk of headache recurrence appears to be increased in patients who resume sexual activity in the first few days following an attack [34, 90, 94, 95], so counseling patients to refrain from sexual activity during an attack period or in the days following an attack is advisable. Patients with preorgasmic headache can often prevent or reduce an attack by controlled muscle relaxation, stopping sexual activity at headache onset, or by assuming a more passive role. Attacks can also be treated pre-emptively with indomethacin 50–100 mg taken 30–60 minutes prior to sexual activity. Naratriptan 2.5 mg or ergotamine tartrate can also be used pre-emptively when taken 2 hours prior to sexual activity [68, 81, 96]. Patients with more frequent attacks may require prophylactic therapy. Options for preventive therapy include indomethacin 25 mg three times a day, propranolol 40–240 mg daily, metoprolol 25–50 mg daily, and atenolol 25–50 mg daily [34, 89, 96, 97]. Although effective, beta-blockers can interfere with sexual function and cause impotence, so they should be used judiciously. Calcium channel blockers have been used with mixed results; one case report demonstrated response to diltiazem 60 mg three times a day [98], whereas another demonstrated no benefit from verapamil [81].

References

1. Rasmussen BK. Epidemiology of headache. *Cephalalgia* 1995;**15**:45–68.
2. Pareja JA, Rujiz J, Deisla C, et al. Idiopathic stabbing headache (jabs and jolt syndrome). *Cephalalgia* 1996;**16**:93–6.
3. Sjaastad O, Pettersen H, Bakketeig LS. The Vaga study of headache epidemiology. II. Jabs: clinical manifestations. *Acta Neurol Scand* 2002;**105**:25–31.
4. Fuh JL, Kuo KH, Wang SJ. Primary stabbing headache in a headache clinic. *Cephalalgia* 2007;**27**:1005–9.
5. Raskin NH, Schwartz RK. Icepick-like pain. *Neurology*, 1980;**30**:203–5.
6. Drummand PD, Lance JW. Clinical diagnosis and computer analysis of headache symptoms. *J Neurol Neurosurg Psychiatr* 1984;**47**:128–33.
7. Sjaastad O. *Cluster Headache Syndrome*. Philadelphia, PA: WB Saunders; 1992.
8. Young WB, Silberstein SD. Hemicrania continua and symptomatic medication overuse. *Headache* 1993;**33**:485–7.
9. Mascellino AM, Lay CL, Newman LC. Stabbing headache as the presenting manifestation of intracerebral meningioma: a report of two patients. *Headache* 2001;**41**:599–601.
10. Levy MJ, Matharu MS, Goadsby PJ. Prolactinomas, dopamine agonists and headache: two case reports. *Eur J Neurol* 2003;**10**:169–71.
11. Medina JL, Diamond S. Cluster headache variant: spectrum of a new headache syndrome. *Arch Neurol* 1981;**38**:705–9.
12. Anmache Z, Graber M, Davis P. Idiopathic stabbing headache associated with monocular visual loss. *Arch Neurol* 2001;**57**:745–6.
13. Dodick DW. Indomethacin responsive headache syndromes. *Curr Pain Head Rep* 2004; **8**:19–28.
14. Rozen TD. Melatonin as a treatment for idiopathic stabbing headache. *Headache* 2003; **61**:865–6.
15. Franca MC, Jr., Costa ALC, Maciel JA, Jr. Gabapentin-responsive idiopathic stabbing headache. *Cephalalgia* 2004;**24**:993–6.
16. Evers S, Rahmann A, Schwaag S, et al. Hypnic headache—the first German cases including polysomnography. *Cephalalgia* 2003;**23**:20–3.
17. Grosberg BM, Lipton RB, Solomon S, et al. Hypnic headache in childhood? *Headache* 2004;**44**:497.
18. Dodick DW, Mosek AC, Campbell JK. The hypnic ("alarm clock") headache syndrome. *Cephalalgia* 1998;**18**:152–6.
19. Gould JD, Silberstein SD. Unilateral hypnic headache: a case study. *Neurology* 1997; **49**:1749–51.
20. Newman LC, Mosek AC. The hypnic headache syndrome. In Olesen J, Goadsby PJ, Ramadan NM, Pfelt-Hansen P, & Welch KMA (eds.), *The Headaches* (3rd edn.). Philadelphia: Lippincott Williams & Wilkins; 2006: pp. 847–50.
21. Gould JD, Silberstein SD. Unilateral hypnic headache: a case study. *Cephalalgia* 1997; **17**:310.

22. Ivanez V, Soler R, Barreiro P. Hypnic headache syndrome: a case with good response to indomethacin. *Cephalalgia* 1998;**18**:225–6.

23. Evers S, Dodick DB. Hypnic headache. In Goadsby PJ, Silberstein SD, & Dodick DW (eds.),*Chronic Daily Headache for Clinicians*. London: BC Decker; 2005: pp. 109–15.

24. Mullally WJ, Hall KE. Hypnic headache secondary to haemangioblastoma of the cerebellum. *Cephalalgia* 2010;**30**:887–9.

25. Garza I, Oas KH. Symptomatic hypnic headache secondary to a non-functioning pituitary macroadenoma. *Headache* 2009;**49**:470–2.

26. Valentenis L, Tuniz F, Mucchiut M, et al. Hypnic headache secondary to a growth hormone-secreting pituitary tumor. *Cephalalgia* 2009;**29**:82–4.

27. Gil-Gouveia R, Goadsby PJ. Secondary "hypnic headache." *J Neurol* 2007;**254**:646–54.

28. Peatfield RC, Mendoza ND. Posterior fossa meningioma presenting as hypnic headache. *Neurology* 2003;**43**:1007–8.

29. Freeman WD, Brazis PW, Capobianco DJ, et al. Hypnic headache and intracranial hypotension. *Headache*, 2004;**44**:498.

30. Raskin NH. The indomethacin-responsive syndromes. In Raskin NH (ed.), *Headache*. New York: Churchill Livingstone, 1988: pp. 255–68.

31. Treiser SL, Cascio CS, O'Donohue TL, Thoa NB, Jacobowitz DM, Kellar KJ. Lithium increases serotonin release and decreases serotonin receptors in the hippocampus. *Science* 1981;**213**:1529–37.

32. Lewis AJ, Kerenyi NA, Feuer G. Neuropharmacology of pineal secretion. *Drug Metab Drug Interact* 1990;**8**:247–312.

33. Somers VK, Dyken ME, Mark AL, Abboud FM. Sympathetic-nerve activity during sleep in normal subjects. *N Engl J Med* 1993;**328**:303–7.

34. Porter M, Jancovic J. Benign coital cephalalgia. Differential diagnosis and treatment. *Arch Neurol* 1981;**38**:710–12.

35. Morales-Asin F, Mauri JA, Iniguez C, et al. The hypnic headache syndrome: report of three new cases. *Cephalalgia* 1998;**18**:157–8.

36. Dodick DW. Polysomnography in hypnic headache syndrome. *Headache* 2000;**40**:748–52.

37. Evers S, Goadsby PJ. Hypnic headache: clinical features, pathophysiology, and treatment. *Neurology* 2003;**60**:905–9.

38. Pinessi L, Rainero I, Cicolin A, et al. Hypnic headache syndrome: association of the attacks with REM sleep. *Cephalalgia* 2003;**23**:150–4.

39. Manni R, Sances G, Terzaghi M, et al. Hypnic headache: PSG evidence of both REM- and NREM-related attacks. *Neurology* 2004;**62**:1411–3.

40. Vieiera-Dias M, Esperanca P. Hypnic headache: report of two cases. *Headache* 2001;**41**:726–7.

41. Raskin NH. The hypnic headache syndrome. *Headache* 1988;**28**:534–6.

42. Newman LC, Lipton RB, Solomon S. The hypnic headache syndrome: a benign headache disorder of the elderly. *Neurology* 1990;**40**:1904–5.

43. Fischer CM. Painful states: a neurological commentary. *Clin Neurosurg* 1984;**31**:32–53.

44. Jones JM, Dodick DW. Hypnic headache: another indomethacin responsive headache syndrome. *Headache* 2000;**40**:412.

45. Dodick DW, Jones JM, Capobianco DJ. Hypnic headache: another indomethacin-responsive headache syndrome? *Headache* 2000;**40**:830–5.

46. Schwedt TJ, Matharu MS, Dodick DW. Thunderclap headache. *Lancet Neurol* 2006;**5**:621–31.

47. Dodick DW. Thunderclap headache. *Current Pain Headache Rep* 2002;**6**:226–32.

48. Slivka A, Philbrook B. Clinical and angiographic features of thunderclap headache. *Headache* 1995;**35**:1–6.

49. Heo YE, Kwon HM, Nam HW. Thunderclap headache as an initial manifestation of phaeochromocytoma. *Cephalalgia* 2008;**29**:388–90.

50. Mucchiut M, Valentinis L, Tuniz F, et al. Adult aqueductal stenosis presenting as a thunderclap headache: a case report. *Cephalalgia* 2007;**27**:1171–3.

51. McGeeney BE, Barest G, Grillone G. Thunderclap headache from complicated sinusitis. *Headache* 2006;**46**:517–20.

52. Cho JH, Ahn JY, Byeon SH, Huh JS. Thunderclap headache as initial manifestation of Vogt-Koyanagi-Harada disease. *Headache* 2008;**48**:153–5.

53. Dalzell JR, Jackson CE, Robertson KE, McEntegart MB, Hogg KJ. A case of the heart ruling the head: acute myocardial infarction presenting with thunderclap headache. *Resuscitation* 2009;**80**:608–9.

54. Broner S, Lay C, Newman L, Swerdlow M. Thunderclap headache as the presenting symptom of myocardial infarction. *Headache* 2007;**47**:724–5.

55. Day JW, Raskin NH. Thunderclap headache: symptom of unruptured cerebral aneurysm. *Lancet* 1986;**2**:1247–8.

56. Dodick DW, Brown RD, Britton JE, Huston J, 3rd. Nonaneurysmal thunderclap headache with diffuse, multifocal, segmental, and reversible vasospasm. *Cephalalgia* 1999;**19**:118–23.

57. Chen SP, Fuh JL, Lirng JF, et al. Recurrent primary thunderclap headache and benign CNS angiopathy: spectra of the same disorder? *Neurology* 2006;**67**:2164–9.

58. Strum JS, Macdonell RA. Recurrent thunderclap headache associated with reversible intracerebral vasospasm causing stroke. *Cephalalgia* 2000;**20**:132–5.

59. Nowak DA, Rodiek SO, Henneken S, et al. Reversible segmental cerebral vasoconstriction (Call-Fleming syndrome): are calcium channel inhibitors a potential treatment option? *Cephalalgia* 2003;**23**:218–22.

60. Lu SR, Liao YC, Fuh JL, et al. Nimodipine for treatment of primary thunderclap headache. *Neurology* 2004;**62**:1414–6.

61. Rasmussen BK, Olesen J. Symptomatic and nonsymptomatic headaches in a general population. *Neurology* 1992;**42**:1225–31.

62. Pasqual J. Primary cough headache. *Curr Pain Head Rep* 2005;**4**:124–8.

63. Headache Classification Committee of the International Headache Society. The International Classification of Headache Disorders: 2nd edition. *Cephalalgia* 2004;**24**(Suppl. 1):9–160.

64. Diamond S. Prolonged benign exertional headache: its clinical characteristics and response to indomethacin. *Headache* 1982;**22**:96–8.

65. Wang SJ, Fuh JL, Lu SR. Benign cough headache is responsive to acetazolamide. *Neurology* 2000;**55**:149–50.

66. Raskin NH. The cough headache syndrome: treatment. *Neurology* 1995;**45**:1784.

67. Chen YY, Ling JF, Sealfon S, et al. Primary cough headache is associated with posterior fossa crowdedness: a morphometric MRI study. *Cephalalgia* 2004;**24**:694–9.

68. Pascual J, Iglesias F, Oterino A, et al. Exertional and sexual headaches: an analysis of 72 benign and symptomatic cases. *Neurology* 1996;**46**:1520–4.

69. Evans RW, Boes CJ. Spontaneous low cerebrospinal fluid pressure syndrome can mimic primary cough headache. *Headache* 2005;**45**:374–7.

70. Chen PK, Fuh JL, Wang SJ. Cough headache: a study of 83 consecutive patients. *Cephalalgia* 2009;**29**:1079–85.

71. Calandre L, Hernandez-Lain A, Lopez-Valdes E, et al. Benign Valsalva's maneuver-related headache: an MRI study of six cases. *Headache* 1996;**36**:251–3.

72. Medrano V, Jmallada J, Sempere AP, et al. Primary cough headache responsive to topiramate. *Cephalalgia* 2005;**25**:627–8.

73. Sjaastad O, Bakketeig LS. Exertional headache. II. Clinical features Vaga study of headache epidemiology. *Cephalalgia* 2003;**23**:803–7.

74. Chen SP, Fuh JL, Lu SR, Wang SJ. Exertional headache—a survey of 1963 adolescents. *Cephalalgia* 2008;**29**:401–7.

75. Dalessio DJ. Effort migraine. *Headache* 1974;**14**:53.

76. Paulson GW. Weightlifter's headache. *Headache* 1983;**23**:193–4.

77. Indo T, Takahashi A. Swimmer's headache. *Headache* 1990;**30**:485–7.

78. Buzzi MG, Bonamini M, Moskowitz MA. Neurogenic model of migraine. *Cephalalgia* 1995;**15**:277–80.

79. Lambert RW, Burnet DL. Prevention of exercise induced migraine by quantitative warm-up. *Headache* 1985;**25**:317–9.

80. Lane JC, Gulevich S. Exertional, cough, and sexual headaches. *Curr Treat Options Neurol* 2002;**4**:375–81.

81. Evans RW, Pascual J. Orgasmic headaches: clinical features, diagnosis and management. *Headache* 2000;**40**:491–4.

82. Diamond S, Medina JL. Benign exertional headache: successful treatment with indomethacin. *Headache* 1979;**19**:249.

83. Frese A, Eikermann A, Frese K, et al. Headache associated with sexual activity. Demography, clinical features, and comorbidity. *Neurology* 2003;**61**:796–800.

84. Kritz K. Coitus as a factor in the pathogenesis of neurological complications. *Cesk Neurol Neurochir* 1970;**33**:162–7.

85. Lance JW. Headaches related to sexual activity. *J Neurol Neurosurg Psychiatr* 1976;**39**:1226–30.

86. Robbins L. Masturbatory-orgasmic extracephalalgic pain. *Headache* 1994;**34**:214–6.

87. Jacome DE. Masturbatory-orgasmic extracephalalgic pain. *Headache* 1998;**38**:138–41.

88. Headache Classification Committee of the International Headache Society. Classification and diagnostic criteria for headache disorders, cranial neuralgias, and facial pain. *Cephalalgia* 1988;**8**(Suppl. 7.):1–96.

89. Silbert PL, Edis RH, Stewart-Wynn EG, Gubbay SS. Benign vascular sexual headache and exertional headache: inter-relationships and long-term prognosis. *J Neurol Neurosurg Psychiat* 1991;**54**:417–21.

90. Lance JW. Benign coital headache. *Cephalalgia* 1992;**12**:339.

91. Queiroz LP. Symptoms and therapies: exertional and sexual headaches. *Curr Pain Headache Rep* 2001;**5**:275–8.

92. Pascual J, Gonzalez-Mandly A, Martin R, Oterino A. Headaches precipitated by cough, prolonged exercise or sexual activity: a prospective etiological and clinical study. *J Headache Pain*, 2008;**9**:259–66.

93. Selwyn DL. A study of coital related headaches in 32 patients. *Cephalalgia* 1985;**5**(Suppl. 3):300–1.

94. Edis RH, Silbert PL. Sequential benign sexual headache and exertional headache. *Lancet* 1988;**1**:993.

95. Kim JS. Swimming headache followed by exertional and coital headaches. *J Korean Med Sci* 1992;**7**:276–9.

96. Kumar KL, Reuler JB. Uncommon headaches: diagnosis and treatment. *J Gen Int Med* 1993;**8**:333–41.

97. Frese A, Frese K, Scwaag S, et al. Prophylactic treatment and course of the disease in headache associated with sexual activity. In Olesen J, Silberstein S, & Tfelt-Hansen P (eds.), *Preventive Pharmacotherapy of Headache Disorders*. Oxford: Oxford University Press; 2004: pp. 50–4.

98. Akpunonu BE, Ahrens J. Sexual headaches: case report, review, and treatment with calcium channel blocker. *Headache* 1991;**31**:141–5.

Part VI

Management of Headache in Specific Patient Populations

Management of Headache in Women

Elizabeth W. Loder[1], Dawn C. Buse[2], Vince Martin[3], Luzma Cardona[1], and Dawn A. Marcus[4]

[1]Harvard Medical School, Boston, MA, USA
[2]Albert Einstein College of Medicine and Ferkauf Graduate School of Psychology, Bronx, NY, USA
[3]University of Cincinnati, Cincinnati, OH, USA
[4]University of Pittsburgh, Pittsburgh, PA, USA

Introduction

The majority of patients who seek headache treatment are women. This chapter reviews selected topics of importance in treating female patients with headache. It is organized according to the stages of the female reproductive life cycle, and covers the most common sex-specific treatment considerations that arise in headache medicine. The stages and stage-specific matters covered in this chapter are: (1) menarche and the onset of sexual maturity, a period when decisions about contraception must be made and when menstrually or hormonally related headaches may appear; (2) the reproductive years, during which the interaction between pregnancy and headache disorders must be considered; and (3) the peri- and postmenopausal years, during which decisions must be made about the use of hormone replacement therapies and the harm to benefit balance of headache treatments in the context of coexistent medical problems.

Many explanations have been offered for the higher prevalence and impact of headache disorders in women compared with men. These include physiologic factors, such as the putative headache-provocative effects of cycling ovarian steroid hormones, and psychosocial influences, including behavioral factors like sex-specific coping strategies or symptom-reporting thresholds. Women may experience high levels of stress and juggle multiple role responsibilities. Women also are more likely than men to have coexisting medical and psychiatric disorders that may aggravate, provoke, or interfere with the treatment of headache disorders. These include eating disorders, pain syndromes such as fibromyalgia and irritable bowel syndrome, mood disorders including affective disorders such as depression or premenstrual dysphoric disorder, and anxiety disorders.

Menarche and the onset of sexual maturity

The prevalence of benign recurrent headache disorders such as migraine is similar in prepubertal boys and girls, but with the onset of sexual maturity this changes. The prevalence of migraine increases more rapidly in girls than boys following the onset of puberty, when adolescent girls may begin to experience a more adult pattern of migraine [1]. Once regular cycles are established, a subset of women with migraine will note a connection between their menstrual cycles and the occurrence of headaches. Headaches that occur

Headache, First Edition. Edited by Matthew S. Robbins, Brian M. Grosberg, and Richard B. Lipton.
© 2013 John Wiley & Sons, Ltd. Published 2013 by John Wiley & Sons, Ltd.

in predictable relation to the menstrual cycle are termed "menstrual migraines" and usually occur around the time of menstrual bleeding. Good-quality evidence links the occurrence of menstrual headache to the late luteal phase decline in estradiol levels that occurs during the natural menstrual cycle [2, 3, 4].

Menstrual migraine

The second edition of the International Classification of Headache Disorders (ICHD-2) identifies a window of 2 days before to 3 days after the onset of menstrual bleeding during which migraine headache must occur in order to be attributed to menstruation. Diagnostic criteria distinguish between "pure menstrual migraine," in which headaches occur predictably and only during this window, and "menstrually related migraine," in which headache occurs predictably during this window but also at other times of the month.

SCIENCE REVISITED

The diagnosis and management of menstrually associated headaches must be based upon an understanding of the physiologic mechanisms involved in the regulation of the normal menstrual cycle. This cycle averages 28 days in length and is divided into two phases: the follicular phase and the luteal phase. The follicular phase of the cycle is initiated by a rise in follicle-stimulating hormone, in response to declining estradiol levels. During the follicular phase, a single, dominant ovarian follicle matures over 10–14 days and then ruptures in response to a complex series of hormonal events, releasing an ovum. Estrogen levels are low during the early to mid-follicular phase and then rise abruptly during the later part of the phase, while progesterone levels are low during the entire follicular phase. Ovum release, termed ovulation, is triggered by a surge in luteinizing hormone that results from a rapid rise in serum estradiol levels. If the ovum does not become fertilized, the remnant forms the corpus luteum, which

produces progesterone. Ovulation is followed by the luteal phase of the menstrual cycle, during which progesterone increases and estradiol levels remain elevated. If the ovum is not fertilized, estrogen and progesterone levels decline and the uterine lining is shed, with the onset of bleeding around day 28.

If the patient desires targeted or specific treatment of her menstrually connected headaches, it is important to have precise information about the timing of such headaches and the regularity of the menstrual cycle. Recent research suggests that considerable care must be taken in order to correctly identify a menstrual trigger for headaches. Self-reporting and review of patient-completed headache calendars might lead to an incorrect diagnosis of menstrual migraine because of low patient compliance with record-keeping. Generally, the more formal use of daily diary recordings for 2–3 months, with strict adherence emphasized, is essential to be confident about a menstrual link. A statistical analysis of self-reporting of menstrual migraine compared with a diagnosis of menstrual migraine by ICHD-2 criteria showed that roughly 20% of women who self-report menstrual migraine do not meet either ICHD-2 or strict probability-based criteria for a diagnosis of menstrual migraine based on careful diary recordings [5].

Once the diagnosis of headaches connected to the menstrual cycle is established, the patient must decide what sort of treatment she prefers. For many women, the same abortive treatments that are used to treat nonhormonal headaches will work well for hormonally triggered attacks, and no special treatment strategies aimed at headaches related to the menses are needed. There is good evidence, for example, that triptans, ergotamine preparations, and combination analgesics all work well for menstrual migraine attacks [6]. In addition, a recent randomized-controlled study also found that a combination of sumatriptan and naproxen was effective in the abortive treatment of attacks of menstrual migraine with accompanying dysmenorrhea [7].

In women with frequent headaches throughout the menstrual cycle, daily preventive treatment may successfully reduce the number or severity of headache attacks overall, but it seems to be less effective in reducing the frequency of attacks of menstrual migraine. For some women, however, headache attacks with hormonal triggers last longer, are more severe, and are less likely to respond to acute or preventive treatment than are nonhormonal attacks. Additionally, menstrually connected attacks are more predictable than are other headaches, and women may wish to exploit this by trying to pre-empt them entirely.

The general strategy in pre-emptive treatment depends upon beginning treatment *before* the expected menstrual migraine begins and continuing it through the period of expected headache susceptibility (usually 4–5 days in total). If the menstrual cycles are irregular, the correct timing of treatment onset can be difficult. In one trial of pre-emptive therapy for menstrual migraine, for example, only about two-thirds of women were able to time the treatment correctly [8].

★ TIPS AND TRICKS

Effective pre-emptive menstrual migraine treatments depend on being able to accurately predict menses. Most such regimens work best when they are begun a day or two before the expected onset of menstruation and the associated headache. Women with irregular menstrual periods may benefit from the use of ovulation prediction kits that can be purchased in any drugstore without a prescription. Although the follicular phase of the menstrual cycle can vary considerably in length, the time from ovulation to the onset of menstrual bleeding is consistently very close to 14 days. Hence, once ovulation has occurred, a woman can expect that menstrual bleeding will commence 14 days later [9].

Nonsteroidal anti-inflammatory drugs (NSAIDs) such as naproxen sodium are first-line treatments for menstrual migraine because they are generally inexpensive and are also useful for treating other menstrual-associated symptoms such as cramping. A common regimen is naproxen sodium 550 mg twice daily for 5–7 days, beginning 1–2 days before the expected onset of the headache [10, 11].

For women whose headaches do not respond to pre-emptive treatment with NSAIDs, or who do not tolerate them, pre-emptive treatment with triptans can be considered, although triptans are not approved by the US Food and Drug Administration (FDA) for this purpose. Randomized-controlled trials support a modest efficacy for both naratriptan and frovatriptan when used in this manner. A common regimen is naratriptan 1 mg orally twice a day for 5–7 days, or frovatriptan 2.5 mg orally four times a day or 2.5 mg orally twice a day for 5–7 days. In clinical trials of frovatriptan with a twice-daily dosing regimen, a loading dose of 5 mg orally twice a day was given on the first day of treatment, with 2.5 mg orally administered twice a day for the next 5 days [8, 12].

There is some evidence that an extended duration use of oral contraceptives (e.g., skipping the placebo pill week) might be helpful for menstrual migraine. However, no controlled trials have examined this hypothesis, and this approach is further complicated by the fact that use of estrogen-containing contraceptives is medically contraindicated in some women with migraine. For these reasons, the use of hormonal contraceptives solely to treat migraine is not generally advised; however, for women with migraine who desire contraception and have no medical contraindications to its use, extended-duration hormonal contraception may offer modest headache benefits. The use of medical oophorectomy with gonadotropins, with or without add-back estrogen, is sometimes used to treat women with refractory menstrual migraine, but at present large-scale trials to support such treatment are lacking, and this approach should be considered to be experimental.

Hormonal factors

Although many women with menstrually triggered headaches wonder whether there is "something wrong with my hormones," there is no evidence that hormonal levels are abnormal in women with this problem. Rather, their migraine-prone nervous system is unusually sensitive to ordinary hormonal fluctuations. Tests of hormonal levels are rarely useful in diagnosing or treating headaches connected with the menstrual cycle.

Headache can be a prominent feature of affective disorders that occur in relation to the menstrual cycle, and occasionally women or their healthcare providers may have difficulty distinguishing between menstrual migraine or headache occurring as part of the premenstrual syndrome (PMS) or premenstrual dysphoric disorder (PMDD). PMS is marked by physical and emotional symptoms that occur during the luteal phase of the menstrual cycle and symptoms are typically *relieved* by the onset of menstruation. Menstrual migraine, in contrast, may begin during the late luteal phase of the menstrual cycle, but often persists well after bleeding is established [13, 14]. Several medications, including magnesium supplementation of 200–400 mg/day, may have efficacy in both PMS/PMDD and hormonally triggered migraines.

Contraceptive choices for women with headache

Among the common recurrent headache disorders of migraine, tension-type, and cluster headache, only a diagnosis of migraine poses challenges when making contraceptive choices. These include both safety and tolerability concerns. Migraine is not a contraindication to the use of nonhormonal contraceptives or to the use of progestin-only hormonal contraception, but the decision to use estrogen-containing contraceptives in women with migraine must be carefully considered.

Safety worries arise because of evidence that migraine, especially migraine with aura, increases the risk of ischemic stroke, as does the use of exogenous estrogens. The risk of stroke is generally judged to be higher in women with aura regardless of age, and in women without aura who have other risk factors for stroke such as age over 35 or smoking. These views are codified in guidelines from the American College of Obstetrics and Gynecology and the World Health Organization, as well as recommendations from a task force of the International Headache Society. All recommend against the use of estrogen-containing contraceptives in women with any type of migraine who are over the age of 35, and in women of any age who have migraine with aura [15, 16, 17].

Separate from the matter of safety is the tolerability of estrogen-containing contraceptives in women with migraine. The impact of estrogen-containing contraceptives on migraine is not predictable. Because the incidence (the number of new-onset cases) of migraine is very high in the age group of women most likely to be starting contraception, it can be difficult to know whether headaches are causally or just coincidentally related to hormonal contraception. In some cases, migraine may be most troublesome during the pill-free week of traditional oral contraceptive regimens. Along with other estrogen withdrawal symptoms, it may respond to regimens that minimize or eliminate the pill-free interlude. Switching to another brand of contraceptive is sometimes also helpful; however, trial and error is necessary because evidence is lacking regarding which if any preparations are least likely to provoke headache. For some women, the prevention will be an overriding consideration, and they may be reluctant to abandon the use of estrogen-containing contraception. It must always be remembered that, for all women under age 35, the morbidity and mortality of pregnancy exceeds that associated with OCs.

> ### ★ TIPS AND TRICKS
>
> A frequent clinical dilemma is whether estrogen-containing contraception should be recommended or approved for young women with migraine, especially a woman with aura who has a strong desire to use estrogen-containing contraception despite the increased risk of stroke. This commonly occurs in young women with severe endometriosis who wish to preserve their fertility. It also occurs occasionally in women who simply prefer estrogen-containing contraception to any other alternative because it is the most effective reversible form of pregnancy prevention. In our view, safety and tolerability concerns should not be a deterrent to providing estrogen-containing contraception in such circumstances as long as the women are willing to accept a small increased risk of

stroke. Our clinical experience is that worsening migraine may be less of a risk and a less urgent problem for a young woman than leaving her unprotected from pregnancy. Additionally, the stroke risk of pregnancy far exceeds that imparted by migraine or estrogen-containing contraceptives. The need for contraception should take precedence.

The reproductive years

The selection of pharmacologic treatment for headache during the reproductive years must be made with care, even in women who do not intend to become pregnant. Unintended pregnancy is common and can occur even in women who are taking appropriate contraceptive measures. The majority of pregnancies in the USA are unplanned, and women often do not know that they are pregnant until several weeks into the pregnancy. A number of medications in common use for headache treatment may be problematic when used during pregnancy. As a general rule, medications that might cause pregnancy problems should be used with caution in women of childbearing age. For example, although divalproex sodium is an effective preventive drug for migraine headaches, first-trimester pregnancy exposure increases the risk of neural tube defects. For this reason, it would not be an appropriate first choice for prevention in a young woman who had not previously tried medications that are not known causes of birth defects.

★ TIPS AND TRICKS

Women with migraine, like all women of reproductive age, should be counselled to take a daily supplement of at least 400 μg (0.4 mg) of folic acid, to reduce the risk of neural tube defects in any pregnancy that might occur [18]. Some headache medications interfere with folate metabolism, particularly divalproex sodium and barbiturates, and it is especially prudent to recommend supplementation if they are prescribed to women of childbearing potential [19].

Larger numbers of women are currently exposed to the complex hormonal regimens used to treat infertility, and headache is a common side effect, particularly in women who already suffer from migraine. Headache seems to be most common during and after the periods of estrogen withdrawal associated with such treatments [20].

Because the pregnancy effects of many commonly used headache medications are not completely known, many women would prefer to discontinue most or all medications prior to pregnancy. Obviously, this is only possible when pregnancies are planned, making it important that physicians discuss pregnancy plans with all headache patients who might become pregnant. There is no need to discontinue medications for long periods of time before attempting pregnancy, so women may attempt pregnancy as soon as they like after stopping the drugs [21]. It is important to remember, however, that although most women would prefer to avoid medications during pregnancy, most women do end up using medications while pregnant. Therefore, advice about safe choices is needed, even for women stating a plan to remain medication-free.

The time around conception and pregnancy is an especially important time to recommend biobehavioral approaches to headache management, which includes relaxation techniques, biofeedback, and cognitive-behavioural therapy. Ideally, such treatments should be initiated when women first discuss a desire for later contraception so that these skills can be mastered and medications minimized prior to attempted conception.

The majority of women with recurrent headache problems, particularly migraine, report that their headaches improve during pregnancy, so many women will use little or no medication for headache during this time. If headaches are mild or occasional, many women are motivated to avoid pharmacologic treatment of headaches, or will be able to manage using acetaminophen or other reasonably safe medications on occasion. Women whose headaches do not improve, however, pose a clinical challenge. Few problems in headache medicine are as anxiety-provoking as the management of headache disorders that persist during pregnancy. The physician must not only distinguish persistent benign headaches from more sinister causes of headache, but also often make headache treatment recommendations in the absence of high-quality evidence of their harm to benefit balance. Not infrequently, otherwise confident and experienced obstetricians or headache medicine specialists find themselves uncertain about the best treatment choices for a pregnant woman with severe, disabling headaches.

A detailed discussion of all aspects of headache management in pregnancy is beyond the scope of this chapter, but several treatment principles should be borne in mind. The first is that although it is ideal to avoid the use of medication in pregnancy, it is not always feasible. Prolonged headaches with nausea or vomiting may produce serious dehydration or disability in the mother; if help is not forthcoming from her physician, she may turn to self-medication.

Treatment during pregnancy

Generally, there are inadequate data to provide definitive proof that a drug is safe in pregnancy, and clinicians typically need to rely on incomplete information from several sources, including post-marketing surveillance studies, case reports, and pregnancy registries. Among newer headache drugs, only sumatriptan has substantial evidence derived from a pregnancy registry. This, combined with other sources of information, has not identified teratogenicity with first-trimester exposure to sumatriptan; however, small increases in the risk of single birth defects cannot be ruled out due to the relatively small sample of exposed babies available for analysis. Clinically, this means that women with unplanned first-trimester exposure to sumatriptan can be reassured that the likelihood of problems is extremely low. Since evidence is incomplete, however, routine use during pregnancy is probably not wise [22, 23, 24, 25, 26].

A second treatment principle is that treatment, if necessary, should consist of drugs that have a longer track record of use during pregnancy and incorporate current evidence about possible adverse effects and teratogenicity. The FDA use-in-pregnancy categories are not especially helpful. A large proportion of drugs have not been assigned a pregnancy rating, and of those that do have one, most are classified as Category C, which unhelpfully suggests use only if benefits are likely to outweigh side effects.

Teratogen Information Service (TERIS) ratings are usually more clinically helpful because they incorporate clinical factors and experience with the drug into the recommendations, although access to the regularly updated online TERIS database requires a subscription. The seven categories of TERIS ratings are meant to identify teratogenic risk, unlike FDA categories, which attempt to balance benefits and harms. TERIS risk categories are None, Minimal, Small, Moderate, High, Undetermined, or Unlikely, and these are assigned based on a consensus of expert opinion and the literature. Agreement between TERIS and FDA ratings is no better than chance [27]. Women and their partners should understand that while the absolute safety of any drug used in pregnancy cannot be guaranteed, the likelihood of problems is low if drugs are chosen and used carefully.

✋ CAUTION!

Divalproex sodium, lisinopril, candesartan and ergotamine-containing drugs are headache medicines known to cause birth defects or other serious problems. Exposure to divalproex sodium is associated with an increased risk of a neural tube defect, while lisinopril and candesartan taken during the third trimester can cause fetal kidney problems. Ergotamine-containing drugs have abortifacient properties and have been associated with birth defects [28, 29, 30, 31].

Finally, the use of nondrug strategies to help control headaches is especially important in pregnant patients. Nondrug strategies include biofeedback, relaxation and stress management training, cognitive-behavioral therapies, and physical methods of treatment such as the use of heat, ice, and massage [32, 33]. Changing schedules to reduce stress and the development of effective coping techniques may also be helpful.

Women with migraine have an increased risk of pregnancy complications such as preeclampsia and postpartum stroke. Migraine may be a risk factor for the occurrence of postpartum cerebral vasoconstrictive syndromes as well [34, 35]. Headache following delivery occurs in about a third of women, and it can be difficult to distinguish recurrence of benign headaches from dangerous causes of headache such as cerebral venous thrombosis [36].

Therefore, migraine-specific therapies such as triptans and ergots, which rarely provoke vasospasm, might be avoided in patients with headache attacks that are atypical (e.g., different headache characteristics from past headaches or new neurologic signs or symptoms). Nonspecific therapies such as non-opioid and opioid analgesics can be used with little fear of aggravating or masking underlying serious conditions.

Breastfeeding offers important benefits to mother and baby and does not appear to have a major impact on headache activity [37]. Migraine, even migraine that requires treatment, is not a contraindication to breastfeeding. The American Academy of Pediatrics considers sumatriptan and many other medications to be compatible with breastfeeding, and their current recommendations regarding medications should be consulted if headache treatment is needed during lactation.

☙ SCIENCE REVISITED

The lipid solubility of a drug determines how much of it appears in breast milk. Drugs that are not very lipid-soluble (such as sumatriptan) are present in negligible amounts, and pumping and discarding milk after a dose ("pump and dump") recommendations are not needed. Following a 6 mg dose of subcutaneous sumatriptan, the peak breast milk concentration of the drug was very low (87.2 µg/L), occurred about 2.5 hours after ingestion, and declined quickly over the following 6 hours. The weight-adjusted infant dose was thus calculated to be only 0.5% of the oral maternal dose [38].

For drugs that are excreted in appreciable quantities in breast milk, the frequency of nursing and the time interval between taking the drug and nursing influence drug levels. In these situations, the timing of medication intake or nursing, or discarding breast milk and substituting it with stored breast milk or commercial infant formula may be a useful strategy [39].

The peri- and postmenopausal years

There has been relatively little study of how the perimenopause and the perimenopausal transition might influence pre-existing headache disorders. Throughout the usual period of life identified with perimenopause, a number of physiologic changes take place that might reasonably be expected to have an impact on headache disorders. Menstrual cycles become less predictable and eventually cease. In clinical practice, many women with migraine note that their headaches may become more active and difficult to treat during the perimenopause, perhaps because of exaggerated hormonal fluctuations. Worsening of headaches can occur even in women whose headaches were under good control [40].

A number of factors may play a role in headache exacerbation during this stage of life. Estrogen levels are sometimes higher during the early years of the perimenopause than during the premenopausal years, so that headache-provocative drops may be more pronounced. Mood disorders including depression and anxiety disorders (e.g., generalized anxiety disorder or panic disorder) also are common in postmenopausal women, and migraine is a risk factor for their occurrence [41].

Once menopause is well established and ovarian steroid hormonal cycling has ceased, many women with migraine report an improvement in their headaches. A sizeable minority, however, still have headache. In one study, the prevalence of migraine in postmenopausal women was roughly 13%, and the majority of those women had premenopausal headaches. Two-thirds of them reported an improvement in headaches after menopause, although the headaches did not disappear [40].

While the use of postmenopausal hormone replacement therapy was common until recently, new evidence has raised worries about its effect on breast cancer and vascular conditions such as heart attack and stroke. At present, it is not clear whether these harms are related to the timing of initiation of hormone replacement therapy, and we cannot clearly identify subgroups of women at low risk from the use of hormone replacement therapy. For these reasons, the prevailing attitude to hormone replacement therapy in women without a definite medical indication for it (such as severe osteoporosis) can be summed up by the phrase "the least amount for the shortest period of time." There is a consensus that women with unbearable estrogen withdrawal symptoms may reasonably use small doses for several years in order to improve their quality of life, but the ultimate goal is usually to discontinue treatment.

Despite the decrease in the use of hormone replacement therapy, some women with headache problems still might contemplate its use and seek advice about its effect on headache. Unfortunately, the effects of estrogen-only replacement or combined estrogen–progestin hormone replacement therapy on migraine are not entirely clear. One population-based study found a worsening of migraine on replacement therapy, while another did not [40, 42, 43].

A retrospective study of patients with migraine showed worsening in about half of patients, but no effect or improvement in the other half who used estrogen replacement therapy (ERT). A cohort of 504 women attending a headache clinic showed that a quarter with migraine reported that they were worse on ERT [44, 45]. The only randomized-controlled study that has been done to date (which followed 1006 women over 5 years) showed no influence on headache of oral ERT compared with no ERT [46].

Estrogen delivered through transdermal patches may be less likely to provoke headache than oral therapy, perhaps because the "first-pass" effect of liver metabolism is avoided and transdermal administration allows for more stable drug levels [47]. In fact, one study identified a 33% decrease in headache index from baseline in women receiving an estrogen patch, while the placebo group experienced a 5% increase in headache index [48]. A common clinical practice if women require the use of replacement is to use continuous, uninterrupted transdermal regimens where feasible. Estrogen is used alone in women without a uterus, but it must be combined with a progestin if the uterus remains.

The administration of progestins along with ERT can also modulate headache activity. Regimens that administer progestins for 14 days per month are associated with an increase in the frequency of migraine compared to those that give them daily [49]. Another study found that conjugated estrogens combined with 14 days per month of medroxyprogestone worsened the frequency of migraine attacks, while daily transder-

mal estrogen with daily medroxyprogesterone led to no changes in headache outcome measures [47]. It is unclear whether the administration of conjugated estrogens or the use of cyclic progestin therapy worsened the frequency of the migraine attacks.

Conclusion

Many primary headache disorders, including migraine, are more common in female patients. Treating female patients requires an awareness of hormonal factors, medical and psychological comorbidities, and social demands and challenges. One method of effective treatment is to tailor treatment based on the stages of the female reproductive life cycle. Data regarding the efficacy and safety of various treatment approaches are often conflicting; so that the treatment decision must often be made based on a thoughtful balance of risks and benefits. In addition to pharmacologic treatments, female patients may also benefit from nonpharmacologic approaches throughout all stages of life.

References

1. Stewart WF, Lipton RB, Celentano DD, Reed ML. Prevalence of migraine headache in the United States. Relation to age, income, race, and other sociodemographic factors. *JAMA* 1992;**267**(1):64–9.

2. MacGregor EA, Frith A, Ellis J, Aspinall L, Hackshaw A. Incidence of migraine relative to menstrual cycle phases of rising and falling estrogen. *Neurology* 2006;**67**(12):2154–8.

3. Somerville BW. Estrogen-withdrawal migraine. I. Duration of exposure required and attempted prophylaxis by premenstrual estrogen administration. *Neurology* 1975; **25**(3):239–44.

4. Somerville BW. Estrogen-withdrawal migraine. II. Attempted prophylaxis by continuous estradiol administration. *Neurology* 1975;**25**(3):245–50.

5. Marcus DA, Bernstein CD, Sullivan EA, Rudy TE. A prospective comparison between ICHD-II and probability menstrual migraine diagnostic criteria. *Headache* 2010;**50**(4): 539–50.

6. Martin VT. Menstrual migraine: a review of prophylactic therapies. *Curr Pain Headache Rep* 2004;**8**(3):229–37.

7. Mannix LK, Martin VT, Cady RK, et al. Combination treatment for menstrual migraine and dysmenorrhea using sumatriptan-naproxen: two randomized controlled trials. *Obstet Gynecol* 2009;**114**(1):106–13.

8. Silberstein SD, Elkind AH, Schreiber C, Keywood C. A randomized trial of frovatriptan for the intermittent prevention of menstrual migraine. *Neurology* 2004;**63**(2):261–9.

9. MacGregor EA, Frith A, Ellis J, Aspinall L. Predicting menstrual migraine with a home-use fertility monitor. *Neurology* 2005;**64**(3): 561–3.

10. Szekely B, Merryman S, Croft H, Post G. Prophylactic effects of naproxen sodium on perimenstrual headache: a double-blind, placebo-controlled study. *Cephalalgia* 1989; **9**(Suppl. 10):452–3.

11. Sances G, Martignoni E, Fioroni L, Blandini F, Facchinetti F, Nappi G. Naproxen sodium in menstrual migraine prophylaxis: a double-blind placebo controlled study. *Headache* 1990;**30**(11):705–9.

12. Newman L, Mannix LK, Landy S, et al. Naratriptan as short-term prophylaxis of menstrually associated migraine: a randomized, double-blind, placebo-controlled study. *Headache* 2001;**41**(3):248–56.

13. Moline ML, Zendell SM. Evaluating and managing premenstrual syndrome. *Medscape Womens Health* 2000;**5**(2):1.

14. Dickerson LM, Mazyck PJ, Hunter MH. Premenstrual syndrome. *Am Fam Physician* 2003;**67**(8):1743–52.

15. Magos AL, Zilkha KJ, Studd JW. Treatment of menstrual migraine by oestradiol implants. *J Neurol Neurosurg Psychiatry* 1983;**46**(11): 1044–6.

16. de Lignieres B, Vincens M, Mauvais-Jarvis P, Mas JL, Touboul PJ, Bousser MG. Prevention of menstrual migraine by percutaneous oestradiol. *Br Med J (Clin Res Ed)* 1986; **293**(6561):1540.

17. ACOG Committee on Practice Bulletins-Gynecology. ACOG Practice Bulletin. The use of hormonal contraception in women with coexisting medical conditions. Number 18, July 2000. *Int J Gynaecol Obstet* 2001; **75**(1):93–106.

18. Czeizel AE. Periconceptional folic acid and multivitamin supplementation for the pre- vention of neural tube defects and other congenital abnormalities. *Birth Defects Res A Clin Mol Teratol* 2009;**85**(4):260–8.

19. Alsdorf R, Wyszynski DF. Teratogenicity of sodium valproate. *Expert Opin Drug Saf* 2005;**4**(2):345–53.

20. Amir BY, Yaacov B, Guy B, Gad P, Itzhak W, Gal I. Headaches in women undergoing in vitro fertilization and embryo-transfer treatment. *Headache* 2005;**45**(3):215–9.

21. Mannix LK, Diamond M, Loder E. Women and headache: a treatment approach based on life stages. *Cleve Clin J Med* 2002; **69**(6):488–500.

22. Kallen B, Lygner PE. Delivery outcome in women who used drugs for migraine during pregnancy with special reference to sumatriptan. *Headache* 2001;**41**(4):351–6.

23. Olesen C, Steffensen FH, Sorensen HT, Nielsen GL, Olsen J. Pregnancy outcome following prescription for sumatriptan. *Headache* 2000;**40**(1):20–4.

24. Shuhaiber S, Pastuszak A, Schick B, et al. Pregnancy outcome following first trimester exposure to sumatriptan. *Neurology* 1998; **51**(2):581–3.

25. O'Quinn S, Ephross SA, Williams V, Davis RL, Gutterman DL, Fox AW. Pregnancy and perinatal outcomes in migraineurs using sumatriptan: a prospective study. *Arch Gynecol Obstet* 1999;**263**(1–2):7–12.

26. Loder E. Safety of sumatriptan in pregnancy: a review of the data so far. *CNS Drugs* 2003;**17**(1):1–7.

27. Friedman JM, Little BB, Brent RL, Cordero JF, Hanson JW, Shepard TH. Potential human teratogenicity of frequently prescribed drugs. *Obstet Gynecol* 1990;**75**(4):594–9.

28. Holmes LB, Harvey EA, Coull BA, et al. The teratogenicity of anticonvulsant drugs. *N Engl J Med* 2001;**344**(15):1132–8.

29. Wegner C, Nau H. Alteration of embryonic folate metabolism by valproic acid during organogenesis: implications for mechanism of teratogenesis. *Neurology* 1992;**42**(4 Suppl. 5):17–24.

30. Koren G, Pastuszak A, Ito S. Drugs in pregnancy. *N Engl J Med* 1998;**338**(16): 1128–37.

31. Schrader H, Stovner LJ, Helde G, Sand T, Bovim G. Prophylactic treatment of migraine

with angiotensin converting enzyme inhibitor (lisinopril): randomised, placebo controlled, crossover study. *BMJ* 2001;**322**(7277): 19–22.

32. Marcus DA, Scharff L, Turk DC. Nonpharmacological management of headaches during pregnancy. *Psychosom Med* 1995;**57**(6): 527–35.

33. Scharff L, Marcus DA, Turk DC. Maintenance of effects in the nonmedical treatment of headaches during pregnancy. *Headache* 1996;**36**(5):285–90.

34. Kittner SJ, Stern BJ, Feeser BR, et al. Pregnancy and the risk of stroke. *N Engl J Med* 1996;**335**(11):768–74.

35. James AH, Bushnell CD, Jamison MG, Myers ER. Incidence and risk factors for stroke in pregnancy and the puerperium. *Obstet Gynecol* 2005;**106**(3):509–16.

36. Stein GS. Headaches in the first post partum week and their relationship to migraine. *Headache* 1981;**21**(5):201–5.

37. Wall VR. Breastfeeding and migraine headaches. *J Hum Lact* 1992;**8**(4):209–12.

38. Wojnar-Horton RE, Hackett LP, Yapp P, Dusci LJ, Paech M, Ilett KF. Distribution and excretion of sumatriptan in human milk. *Br J Clin Pharmacol* 1996;**41**(3):217–21.

39. American Academy of Pediatrics Committee on Drugs. Transfer of drugs and other chemicals into human milk. *Pediatrics* 2001;**108**(3): 776–89.

40. Wang SJ, Fuh JL, Lu SR, Juang KD, Wang PH. Migraine prevalence during menopausal transition. *Headache* 2003;**43**(5):470–8.

41. Smoller JW, Pollack MH, Wassertheil-Smoller S, et al. Prevalence and correlates of panic attacks in postmenopausal women: results from an ancillary study to the Women's Health Initiative. *Arch Intern Med* 2003; **163**(17):2041–50.

42. Li C, Wilawan K, Samsioe G, Lidfeldt J, Agardh CD, Nerbrand C. Health profile of middle-aged women: the Women's Health in the Lund Area (WHILA) study. *Hum Reprod* 2002;**17**(5):1379–85.

43. Mattsson P. Hormonal factors in migraine: a population-based study of women aged 40 to 74 years. *Headache* 2003;**43**(1):27–35.

44. MacGregor EA. Menstruation, sex hormones, and migraine. *Neurol Clin* 1997;**15**(1): 125–41.

45. Kelman L. Women's issues of migraine in tertiary care. *Headache* 2004;**44**(1):2–7.

46. Vestergaard P, Hermann AP, Stilgren L, et al. Effects of 5 years of hormonal replacement therapy on menopausal symptoms and blood pressure—a randomised controlled study. *Maturitas* 2003;**46**(2): 123–32.

47. Nappi RE, Cagnacci A, Granella F, Piccinini F, Polatti F, Facchinetti F. Course of primary headaches during hormone replacement therapy. *Maturitas* 2001;**38**(2):157–63.

48. Martin V, Wernke S, Mandell K, et al. Medical oophorectomy with and without estrogen add-back therapy in the prevention of migraine headache. *Headache* 2003;**43**(4): 309–21.

49. Facchinetti F, Nappi RE, Tirelli A, Polatti F, Nappi G, Sances G. Hormone supplementation differently affects migraine in postmenopausal women. *Headache* 2002;**42**(9): 924–9.

Management of Headache in Children

Oranee Sanmaneechai[1,2] and Karen Ballaban-Gil[2]

[1]Siriraj Hospital, Mahidol University, Bangkok, Thailand
[2]Albert Einstein College of Medicine, Montefiore Medical Center, Bronx, NY, USA

Introduction

Headache is one of the most common problems in children, particularly in adolescents, both in the pediatrician's office and in emergency room settings. Unique challenges to diagnosing headaches in children include the fact that young children may have difficulty describing and recalling their headache and associated symptoms. Therefore, headache in children is often unrecognized, underdiagnosed, and undertreated. An awareness of common primary headache syndromes in children combined with careful history-taking from parents, including behavioral observations, is crucial.

Etiologies of headache in children are divided into primary and secondary headache. Recurrent episodic headaches are most likely primary headaches, and the majority of primary headaches in children are migraine or tension-type headache (TTH). In children with acute or chronic progressive headaches, physicians should consider secondary headaches from specific etiologies, such as infections, brain tumors, or other systemic illness. Diagnosis is usually dependent on careful history-taking and physical examination; less often, further investigations may be required. The focus of this chapter will be the management of primary headaches in children.

Primary headaches in children

Epidemiology

Headache in children is one of the most common complaints in both general pediatrics and pediatric neurology clinics. Primary headaches in children are not rare: in fact, headache is at least as common in the pediatric population as in the adult population. Primary headaches commonly start in childhood and adolescence, which may explain the high prevalence of headache in this age group. The prevalence of TTH in children and adolescents (aged 7–19 years old) is 10%–25% [1, 2, 3, 4, 5]. The prevalence of migraine in children and adolescents (aged 7–19 years old) is 6%–14% [5, 6, 7, 8, 9]. The prevalence increases with age and peaks during adolescence. Migraine may be more prevalent in boys than girls in the prepubertal population, but more common in girls than boys after puberty [10]. Migraine or its variants (childhood periodic syndromes) can occur at any age, although most studies of childhood migraine use 3 years old as the lower age limit for inclusion.

Headache, First Edition. Edited by Matthew S. Robbins, Brian M. Grosberg, and Richard B. Lipton.
© 2013 John Wiley & Sons, Ltd. Published 2013 by John Wiley & Sons, Ltd.

Table 22.1. 2004 IHS classifications of headache disorders for pediatric migraine without aura

A. At least 5 attacks fulfilling criteria B–D
B. Headache attacks lasting 1–72 hours
C. Headache has at least two of the following four features:
   1. Either bilateral or unilateral (frontal/temporal) location
   2. Pulsating quality
   3. Moderate or severe pain intensity
   4. Aggravation by routine physical activities
D. At least one of the following accompanies headache:
   1. Nausea and/or vomiting
   2. Photophobia and phonophobia (may be inferred from their behavior)
E. Not attributed to another disorder

Reproduced with permission from Lewis D, Ashwal S, Hershey A, et al. Practice parameter: pharmacological treatment of migraine headache in children and adolescents: report of the American Academy of Neurology Quality Standards Subcommittee and the Practice Committee of the Child Neurology Society. *Neurology* 2004;63:2215–24.

Migraine

Clinical manifestations

Migraine is characterized by headaches with specific features and associated symptoms, as defined by the International Headache Society (IHS) criteria for migraine diagnosis in children (Table 22.1) [11]. Establishing a diagnosis of migraine in children can be particularly challenging. Younger children may have difficulty describing and recalling their headaches and associated symptoms; therefore, a history from parental observation of children's behavior is necessary. Additionally, many disorders in childhood have symptoms similar to those of migraine, including allergies, infectious diseases, and gastrointestinal disorders.

Migraines in children may have features that are different from those of migraines in adults, including a bilateral location, a shorter duration, and nonspecific associated symptoms [12]. Characteristics of migraine include pulsation or a throbbing quality, a moderate to severe intensity, aggravation by routine physical activity, and a unilateral or bilateral location. Migraine headaches in childhood are more likely to be bilateral, often frontotemporal, unlike migraine in late adolescence or adulthood, in which the pain is typically unilateral. If the location of the headache is exclusively occipital, structural lesions should be ruled out [11]. The duration of migraines in children is often shorter than in adults, ranging from 1 to 72 hours. It has been proposed that the duration of sleep should be included as part of the headache duration when determining the total duration of the attack if the child falls asleep during the migraine and wakes up without it [2], although the IHS has not yet accepted this criterion.

Constitutional associated symptoms in children with migraine may be more nonspecific than in adults, including nausea, vomiting, and/or photophobia, phonophobia, difficulty concentrating, lightheadedness, or fatigue. In younger children, many of these symptoms may have to be inferred by the parents, based on the child's behavior [13]. Again, it has been proposed that the IHS criteria for migraine in children should be expanded to formally include these more nonspecific features in the definition of pediatric migraine, but these have not yet been adopted [2].

Migraine classification

Migraine can be divided into many subtypes, but the most common subtypes seen in the pediatric population are migraine without aura, migraine with aura, and childhood periodic syndromes, which are commonly precursors of migraine.

Migraine without aura is the more common subtype of migraine in children. These tend to occur more frequently and be more disabling than migraine with aura [11]. Migraine with aura is characterized by the presence of focal neurologic symptoms that accompany the headache. Auras can be visual, sensory, speech, or motor, a change in level of consciousness, or brainstem symptoms that occur before or at the onset of headache with a duration of 5–60 minutes. Age can also influence the manifestations and types of aura experienced during a migraine. Common visual auras in adults include scintillating scotomas, flashes of light, and zigzagging patterns. In contrast, visual distortions including metamorphopsia, micropsia, or macropsia are more common in children. Basilar-type migraines, which are migraines with brainstem symptoms, including dysarthria, vertigo, tinnitus, decreased hearing, double vision, ataxia, and a decreased level of consciousness, occur most commonly in adolescents and young adults.

Childhood periodic syndromes

Childhood periodic syndromes have been classified as a subtype of migraines by the IHS [11]. These include cyclical vomiting, abdominal migraine, and benign paroxysmal vertigo of childhood. Benign paroxysmal torticollis is not included in these syndromes, but is included in the IHS Appendix and is currently thought to be a precursor to migraine as well. The characteristic features of these syndromes are similar to those of migraine, including that they are have a recurrent, episodic, sudden onset of stereotypic symptoms. The child may look extremely sick during the attack, especially in abdominal migraine and cyclical vomiting, but the attacks resolve spontaneously and the child will be completely healthy and have a normal neurologic examination between the attacks.

Clinical presentations differ depending upon the particular syndrome, as summarized in Table 22.2. Manifestations include vertigo, torticollis, and gastrointestinal symptoms including abdominal pain, nausea, vomiting, and anorexia. The attacks tend to occur more frequently when they first begin and then become less frequent as the patient gets older. Headache may be minimal or absent during attacks. Children with periodic syndromes frequently have a family history of migraine [14, 15]. Additionally, patients with cyclical vomiting or abdominal migraine may also have a family history of motion sickness. Most children with periodic syndromes develop migraine headaches: 70% of children with abdominal migraine develop typical migraine headaches within 10 years [16], and 75% percent of patients with cyclical vomiting develop migraines by age 18 years [17].

These periodic syndromes may be difficult to diagnose because of the absence of headaches and the nonspecific and at times severe nature of the symptoms. The differential diagnosis of these syndromes includes metabolic disorders (i.e., inborn errors of metabolism and mitochondrial disorders), epilepsy, ischemic episodes, gastrointestinal disorders, and psychological disorders. These other potential etiologies must be thoroughly investigated and ruled out prior to diagnosing a child with periodic childhood syndrome.

Supportive treatment with fluid and electrolyte replacement is crucial during acute attacks. Symptomatic treatments may be used, such as antiemetic medication for nausea and vomiting. Prophylactic migraine medication may be used to prevent recurrent attacks: in younger children cyproheptadine or propanolol may be considered, and in older children propanolol or amitriptyline may be useful. However, these treatments are empiric rather than evidence-based, as there are no controlled treatment trials in these syndromes. Reassurance and lifestyle adjustment are also essential to the treatment.

Impact and comorbidity of migraines in children

Migraine is a chronic recurrent disease that affects an individual's quality of life. The World Health Organization rates migraine to be one of the most disabling chronic disorders, together with quadriplegia, psychosis, and dementia [18]. In adults, migraine can affect work, social functioning, and family life. Similarly, childhood migraines may have a significant negative impact on a child's life and family, including school performance, daily activities, and peer relationships. The onset of migraines in childhood or adolescence may thus lead to a longer duration of the negative impact on the quality of life of an individual than an adult onset. The Pediatric Migraine Disability Assessment (Ped MIDAS) can be used to assess the degree of disability and the need for prophylactic treatment, and can be used to monitor the response to treatment.

Children with migraine may have a variety of comorbid medical conditions, including epilepsy, sleep disorders, obesity, asthma, allergies, and psychological disorders. These disorders may complicate migraine management in terms of diagnosis, decisions about medication choices, and long-term outcome. For instance, comorbid conditions can affect medication choices: antiepileptic drugs should be considered in patients with comorbid epilepsy, antidepressants in those with depression or anxiety, etc. Additionally,

Table 22.2. Childhood periodic syndromes

Syndrome	Age of onset	Clinical criteria	Age improve	Differential diagnosis
Benign paroxysmal torticollis of infancy	2–8 months	Sudden onset of head tilt, with vomiting, ataxia pallor, irritability, or malaise. Lasting for hours to days (rarely minutes). Frequency: monthly. Positive family history of migraine, motion sickness	3–5 years	Posterior fossa tumors. Craniocervical tumor/lesion. Gastroesophageal reflux. Complex partial seizure. Idiopathic torsional dystonia
Benign paroxysmal vertigo	2–4 years	Sudden onset of vertigo, ataxia, nystagmus accompanied by an inability to stand without support (unexplained fright, imbalance, falls). Lasting minutes (rarely hours). Frequency: once a day to once every 1–3 months. Positive family history of migraine, motion sickness	5 years	Pontocerebellar angle tumor. Episodic ataxia. Benign positional vertigo. Epilepsy. Acute vestibulitis
Cyclic vomiting	4–5 years	Recurrent paroxysmal severe vomiting, nausea, extremely sick and electrolyte imbalance during attack. Lasting for 1 hour to 5 days. Frequency: occurring at regular intervals 4–12 episodes per year	75% develop migraine later	GI: gastroesophageal reflux, bowel obstruction, gallbladder disease, hepatitis, pancreatitis, GU: ureteropelvic junction obstruction. Metabolic disorders. Increased intracranial pressure
Abdominal migraine	7–10 years	Recurrent acute noncolicky midline abdominal pain accompanied by pallor, anorexia, nausea, or vomiting. Trigger factors: stress, skipped meal, sleep deprivation, and exercise. Lasting for 1–72 hours	70% develop migraine later	GI: irritable bowel syndrome, peptic ulcer, Crohn's disease, gastroesophageal reflux. GU: ureteropelvic junction obstruction. Systemic diseases: porphyria

Reproduced from Cuvellier JC, Lepine A. Childhood periodic syndromes. *Pediatr Neurol* 2010;42(1):1–11. GI, gastrointestinal disorders; GU, genitourinary disorders.

comorbid conditions may steer a practitioner away from using certain medications; for example, beta-blockers should be avoided in children with asthma or depression, and medications associated with weight gain should be avoided in obese patients. As part of migraine management, it is important for physicians to address those comorbid conditions which may be contributing to or worsening migraines. Appropriate sleep and exercise as well as a proper diet is also essential to migraine treatment.

Tension-type headache

TTH commonly begins at approximately 7 years of age [19]. It is characterized by a bilateral pressure-like headache without autonomic or migrainous associated symptoms. TTH should be considered in children with normal neurologic examinations and headaches that are not associated with a throbbing quality, unilateral pain, nausea, vomiting, photophobia, phonophobia, aggravation by routine activity, or autonomic symptoms [20]. TTH can be divided into episodic and chronic subtypes, defined by the frequency of the headache attacks—more than 15 headache days per month for longer than 3 months is consistent with chronic TTH [21]. As in migraine headaches, the treatment in TTH includes acute treatment and preventive treatment, with preventive therapies being used for those children with chronic TTH. Behavioral treatments must be combined with medication therapies for the successful management of TTH [20].

Evaluation of children with headache

When evaluating children with headaches, it is essential to differentiate primary from secondary headaches. The history and physical examination are key in diagnosing primary headaches in children. Important historical features include the headache characteristics, frequency, pain intensity, duration, associated symptoms, aggravating and alleviating factors, radiation of pain, and presence or absence of symptoms that suggest neurologic dysfunction. In addition, prior pain medications, including the type and number that have been used and the response to these therapies, should be reviewed. Since the majority of children with migraine have a family history of migraine, the family history should also

be investigated. A complete physical and neurologic examination is necessary to rule out headaches secondary to systemic diseases or intracranial structural lesions.

Physicians can usually diagnose primary headaches in children on a clinical basis, without the need for additional testing. Although secondary headaches may occur in children, they are more common in the adult population, and thus the evaluation in children may differ from that in adults. Neuroimaging is not typically necessary in the evaluation of primary headaches in children who experience chronic, recurrent, nonprogressive headaches with a normal neurologic examination [22]. Neuroimaging is indicated if the history and/or physical examination are suggestive of secondary headache. Concerning historical features that suggest CNS disease include an occipital location, chronic progressive headaches, a recent onset of severe headaches, a change in the type of headache, coexistent seizures, or associated symptoms that suggest focal neurologic dysfunction or increased intracranial pressure (such as headaches when lying down and headaches that wake the child out of sleep). Concerning features on neurologic examination include focal neurologic deficits, signs of increased intracranial pressure, and significant alteration of consciousness. If neuroimaging is considered, MRI is the recommended study [22]. If a vascular disorder is suspected, magnetic resonance angiography may be added. Variables that predict the presence of a space-occupying lesion included: (1) headache of less than 1 month's duration; (2) an absence of a family history of migraine; (3) abnormal neurologic findings on examination; (4) gait abnormalities; and (5) the occurrence of seizures [22].

Treatment of migraine in children

The goal of treatment is to reduce the frequency of headache attacks, relieve headaches as rapidly as possible, and decrease the impact of headache on quality of life, including school performance and relationships with peers and family, as well as to prevent progression to long-term comorbidities [23, 24]. The treatment of migraine can be divided into pharmacologic treatment, including acute therapy and prophylactic treatments, and nonpharmacologic or biobehavioral interventions.

Acute migraine treatment

Acute migraine treatment refers to medication taken during the attack with the aim of aborting the headache attack rapidly without recurrence and enabling a return to normal activity. Ideally, effective medications for the abortive treatment of migraines should be able to be given quickly at the beginning of an attack and have a rapid onset of action. In the outpatient setting, there are many different over-the-counter and prescription medications used to treat migraines. While some of these medications have been approved for use in children, very few have been approved for use specifically in the treatment of headaches in the pediatric population. In fact, most medications that are used in the acute treatment of migraines in the pediatric population are off-label use.

While acetaminophen, ibuprofen, acetaminophen, aspirin, and caffeine compound (Excedrin), naproxen with sumatriptan, diclofenac potassium, triptans, and ergotamine have been approved by the US Food and Drug Administration (FDA) for the treatment of migraines in adults, only almotriptan has been approved by the FDA for the treatment of migraine headaches in adolescents age 12–17 years. No medication has an FDA indication for the treatment of migraine headache in children under the age of 12 years. Nasal sumatriptan and oral zolmitriptan have been approved in Europe for the treatment of migraines in the pediatric population. Additionally, in the 2004 practice parameter on pharmacologic treatment of migraine in children and adolescents, the American Academy of Neurology (AAN) concluded that ibuprofen is effective and acetaminophen is probably effective, and stated that both should be considered for the acute treatment of migraine in children older than 6 years old [24]. For adolescents with migraine (ages 12 and above), they concluded that nasal spray sumatriptan is effective and should be considered for the acute treatment of migraine [24]. Although there are some trials of the use of other antimigraine medications in the pediatric population, the other triptans and dihydroergotamine (DHE) lack sufficient data for their use in the pediatric population, and further studies of their use are needed.

The dosage of medications that can be used for the treatment of childhood migraine and their side effects are summarized in Table 22.3. As previously noted, most of these are off-label usage. Nonsteroidal anti-inflammatory drugs (NSAIDs) and non-opiate analgesics are often used in pediatric migraine. Dosages for children are 15 mg/kg per dose for acetaminophen and 7.5–10 mg/kg per dose for ibuprofen. Naproxen is frequently used and probably effective in children, but there are no randomized-controlled trials in the treatment of pediatric migraines. In order to avoid medication overuse or rebound headaches, the use of these agents should be limited to no more than two or three headaches per week.

For more severe migraine attacks, or in patients who have either a partial response or no response to NSAIDs/analgesic drugs, migraine-specific medications such as triptans and ergotamine can be considered. The oral triptan preparations may not be as effective in children during acute migraine attacks because nausea, vomiting, and gastric stasis can delay drug absorption. Ergot alkaloids are another specific migraine medication that can be used in the treatment of moderate to severe migraine attacks. DHE is available as a nasal spray, oral preparation, and intravenous (i.v.) injection. There are no prospective trials of DHE in the pediatric population.

Patients who present to the emergency department with migraines may have status migrainosus (a prolonged severe migraine headache lasting >72 hours) or refractory migraines (a failure to respond to home medication treatment). These patients may suffer from severe headaches, nausea, and vomiting and be unable to eat or drink, often having dehydration at the time of the emergency room visit. These patients should be placed in a dark and quiet room so as not to exacerbate their photophobia and phonophobia. Intravenous fluid hydration with a normal saline bolus and electrolyte correction should be given, and if the vomiting is severe, the physician should consider parenteral antiemetic drugs.

For pain management, parenteral medications such as dopamine-blocking medications combined with NSAIDs can be given. Antiemetics or dopamine-blocking medications are effective both for the antiemetic effects as well as for aborting the migraine attack. These agents include metoclopramide 10 mg intramuscularly (i.m.), i.v., or per rectum, prochlorperazine 10 mg i.m., i.v., or per rectum, and chlorpromazine

Table 22.3. Abortive medications in pediatric migraine

Drug name	Dosing (mg/kg/dose) and maximum dose	Brand name	Side effect	Study class	n^a	Subjects' ages (years)	Efficacy[b]	Reference
Acetaminophen	15 mg/kg/dose Max 100 mg/kg/day Max 4 g/day	Tylenol	Hypersensitivity	RCT	88	4–16	+	[74]
NSAID								
Ibuprofen	7.5–10 mg/kg/dose Max 40 mg/kg/day or 2400 mg/day	Advil, Motrin	GI distress, rash, dizziness, hypersensitivity	2 RCTs	172	4–16	+	[74, 75]
Naproxen sodium	5 mg/kg/dose 220 mg twice a day Max 1100 mg/day	Aleve	GI distress, dizziness, hypersensitivity					No study
Ketorolac i.v.	0.5 mg/kg/dose 30 mg i.v. every 6 hours Max 120 mg/day	Toradol	GI distress, anemia, dizziness, edema, rash, bronchospasm, hypersensitivity	RCT	62	5–18	+	[25]
Triptans								
Almotriptan	12.5 mg	Axert	Nausea, dizziness, somnolence	RCT	866	12–17	+	[76]
Sumatriptan nasal spray	5–10 mg (weight 20–40 kg) 20 mg (weight >40 kg) Max 40 mg/day	Imitrex NS	Taste disturbance, nausea, vomiting	4 RCTs	111	6–17	+	[77, 78, 79, 80]
Sumatriptan subcutaneous	0.06 mg/kg/dose 3–6 mg Max 12 mg/day	Imitrex SC	Drowsiness, neck and chest discomfort, dizziness, paresthesia	2 OLs	65	6–18	+	[81, 82]
Sumatriptan oral	25–100 mg Max 200 mg/day	Imitrex	Head, neck and chest discomfort, dizziness, paresthesia	RCT	23	8–16	–	[83]
Rizatriptan	5 mg	Maxalt	Asthenia, dizziness, dry mouth	RCT	296	12–17	–	[84]
Zolmitriptan	2.5 mg	Zomig	Dizziness, somnolence	RCT [84] OL [85]	70	6–18	+	[85, 86]

(Continued)

Table 22.3. (Continued)

Drug name	Dosing (mg/kg/dose) and maximum dose	Brand name	Side effect	Study class	n^a	Subjects' ages (years)	Efficacy[b]	Reference
Antiemetics, antidopaminergics								
Prochlorperazine	0.15 mg/kg/dose 5–10 mg i.v., i.m. every 6–8 hours Max 20 mg/day	Compazine	Dizziness, dystonia, somnolence, prolonged QT interval	1	62	5–18	+	[25]
Metoclopramide	1–2 mg/kg/dose 10–20 mg i.v., i.m. every 4–6 hours	Reglan	Acute dystonia, seizure, hypertension					No study
Chlorpromazine	0.55 mg/kg 12.5 mg i.v., i.m. every 6–8 hours max 75 mg/day	Thorazine	Postural hypotension, drowsiness					No study
DHE mesylate								
Ergotamine oral DHE	20 µg/kg		Nausea, vomiting	RCT	12	5–15	+	[87]
DHE nasal spray	0.5– mg Max 3 mg/day		Rhinitis, taste change, nausea, vomiting					No study
DHE i.v./i.m.	0.1–0.5 mg i.v., i.m. Max 2 mg i.v./dose		Nausea, vomiting, chest pain, vasoconstriction. Avoid in basilar migraine and hemiplegic migraine	2 RCRs	62	5–18	+	[26, 88]
Valproate	300–500 mg i.v.	Depakote	Avoid in pregnancy and hepatic diseases	RCR	31	13–17	+	[27]

aTotal number of subjects in all studies combined.
b+, studies showing positive results or consistent positive results in all studies; −, studies showing negative results or consistent negative results in all studies.

GI, gastrointestinal; OL, open-label; RCR, retrospective chart review; RCT, randomized, double-blind, placebo-controlled study.

12.5 mg i.m. or i.v. Side effects of dopamine-blocking medications include somnolence, dizziness, arrhythmias, acute dystonia, and extrapyramidal effects. In order to prevent the extrapyramidal side effects, the patient can be premedicated with anticholinergic drugs, including diphenhydramine 12.5–25 mg i.m. or i.v. (maximum 300 mg/day) or benztropine 0.02–0.05 mg/kg i.m. or i.v. Ketorolac 0.5 mg/kg i.m. or i.v. (to a maximum of 30 mg) can be used together with the dopamine-blocking medications. Prochlorperazine intravenously (which gives an 84% response rate) was superior to i.v. ketorolac (a 55% response rate) in the acute treatment of migraine headaches in children in a randomized-controlled trial [25].

In patients with persisting headaches despite the above treatment, one can consider treatment with DHE. Although not indicated by the FDA for the pediatric population, i.v. or i.m. DHE has been demonstrated to be effective in the treatment of status migrainous in adolescents in a retrospective study [26]. The recommended dosage is lower than in adults, beginning with 0.1 mg, which can be repeated in 1 hour if necessary and if tolerated, followed by 0.25 mg and then 0.5 mg every 8 hours. The maximum single dose is 1 mg. Potential side effects include nausea, vomiting, chest pain, diarrhea, abdominal cramps, leg pain, and vasoconstriction. Premedication with antiemetic drugs such as metoclopramide 10 mg i.v. or orally, or prochlorperazine 10 mg i.v., approximately 30 minutes prior to administering DHE is recommended. Anticholinergic drugs are also recommended when using antiemetic drugs (diphenhydramine or benztropine), to prevent extrapyramidal side effects. DHE is contraindicated in patients with basilar or hemiplegic migraine, pregnancy, severe peripheral vascular disease, coronary artery disease, or cerebrovascular disease. DHE should not be used if another ergotamine or triptan has been used within the previous 24 hours.

Valproate, 300–500 mg i.v., was also shown to be effective in a retrospective review in children [27]. The advantage of valproate is that there are no cardiovascular side effects, no sedation, no interaction with ergotamines and triptans, and no vasoconstrictive side effects. However, it should not used in pregnant patients or those with hepatic disease.

Steroids (dexamethasone 10–20 mg i.v.) may be used as adjunctive therapy with other abortive drugs for status migrainosus [28]. Opioids should be avoided in acute migraine treatment, especially in adolescents, because of the risk of drug addiction and because they tend not to be effective [29].

> ★ **TIPS AND TRICKS**
>
> Treatment of childhood migraine starts with ibuprofen 10 mg/kg or acetaminophen 15 mg/kg. In severe migraine or if there is incomplete relief with nonspecific migraine medications, consider treating with migraine-specific drugs including triptans (almotriptan 12.5 mg or sumatriptan nasal spray 10–20 mg) or ergotamine (DHE nasal spray 0.5–1 mg). If treatment at home is not effective, treatment in the emergency room with dopamine-blocking agents (i.e., metoclopramide 10 mg i.v./i.m. or prochlorperazine 10 mg i.v./i.m.) and ketorolac 0.5 mg/kg is recommended. Alternatively, valproate 500 mg i.v. may be used as well. If emergency room treatment fails, admit the patient and consider treatment with DHE 0.1–0.5 mg i.m./i.v.

Prophylactic migraine treatment

Prophylactic or preventive migraine treatment refers to medication given every day even in the absence of headache, with the aim of decreasing the frequency, severity, and duration of headaches in order to reduce disability and improve functioning. Preventive medications should be considered in patients with migraine attacks occurring more than five times per month, in those who experience severe or prolonged migraine attacks or recurrent migraines with debilitating auras (i.e.. basilar-type migraine or hemiplegic migraine), and in those in whom acute migraine treatment is ineffective [13]. In addition, patients with medication overuse may benefit from prophylactic treatment. In the experience and opinion of the authors, the threshold for starting preventive treatment in children may be higher than in the adult population because of concerns regarding the safety and tolerability of the medications in the pediatric population, as well as the fact that no medications have an FDA indication for the prevention of headaches in the pediatric population. However, preventive medication should be considered in children with significant disability due to severe headaches that interfere with their daily activities or cause them to miss school frequently.

The decision about which preventive treatment to use should be individualized for each patient, after a complete discussion with the parents and patient about the potential side effects and benefits of medication. Several classes of medications are used for migraine prophylaxis in children, including beta-blockers (propranolol), tricyclic antidepressants (amitriptyline), antiepileptic drugs (valproic acid and topiramate), and antihistamines (cyproheptadine). Physicians should choose medications based on available evidence about efficacy and side effects, and should also consider comorbid conditions. Comorbid conditions may influence the choice of one medication over another. For example, the clinician may choose a medication that can treat both the headaches and the comorbid conditions. In addition, clinicians must avoid medications that can worsen comorbid conditions and must consider potential drug interactions. Some prophylactic medications, such as valproate, may have teratogenic effects that need to be considered in adolescent girls.

The FDA has approved five preventive agents in adults, including propranolol, timolol, valproate, topiramate, and OnabotulinumtoxinA (for chronic migraine). There are no FDA-approved medications for migraine prevention in children. Flunarizine is the only medication that had sufficient evidence of efficacy in pediatric migraine prophylaxis to be recommended by the AAN as probably effective [24]. Flunarizine is approved for use in Europe but is not available in the USA. Despite the lack of available studies and the absence of indicated medications for the prevention of migraine in pediatric patients, practitioners faced with children and adolescents with frequent, disabling recurrent headaches nonetheless often do chose to use off-label treatments for the prevention of migraines. If they are initiated, medications should be initiated at a low dose and slowly titrated up to clinical response or toxicity. It can take up to 2–3 months to achieve complete clinical benefit from prophylactic medication, and it is important that patients and families are informed of this time-frame.

Preventive medication can be discontinued if headaches become well controlled with an average of one or two headaches or less per month for 4–6 months. The clinician may choose to wait to discontinue prophylactic medication in children until summer break, since children typically show an improvement in headaches over the summer and worsening headaches during the school year [13]. The dosage of medications that can be used for the prophylactic treatment of childhood migraines and their side effects are summarized in Table 22.4.

Antiepileptic medications

Antiepileptic drugs may be useful for migraine patients with comorbid epilepsy. However, the dose for migraine prevention is lower than the dosage used in treating epilepsy. In adults, topiramate is FDA-approved for the prevention of migraine headaches. There are three randomized-controlled trials and one open-label study of the use of topiramate in pediatric migraine in children ranging in age from 6 to 17 years old. The results demonstrated an improvement in headache frequency and an improvement in Ped MIDAS score [30, 31, 32, 33]. The dosage used for migraine prophylaxis (2 mg/kg per day) is considerably lower than that used in the treatment of epilepsy (5–10 mg/kg per day). Topiramate may be particularly beneficial in patients with comorbid epilepsy or obesity. However, the cognitive side effects can be particularly problematic in the pediatric population, as even small changes in cognitive abilities may have a significantly adverse effect on learning and school performance.

Valproate is also approved by the FDA as a prophylactic medication in the treatment of migraine in adults. There are three open-label trials in children ranging in age from 12 to 17 years old. The two smaller trials ($n = 42$ and 10, respectively) demonstrated efficacy, with an improvement in headache in 80%–90% of subjects [34, 35]. However, the larger trial ($n = 305$) found no significant difference in migraine reduction when comparing all treatment groups of valproate (250, 500, and 1000 mg) versus placebo [36]. Valproate may be of benefit in patients with comorbid epilepsy and/or mood disorders. Valproate

Table 22.4. Preventive medications in pediatric migraine

Drug name	Dosing (mg/kg/ dose) max dose	Brand name	Side effects	Study class	n^a	Subjects' ages (years)	Efficacy[b]	Reference
Antiepileptic drugs								[89]
Topiramate	2 mg/kg/day (range 1–10 mg/kg/ day) 50 mg twice a day Max 200 mg/day	Topamax	Paresthesia, weight loss, anorexia, sedation, memory impairment	3 RCTs 1 OL	333	6–17	+	[30, 31, 32]
Valproate	20–40 mg/kg/day 250–500 mg twice a day	Depakote	Nausea, vomiting, weight gain, hair loss, sedation, tremor, polycystic ovarian syndrome, teratogenicity, hematologic and liver abnormalities	3 OLs	357	12–17	+/–	[34, 35, 36]
Levetiracetam	20–40 mg/kg/day 125–750 mg twice a day	Keppra	Somnolence, dizziness, irritability	1 OL 1 RCR	39	3–17	+	[37, 38]
Antidepressants								
Amitriptyline (tricyclic antidepressants)	1 mg/kg/day 10–50 mg at bedtime	Elavil	Sedation, dry mouth, constipation, increased appetite, weight gain, cardiac toxicity, orthostatic hypotension	1 OL 1 RCR	265	3–15	+	[39, 40]

(Continued)

Table 22.4. (*Continued*)

Drug name	Dosing (mg/kg/dose) max dose	Brand name	Side effects	n[a]	Subjects' ages (years)	Efficacy[b]	Reference
Trazodone (serotonin 2 antagonist/reuptake inhibitor)	1 mg/kg/day divided three times a day	Desyrel, Oleptro	Drowsiness, nausea/vomiting, headache, dry mouth, priapism, orthostatic hypotension	35	7–18	+	[41]
Pizotifen (serotonin 2 receptor antagonist)	1 mg divided twice a day	Pizotyline	Drowsiness, weight gain	47	7–14	–	[42]
Antihypertensive							
Beta-blocker							
Propanolol	1–3 mg/kg/day divided two or three times a day 40–120 mg/day	Inderal	Orthostatic hypotension, depression, fatigue, sexual dysfunction	95	6–16	+/–	[45, 46, 47]
Calcium channel blocker							
Flunarizine	5–15 mg/day	Flexyx Sibelium	Constipation, drowsiness, weight gain hypotension, atrioventricular block, nausea, depression, extrapyramidal reactions (tremor)	75	5–13	+	[48, 49]
Nimodipine	10–20 mg three times a day	Nimotop	Hypertension, itching, dizziness	30	7–18	+	[51]
Alpha-2-agonists							
Clonidine	25 μg daily twice a day	Catapres	Fatigue, nausea	100	0–15	–	[52, 53]

Others

Cyproheptadine (antihistamine, serotonin antagonist)	0.25–1.5 mg/kg divided three times a day Max 12–16 mg	Periactin Tablets 4 mg Liquid 2 mg/5 mL	Sedation, increases appetite	1 OL, 1 RCR	49	3.2–18	+	[40, 54]

Natural substances and minerals

Coenzyme Q10	1–3 mg/kg/day	CoQ10	Sedation	OL	252	3–22	+	[55]
Butterbur root extract	50–150 mg/day divided twice a day	Petadolex	Eructation or burping, nausea, stomach ache (rare)	1 OL, 1 partial RCT	166	6–17	+	[57, 58]
Riboflavin (vitamin B$_2$)	200 or 400 mg/day With food		Nausea, vomiting	2 RCT, 1 RCR	85	5–18	+/−	[59, 60, 61, 62]
Magnesium	Magnesium oxide orally 9 mg/kg/day divided into three daily doses with food for 16 weeks 400–600 mg/day			RCT, parallel group	118	3–17	−	[63]
Botulinum toxin type A injections	Migraine and chronic daily headache children for 3–29 months	Botox	Ptosis, blurred vision, hematoma at the injection site, burning	Observational study	12	14–18	+	[66]

[a]Total number of subjects in all studies combined.
[b]+, studies showing positive results or consistent positive results in all studies; −, studies showing negative results or consistent negative results in all studies; +/−, studies showing inconsistent results.
OL, open-label; RCR, retrospective chart review; RCT, randomized; double-blind, placebo-controlled study.

should not be given in patients with liver diseases or thrombocytopenia, and should be used with caution in young women of reproductive age.

There are two uncontrolled trials of levetiracetam (one open-label, the other a retrospective review) in children ranging in age from 3 to 17 years old (total $n = 39$) that have shown efficacy in reducing the frequency of migraine attacks [37, 38].

Although it is used by many practitioners, there are no studies of gabapentin in the prevention of migraines in children.

Antidepressant medications

There are two uncontrolled trials of amitriptyline (one open-label, the other a retrospective review) in children ranging in age from 3 to 15 years old ($n = 192$ and 73, respectively) that have shown efficacy in migraine prophylaxis, with a reduction in headache frequency and severity, although not duration [39, 40]. The dosage recommended for migraine prophylaxis is 10–50 mg or 1 mg/kg/day before bedtime. These doses are considerably lower than the doses used for treating depression (100–200 mg/day). Amitriptyline may be beneficial in patients with sleep disturbances. Amitriptyline should not be given to patients with arrhythmia or a conduction block, and an ECG may be carried out before starting the medication.

There is one double-blind, placebo-controlled crossover trial of trazodone in the treatment of headaches in children. In the first phase, there was an improvement in headache in both the placebo and treatment groups; in the second phase, only the group treated with placebo followed by trazodone had a significant further improvement in their headache [41]. There are no significant differences in the efficacy of pizotifen compared to placebo in double-blind, placebo-controlled crossover trials in children [42].

Some practitioners use selective serotonin reuptake inhibitors (SSRIs), including fluoxetine, sertraline, and escitalopram, for the prevention of headaches. There are no studies of the use of SSRIs in children with migraines. However, several studies have shown that SSRIs are no more efficacious than placebo in adult patients with migraine [43]. Further, the combination of SSRIs with triptans can theoretically lead to serotonin syndrome, although reported cases to date have been questioned [44]. In addition, although some SSRIs do have an FDA indication for use in the pediatric population for the treatment of psychiatric disorders, these medications have a "black box" label warning indicating that they may increase the risk of suicidal thinking and behavior in some children and adolescents with major depressive disorder. The practitioner should therefore be cautious when prescribing these medications in children and adolescents.

Antihypertensive medications

Beta-blockers Propranolol and timolol have been approved by the FDA for migraine prophylaxis in adult patients. Propranolol is one of the most commonly used medications for migraine prevention in children. However, in controlled studies, its efficacy has varied; two out of three randomized double-blind crossover trials failed to demonstrate efficacy [45, 46], while the third demonstrated a significant decrease in headache frequency [47]. Patients with comorbid hypertension may benefit from propranolol, but it is contraindicated in the presence of asthma, diabetes mellitus, bradyarrhythmia, depression, and Raynaud's disease. Special precautions should be taken in athletes, who may experience a lack of stamina and decreased performance, in patients with comorbid mood disorders, who may experience worsened depression, and in adolescent girls, who are particularly prone to orthostatic hypotension. Propranolol has a short half-life and therefore needs to be dosed 2–4 times a day. There are no comparative trials comparing the efficacy of dosing propranolol one versus two versus three times a day. Long-acting betablockers such as nadolol and atenolol can be given once daily, which may improve compliance; however, there are no data from controlled trials available. Metoprolol has fewer side effects than propranolol, but again there are no data available regarding its use in migraine patients.

Calcium channels blockers The mechanism of migraine prevention with calcium channel blockers is not clear, but may relate to direct neuronal effects such as the prevention of intracellular calcium influx, which may play particularly important roles in the propagation of migraine aura. Therefore, calcium channel blockers are commonly used in patients with prolonged auras and migraines with neurologic complications, such as hemiplegic migraine or basilar-type migraine.

Flunarizine is the only medication that has sufficient evidence of efficacy in migraine prevention in children to be recommended as probably effective by the AAN. However, flunarizine is not available in the USA. There are two randomized-controlled trials that have compared flunarizine with placebo (n = 63) and flunarizine with propranolol (n = 32), which have demonstrated headache improvement in both the flunarizine and propranolol groups. In addition, one open-label study and another open-label crossover trial with nimodipine both demonstrated efficacy of flunarizine for migraine prophylaxis in children [48, 49]. In contrast, flunarizine may be not effective for migraine prophylaxis in adults [50]. There are potential drug interactions when flunarizine is used together with beta-blockers. There is a single 8-month, double-blind, placebo-controlled crossover trial of 12 weeks of nimodipine versus placebo for migraine prophylaxis in 37 pediatric patients, ages 7–18 years old. There was no significant difference after treatment 13–20 weeks after the initiation of medication, but a significant difference in headache improvement at follow-up at 33–40 weeks after treatment initiation (P = 0.04) [51].

Alpha-2-agonists Clonidine, an alpha-adrenergic agonist, has been studied in two randomized-controlled trials in children up to 15 years of age (n = 43 and 57, respectively). Neither study demonstrated efficacy in migraine prophylaxis in children [52, 53].

Antihistamine
Cyproheptadine is an antihistamine with both serotonin antagonist and calcium channel blocker actions. It had been widely used in migraine prevention in children younger than 12 year old, because of fewer perceived side effects. However, there are only two uncontrolled trials (one open-label and one retrospective review) in children ranging in age from 3 to 18 years old (total n = 30 and 19, respectively) which showed headache improvement in over 80% of patients [40, 54]. Potential drug interactions may occur with beta-blockers, ergotamine, and DHE.

Natural supplements
Since prophylactic medications may have considerable side effects, there is an interest in the use of natural and mineral supplements as prophylactic agents for migraine. There are few studies of the use of natural supplements for migraine prevention, most of which are in the adult population. There are only rare studies of the use of these agents in children.

There is one open-label observational study of coenzyme Q10 in 1550 children and adolescents with migraines. Coenzyme Q10 levels were measured, and then coenzyme Q10 supplementation was recommended in 1143 patients who had low CoQ10 levels (<0.700 µg/mL). Two hundred and fifty-two patients who took coenzyme Q10 (1–3 mg/kg per day) for 3 months had a normalization of coenzyme Q10 levels, and showed an improvement in headache frequency, quality of life measures, and Ped MIDAS scores. This study suggests that a large majority of migraine patients may have low levels of coenzyme Q10, which has an uncertain relationship to their migraine headache [55].

Butterbur (*Petasites*) root extract has spasmolytic and analgesic effects and is used to treat migraines, back pain, asthma, and urinary tract spasm. The mechanism of migraine relief may come from anti-inflammatory and/or vasodilatory effects [56]. There are two multicenter placebo-controlled butterbur studies in adults showing efficacy in migraine prophylaxis. In a prospective open-label study of 108 children with chronic migraine, aged 6–17 years old, treated with 50–150 mg of the butterbur root extract, headache frequency was reduced by 63%. The major side effect is eructation [57]. There was a subsequent prospective, randomized, partly double-blind, placebo-controlled, parallel-group trial of 12 weeks of treatment with butterbur root extract, placebo, and music therapy in 58 children with migraine, ages 8–12 years old. Headache reduction at 12–20 weeks after the treatment was superior in the music therapy cohort compared to placebo (P = 0.005). During the follow-up period of 32–40 weeks after the treatment, both music therapy and butterbur root extract were superior to placebo (P = 0.018 and P = 0.044, respectively) [58].

Riboflavin (vitamin B$_2$) is also used for migraine prevention. The rationale for using riboflavin in migraine prophylaxis is that the pathogenesis of migraine may involve a defect in brain oxidative metabolism in which riboflavin is a cofactor, involving the mitochondrial electron transport chain and energy production. Therefore, the doses of riboflavin used in migraine prophylaxis are similar to those used in mitochondrial disorders, 100–300 mg/day (100-fold the usual recommended dietary intake). Riboflavin should be taken with food because its absorption is decreased on an empty stomach. Multiple daily doses may be needed because of its short half-life [59].

Studies have demonstrated efficacy and tolerability of high-dose riboflavin in migraine prophylaxis in adults. However, in a double-blind, randomized, placebo-controlled trial of 12 weeks of treatment of high-dose riboflavin for migraine prophylaxis in children (n = 48), there was no significant difference in terms of a 50% reduction in headache between the two groups (placebo, 14/21, 66.6%; riboflavin, 12/27, 44.4%; P = 0.125), although the placebo responder rate was high [60]. Another randomized, placebo-controlled, double-blind, crossover trial of 50 mg/day of riboflavin was studied in 42 children (ages 6–13 years), 14 of whom also had TTH. The results showed no significant difference in the reduction in headache frequency between placebo and riboflavin (P = 0.44). However, a significant difference in the reduction in mean frequency of TTHs was found in the riboflavin-treated group (P = 0.04) [61]. One retrospective chart review did demonstrate efficacy in migraine prevention in children treated with riboflavin [62].

Magnesium may play a role in migraine pathogenesis by modulating the responsiveness of the NMDA receptors to glutamate, which is involved in cortical spreading depression. Some studies have demonstrated an efficacy of magnesium in migraine prophylaxis in adults. However, a randomized, double-blind, placebo-controlled trial of magnesium oxide in children showed no statistically significant difference in frequency or severity of headaches compared to placebo (P = 0.88) [63].

There is a single open-label trial utilizing ginkgolide B/coenzyme-Q10/riboflavin/magnesium complex twice a day for 3 months in 119 school-aged migraine patients (mean age 9.7 ± 1.42). There was a significant decrease in monthly frequency of migraines (9.71 ± 4.33 versus 4.53 ± 3.96 attacks; P = 0.001), and no side effects were reported [64].

Botulinum toxin inhibits acetylcholine release at the neuromuscular junction, leading to muscle weakness. Studies utilizing botulinum toxin in headache treatment have demonstrated no efficacy in the treatment of chronic TTH and inconsistent results in migraine prophylaxis overall, but have demonstrated efficacy in chronic daily headache, largely driven by chronic migraine [65]. One observational study has used botulinum toxin type A for migraine prophylaxis in 12 adolescents, aged 14–18 years, for 3–29 months. Six of the patients who had long-term treatment with botulinum toxin showed an improvement in headache severity and quality of life [66].

Nonpharmacologic treatments for migraine headache

These include education, lifestyle modification, biobehavioral therapy, and acupuncture. Patients and parents should be educated about the natural disease progression of migraine and the plan of treatment, including the proper use of abortive and prophylactic medications, in order to insure good compliance. Lifestyle modification is as important as pharmacologic treatment in the management of migraine headaches. Headache diaries can be useful in identifying triggers and should include foods, situations, and symptoms that are associated with each headache. Specific foods that may trigger migraine headaches in an individual patient include aged cheeses, tyramine-containing foods, alcohol, food preservatives, artificial sweeteners, and cold foods. In addition, patients should limit caffeinated beverages including coffee, tea, chocolate, cocoa, and soda. Adequate nutritional and fluid intake, avoidance of skipping meals, regular exercise, good sleep hygiene, and avoidance of sun exposure [67] are also key to the prevention of migraine headaches.

The relationship between biologic, psychological, and social factors plays a role in pain expression in migraine [68]. Therefore, behavioral and psychological interventions may support pharmacologic treatment and be useful in migraine prophylaxis. Behavioral treatments involve training the patient to identify headache triggers and modify their behavioral response to pain, using self-regulation skills aimed to prevent headache episodes [69]. Behavioral treatments include relaxation training, biofeedback training, cognitive-behavioral therapy, or stress management training and are usually used in combination treatment [70]. Based on the available literature in children, 12 controlled trials demonstrated that relaxation alone or in combination with biofeedback or/and cognitive-behavioral therapy was more effective compared with controls [71]. Behavioral treatment should be considered an option for migraine in children and in patients with contraindications to medication. Issues that may impede the use of behavioral therapies include difficulty in finding affordable, trained mental healthcare providers and the lack of insurance reimbursement for these services.

The Cochrane database includes several studies which suggest that acupuncture is at least as effective as, or possibly more effective than, prophylactic drug treatment and has fewer adverse effects in adults [72]. A single controlled trial in children ($n = 22$) demonstrated a significantly lower headache frequency in the acupuncture group compared to the placebo group [73].

★ TIPS AND TRICKS

If preventive therapy for childhood migraine is required, topiramate and flunarizine have demonstrated efficacy and safety in randomized-controlled trials in pediatric patients. Randomized-controlled trials have shown conflicting results with propanolol. Results with riboflavin are equivocal. Valproate, levetiracetam, amitriptyline, cyproheptadine, coenzyme Q10, and butterbur appear to be effective and safe in uncontrolled trials, including retrospective chart reviews and/or open-label trials. Clonidine, nimodipine, pizotifen, trazodone, and magnesium have been shown to be ineffective in migraine prophylaxis in children. Nonpharmacologic treatments including education, lifestyle modification, biobehavioral therapy, and acupuncture can be combined with medication therapy in the management of headaches in children and may have additive benefits.

☝ CAUTION!

Be careful using multiple vasoconstrictive drugs within one 24-hour period, such as two different triptans or a triptan plus ergotamine,

---

References

1. Ozge A, Bugdayci R, Sasmaz T, et al. The sensitivity and specificity of the case definition criteria in diagnosis of headache: a school-based epidemiological study of 5562 children in Mersin. *Cephalalgia* 2002;**22**(10):791–8.
2. Laurell K, Larsson B, Eeg-Olofsson O. Prevalence of headache in Swedish schoolchildren, with a focus on tension-type headache. *Cephalalgia* 2004;**24**(5):380–8.
3. Zwart JA, Dyb G, Holmen TL, Stovner LJ, Sand T. The prevalence of migraine and tension-type headaches among adolescents in Norway. The Nord-Trondelag Health Study (Head-HUNT-Youth), a large population-based epidemiological study. *Cephalalgia* 2004;**24**(5):373–9.
4. Kaynak Key FN, Donmez S, Tuzun U. Epidemiological and clinical characteristics with psychosocial aspects of tension-type headache in Turkish college students. *Cephalalgia* 2004;**24**(8):669–74.
5. Alp R, Alp SI, Palanci Y, et al. Use of the International Classification of Headache Disorders, Second Edition, criteria in the diagnosis of primary headache in schoolchildren: epidemiology study from eastern Turkey. *Cephalalgia* 2010;**30**(7):868–77.
6. Karli N, Akis N, Zarifoglu M, et al. Headache prevalence in adolescents aged 12 to 17: a student-based epidemiological study in Bursa. *Headache* 2006;**46**(4):649–55.
7. Akyol A, Kiylioglu N, Aydin I, et al. Epidemiology and clinical characteristics of migraine among school children in the Menderes region. *Cephalalgia* 2007;**27**(7):781–7.
8. Fendrich K, Vennemann M, Pfaffenrath V, et al. Headache prevalence among adolescents—the German DMKG headache study. *Cephalalgia* 2007;**27**(4):347–54.
9. Bigal ME, Lipton RB, Winner P, Reed ML, Diamond S, Stewart WF. Migraine in

adolescents: association with socioeconomic status and family history. *Neurology* 2007; **69**(1):16–25.

10. Hershey AD. Current approaches to the diagnosis and management of paediatric migraine. *Lancet Neurol* 2010;**9**(2):190–204.

11. The International Classification of Headache Disorders: 2nd edition. *Cephalalgia* 2004; **24**(Suppl. 1):9–160.

12. Virtanen R, Aromaa M, Rautava P, et al. Changing headache from preschool age to puberty. A controlled study. *Cephalalgia* 2007;**27**(4):294–303.

13. Winner P. Pediatric headache. *Curr Opin Neurol* 2008;**21**(3):316–22.

14. Cuvellier JC, Lepine A. Childhood periodic syndromes. *Pediatr Neurol* 2010;**42**(1):1–11.

15. Cullen KJ, Macdonald WB. The periodic syndrome: its nature and prevalence. *Med J Aust* 1963;**50**(2):167–73.

16. Dignan F, Abu-Arafeh I, Russell G. The prognosis of childhood abdominal migraine. *Arch Dis Child* 2001;**84**(5):415–8.

17. Li BU, Misiewicz L. Cyclic vomiting syndrome: a brain-gut disorder. *Gastroenterol Clin North Am* 2003;**32**(3):997–1019.

18. Menken M, Munsat TL, Toole JF. The global burden of disease study: implications for neurology. *Arch Neurol* 2000;**57**(3):418–20.

19. Anttila P, Metsahonkala L, Aromaa M, et al. Determinants of tension-type headache in children. *Cephalalgia* 2002;**22**(5):401–8.

20. Anttila P. Tension-type headache in childhood and adolescence. *Lancet Neurol* 2006;**5**(3):268–74.

21. Headache Classification Subcommittee of the International Headache Society. The international classification of headache disorders. *Cephalalgia* 2004;**24**(Suppl.):1–160.

22. Lewis DW, Ashwal S, Dahl G, et al. Practice parameter: evaluation of children and adolescents with recurrent headaches: report of the Quality Standards Subcommittee of the American Academy of Neurology and the Practice Committee of the Child Neurology Society. *Neurology* 2002;**59**(4):490–8.

23. Hershey AD. Recent developments in pediatric headache. *Curr Opin Neurol* 2010;**23**(3):249–53.

24. Lewis D, Ashwal S, Hershey A, Hirtz D, Yonker M, Silberstein S. Practice parameter: phar-

macological treatment of migraine headache in children and adolescents: report of the American Academy of Neurology Quality Standards Subcommittee and the Practice Committee of the Child Neurology Society. *Neurology* 2004;**63**(12):2215–24.

25. Brousseau DC, Duffy SJ, Anderson AC, Linakis JG. Treatment of pediatric migraine headaches: a randomized, double-blind trial of prochlorperazine versus ketorolac. *Ann Emerg Med* 2004;**43**(2):256–62.

26. Linder SL. Treatment of childhood headache with dihydroergotamine mesylate. *Headache* 1994;**34**(10):578–80.

27. Reiter PD, Nickisch J, Merritt G. Efficacy and tolerability of intravenous valproic acid in acute adolescent migraine. *Headache* 2005; **45**(7):899–903.

28. Singh A, Alter HJ, Zaia B. Does the addition of dexamethasone to standard therapy for acute migraine headache decrease the incidence of recurrent headache for patients treated in the emergency department? A meta-analysis and systematic review of the literature. *Acad Emerg Med* 2008;**15**(12): 1223–33.

29. Robertson CE, Black DF, Swanson JW. Management of migraine headache in the emergency department. *Semin Neurol* 2010;**30**(2): 201–11.

30. Lewis D, Winner P, Saper J, et al. Randomized, double-blind, placebo-controlled study to evaluate the efficacy and safety of topiramate for migraine prevention in pediatric subjects 12 to 17 years of age. *Pediatrics* 2009;**123**(3): 924–34.

31. Winner P, Pearlman EM, Linder SL, Jordan DM, Fisher AC, Hulihan J. Topiramate for migraine prevention in children: a randomized, double-blind, placebo-controlled trial. *Headache* 2005;**45**(10):1304–12.

32. Lakshmi CV, Singhi P, Malhi P, Ray M. Topiramate in the prophylaxis of pediatric migraine: a double-blind placebo-controlled trial. *J Child Neurol* 2007;**22**(7):829–35.

33. Campistol J, Campos J, Casas C, Herranz JL. Topiramate in the prophylactic treatment of migraine in children. *J Child Neurol* 2005;**20**(3):251–3.

34. Caruso JM, Brown WD, Exil G, Gascon GG. The efficacy of divalproex sodium in the pro-

phylactic treatment of children with migraine. *Headache* 2000;**40**(8):672–6.

35. Serdaroglu G, Erhan E, Tekgul H, et al. Sodium valproate prophylaxis in childhood migraine. *Headache* 2002;**42**(8):819–22.

36. Apostol G, Lewis DW, Laforet GA, et al. Divalproex sodium extended-release for the prophylaxis of migraine headache in adolescents: results of a stand-alone, long-term open-label safety study. *Headache* 2009; **49**(1):45–53.

37. Miller GS. Efficacy and safety of levetiracetam in pediatric migraine. *Headache* 2004;**44**(3):238–43.

38. Pakalnis A, Kring D, Meier L. Levetiracetam prophylaxis in pediatric migraine—an open-label study. *Headache* 2007;**47**(3):427–30.

39. Hershey AD, Powers SW, Bentti AL, deGrauw TJ. Effectiveness of amitriptyline in the prophylactic management of childhood headaches. *Headache* 2000;**40**(7):539–49.

40. Lewis DW, Diamond S, Scott D, Jones V. Prophylactic treatment of pediatric migraine. *Headache* 2004;**44**(3):230–7.

41. Battistella PA, Ruffilli R, Cernetti R, et al. A placebo-controlled crossover trial using trazodone in pediatric migraine. *Headache* 1993;**33**(1):36–9.

42. Gillies D, Sills M, Forsythe I. Pizotifen (Sanomigran) in childhood migraine. A double-blind controlled trial. *Eur Neurol* 1986;**25**(1):32–5.

43. Moja PL, Cusi C, Sterzi RR, Canepari C. Selective serotonin re-uptake inhibitors (SSRIs) for preventing migraine and tension-type headaches. *Cochrane Database Syst Rev* 2005;(3):CD002919.

44. Evans RW, Tepper SJ, Shapiro RE, Sun-Edelstein C, Tietjen GE. The FDA alert on serotonin syndrome with use of triptans combined with selective serotonin reuptake inhibitors or selective serotonin-norepine-phrine reuptake inhibitors: American Headache Society position paper. *Headache* 2010;**50**(6):1089–99.

45. Forsythe WI, Gillies D, Sills MA. Propanolol ('Inderal') in the treatment of childhood migraine. *Dev Med Child Neurol* 1984; **26**(6):737–41.

46. Olness K, MacDonald JT, Uden DL. Comparison of self-hypnosis and propranolol in the treatment of juvenile classic migraine. *Pediatrics* 1987;**79**(4):593–7.

47. Ludvigsson J. Propranolol used in prophylaxis of migraine in children. *Acta Neurol Scand* 1974;**50**(1):109–15.

48. Sorge F, De SR, Marano E, Nolano M, Orefice G, Carrieri P. Flunarizine in prophylaxis of childhood migraine. A double-blind, placebo-controlled, crossover study. *Cephalalgia* 1988;**8**(1):1–6.

49. Guidetti V, Moscato D, Ottaviano S, Fiorentino D, Fornara R. Flunarizine and migraine in childhood. An evaluation of endocrine function. *Cephalalgia* 1987;**7**(4): 263–6.

50. Silberstein SD. Practice parameter: evidence-based guidelines for migraine headache (an evidence-based review): report of the Quality Standards Subcommittee of the American Academy of Neurology. *Neurology* 2000; **55**(6):754–62.

51. Battistella PA, Ruffilli R, Moro R, et al. A placebo-controlled crossover trial of nimodipine in pediatric migraine. *Headache* 1990;**30**(5):264–8.

52. Sills M, Congdon P, Forsythe I. Clonidine and childhood migraine: a pilot and double-blind study. *Dev Med Child Neurol* 1982;**24**(6): 837–41.

53. Sillanpaa M. Clonidine prophylaxis of childhood migraine and other vascular headache. A double blind study of 57 children. *Headache* 1977;**17**(1):28–31.

54. Bille B, Ludvigsson J, Sanner G. Prophylaxis of migraine in children. *Headache* 1977; **17**(2):61–3.

55. Hershey AD, Powers SW, Vockell AL, et al. Coenzyme Q10 deficiency and response to supplementation in pediatric and adolescent migraine. *Headache* 2007;**47**(1):73–80.

56. Scheidegger C, Dahinden C, Wiesmann U. Effects of extracts and of individual components from Petasites on prostaglandin synthesis in cultured skin fibroblasts and on leucotriene synthesis in isolated human peripheral leucocytes. *Pharm Acta Helv* 1998;**72**(6):376–8.

57. Pothmann R, Danesch U. Migraine prevention in children and adolescents: results of an open study with a special butterbur root extract. *Headache* 2005;**45**(3):196–203.

58. Oelkers-Ax R, Leins A, Parzer P, et al. Butterbur root extract and music therapy in the prevention of childhood migraine: an explorative study. *Eur J Pain* 2008;**12**(3):301–13.

59. O'Brien HL, Hershey AD. Vitamins and paediatric migraine: Riboflavin as a preventative medication. *Cephalalgia* 2010;**30**(12):1417–8.

60. MacLennan SC, Wade FM, Forrest KM, Ratanayake PD, Fagan E, Antony J. High-dose riboflavin for migraine prophylaxis in children: a double-blind, randomized, placebo-controlled trial. *J Child Neurol* 2008;**23**(11):1300–4.

61. Bruijn J, Duivenvoorden H, Passchier J, Locher H, Dijkstra N, Arts WF. Medium-dose riboflavin as a prophylactic agent in children with migraine: a preliminary placebo-controlled, randomised, double-blind, crossover trial. *Cephalalgia* 2010;**30**(12):1426–34.

62. Condo M, Posar A, Arbizzani A, Parmeggiani A. Riboflavin prophylaxis in pediatric and adolescent migraine. *J Headache Pain* 2009;**10**(5):361–5.

63. Wang F, Van Den Eeden SK, Ackerson LM, Salk SE, Reince RH, Elin RJ. Oral magnesium oxide prophylaxis of frequent migrainous headache in children: a randomized, double-blind, placebo-controlled trial. *Headache* 2003;**43**(6):601–10.

64. Esposito M, Carotenuto M. Ginkgolide B complex efficacy for brief prophylaxis of migraine in school-aged children: an open-label study. *Neurol Sci* 2010;**32**(1):79–81.

65. Roach ES. Questioning botulinum toxin for headache: reality or illusion. *Arch Neurol* 2008;**65**(1):151–2.

66. Chan VW, McCabe EJ, MacGregor DL. Botox treatment for migraine and chronic daily headache in adolescents. *J Neurosci Nurs* 2009;**41**(5):235–43.

67. Bruni O, Galli F, Guidetti V. Sleep hygiene and migraine in children and adolescents. *Cephalalgia* 1999;**19**(Suppl. 25):57–9.

68. Grazzi L, Andrasik F. Non-pharmacological approaches in migraine prophylaxis: behavioral medicine. *Neurol Sci* 2010;**31**(Suppl. 1):S133–5.

69. Penzien DB, Rains JC, Lipchik GL, Nicholson RA, Lake AE, III, Hursey KG. Future directions in behavioral headache research: applications for an evolving health care environment. *Headache* 2005;**45**(5):526–34.

70. Andrasik F, Buse DC, Grazzi L. Behavioral medicine for migraine and medication overuse headache. *Curr Pain Headache Rep* 2009;**13**(3):241–8.

71. Damen L, Bruijn J, Koes BW, Berger MY, Passchier J, Verhagen AP. Prophylactic treatment of migraine in children. 1. A systematic review of non-pharmacological trials. *Cephalalgia* 2006;**26**(4):373–83.

72. Linde K, Allais G, Brinkhaus B, Manheimer E, Vickers A, White AR. Acupuncture for migraine prophylaxis. *Cochrane Database Syst Rev* 2009;(1):CD001218.

73. Pintov S, Lahat E, Alstein M, Vogel Z, Barg J. Acupuncture and the opioid system: implications in management of migraine. *Pediatr Neurol* 1997;**17**(2):129–33.

74. Hamalainen ML, Hoppu K, Valkeila E, Santavuori P. Ibuprofen or acetaminophen for the acute treatment of migraine in children: a double-blind, randomized, placebo-controlled, crossover study. *Neurology* 1997;**48**(1):103–7.

75. Lewis DW, Kellstein D, Dahl G, et al. Children's ibuprofen suspension for the acute treatment of pediatric migraine. *Headache* 2002;**42**(8):780–6.

76. Linder SL, Mathew NT, Cady RK, Finlayson G, Ishkanian G, Lewis DW. Efficacy and tolerability of almotriptan in adolescents: a randomized, double-blind, placebo-controlled trial. *Headache* 2008;**48**(9):1326–36.

77. Ahonen K, Hamalainen ML, Rantala H, Hoppu K. Nasal sumatriptan is effective in treatment of migraine attacks in children: a randomized trial. *Neurology* 2004;**62**(6):883–7.

78. Ueberall MA, Wenzel D. Intranasal sumatriptan for the acute treatment of migraine in children. *Neurology* 1999;**52**(7):1507–10.

79. Winner P, Rothner AD, Saper J, et al. A randomized, double-blind, placebo-controlled study of sumatriptan nasal spray in the treatment of acute migraine in adolescents. *Pediatrics* 2000;**106**(5):989–97.

80. Winner P, Rothner AD, Wooten JD, Webster C, Ames M. Sumatriptan nasal spray in adolescent migraineurs: a randomized,

double-blind, placebo-controlled, acute study. *Headache* 2006;**46**(2):212–22.

81. Linder SL. Subcutaneous sumatriptan in the clinical setting: the first 50 consecutive patients with acute migraine in a pediatric neurology office practice. *Headache* 1996; **36**(7):419–22.

82. MacDonald JT. Treatment of juvenile migraine with subcutaneous sumatriptan. *Headache* 1994;**34**(10):581–2.

83. Hamalainen ML, Hoppu K, Santavuori P. Sumatriptan for migraine attacks in children: a randomized placebo-controlled study. Do children with migraine respond to oral sumatriptan differently from adults? *Neurology* 1997;**48**(4):1100–3.

84. Winner P, Lewis D, Visser WH, Jiang K, Ahrens S, Evans JK. Rizatriptan 5 mg for the acute treatment of migraine in adolescents: a randomized, double-blind, placebo-controlled study. *Headache* 2002;**42**(1):49–55.

85. Evers S, Rahmann A, Kraemer C, et al. Treatment of childhood migraine attacks with oral zolmitriptan and ibuprofen. *Neurology* 2006;**67**(3):497–9.

86. Linder SL, Dowson AJ. Zolmitriptan provides effective migraine relief in adolescents. *Int J Clin Pract* 2000;**54**(7):466–9.

87. Hamalainen ML, Hoppu K, Santavuori PR. Oral dihydroergotamine for therapy-resistant migraine attacks in children. *Pediatr Neurol* 1997;**16**(2):114–7.

88. Kabbouche MA, Powers SW, Segers A, et al. Inpatient treatment of status migraine with dihydroergotamine in children and adolescents. *Headache* 2009;**49**(1):106–9.

89. Bakola E, Skapinakis P, Tzoufi M, Damigos D, Mavreas V. Anticonvulsant drugs for pediatric migraine prevention: an evidence-based review. *Eur J Pain* 2009;**13**(9):893–901.

Management of Headache in the Elderly

Matthew S. Robbins and Richard B. Lipton

Albert Einstein College of Medicine, Bronx, NY, USA

Introduction

The elderly patient presenting to the practitioner with headache provides a unique management challenge. As secondary disorders are more common in older patients, new-onset headache in this age group is an automatic "red flag" that requires diagnostic vigilance. Incident primary headache disorders are less common in the elderly but do occur. More commonly, headache disorders such as migraine may persist from early and middle life into late life. Even after a primary headache disorder is diagnosed, its management can be complex. Medical comorbidities and polypharmacy often limit choices of acute and preventive medications. The metabolism and clearance of drugs may be altered by derangements of hepatic and renal function.

In this discussion, we will first briefly address secondary headache disorders in the elderly, as incident headache in this group is more commonly attributable to an underlying cause than in persons of younger age. We will then discuss primary headache disorders in the context of their epidemiology, clinical features, and management strategies in the elderly. The treatment approach to headache disorders in the elderly is multifaceted, and includes classes of acute, tran-sitional, and preventive headache medications, as well as interventional treatments, nonpharmacologic techniques, and, particularly for migraine, addressing risk factors for headache chronification.

Secondary headache disorders

New-onset headache in the elderly is attributable to an underlying cause in at least 15% of individuals aged 64 years or over [1]. In the same age group, migraine and giant cell arteritis (GCA) may present to the practitioner in equal proportions [2]. In the elderly, neoplastic and cerebrovascular etiologies may predominate, but a large variety of pathophysiologic categories may be responsible (Table 23.1).

Aside from a careful physical and neurologic examination, adults over age 55 with new-onset headache usually require neuroimaging even with normal examinations. However, imaging abnormalities are more likely to be uncovered in the setting of examination abnormalities, systemic symptoms, signs and symptoms of raised intracranial pressure, early-morning headache, or provocation by Valsalva maneuver. Patients with signs and symptoms of raised intracranial pressure should have a lumbar puncture performed to

Headache, First Edition. Edited by Matthew S. Robbins, Brian M. Grosberg, and Richard B. Lipton.
© 2013 John Wiley & Sons, Ltd. Published 2013 by John Wiley & Sons, Ltd.

Table 23.1. Secondary headache disorders that may occur in the elderly [74, 109]

Ocular/orbital	Intracranial pressure and volume derangements
Acute or subacute angle-closure glaucoma	Postdural puncture headache
Cavernous–carotid fistula	Spontaneous intracranial hypotension
	Idiopathic intracranial hypertension
Traumatic	
Acute or chronic subdural hematoma	**Infections**
Intraparenchymal hemorrhage	Post-herpetic neuralgia
	Lyme disease
Vascular	Meningitis
Acute posterior circulation ischemic stroke	Encephalitis
Hemorrhagic stroke	Brain abscess
GCA	
Cortical vein and venous sinus thrombosis	**Substance-related**
Cardiac cephalalgia	Medications
Cervical artery dissection	Caffeine withdrawal
	Alcohol
Mass lesions	
Primary and metastatic brain tumors	**Disorders of homeostasis**
Sella turcica lesions	Acute severe hypertension
	Obstructive sleep apnea
Bone and structural	Hemodialysis
Skull metastases	Hypothyroidism
Extramedullary hematopoiesis	

evaluate for neoplastic, infectious, and inflammatory etiologies. Conversely, in patients with new headache that is orthostatic or in the setting of a recent spinal surgery or intervention, spontaneous intracranial hypotension or postdural puncture headache should be suspected [3].

Diagnosing GCA is particularly important to prevent the morbidity of irreversible visual loss. Diagnostic certainty must be achieved as the treatment mainstay is corticosteroids, administered over months to even years, exposing the patient to potential adverse effects such as glucose intolerance, hypertension, osteoporosis, and avascular necrosis of the femoral head [4]. In the minority of patients with GCA, the erythrocyte sedimentation rate (ESR) may be below 50 mm/hour [5]. If the clinical suspicion remains high, an elevated C-reactive protein level may be a more sensitive blood test, the patient should be treated empirically with corticosteroids, and a temporal artery biopsy should still be pursued.

We advocate a neuroimaging study and an ESR for all patients over age 55 to exclude intracranial structural disorders and GCA. In addition, the patient's medications should be reviewed to evaluate for the many agents that may induce headache (Table 23.2).

★ TIPS AND TRICKS

The diagnosis of GCA is often confounded by the misconception that the headache must be in the temporal region, as the term "temporal arteritis" is often used interchangeably. Only 25% of patients with biopsy-proven GCA have a strictly temporal headache, and 30% of patients will have a headache sparing the temples altogether [6].

Table 23.2. Medications used in the elderly reported to cause headache

Amantadine	Levodopa
Caffeine	Monoamine oxidase inhibitors
Calcineurin inhibitors (tacrolimus, cyclosporine)	Nicotinic acid
Calcium-channel antagonists	Nitrates
Corticosteroids	NSAIDs (including indomethacin)
Cyclophosphamide	Phenothiazines
Dipyridamole	Phosphodiesterase inhibitors
Dopamine agonists	Sympathomimetic agents
Estrogen	Tamoxifen
Histamine receptor antagonists	Tetracyclines
Hydralazine	Theophylline
Immune globulin	Trimethoprim

Primary headache disorders

As in persons of younger age, the most prevalent primary headache disorder in later life is tension-type headache (TTH), followed by migraine. In the general population, the 1-year prevalence of TTH is 40% [7] and of migraine is 12% [8]. In persons aged 55–94, the prevalence of primary headache disorders is 40.5% overall—47.6% in women, and 31.9% in men [9]. Headache prevalence progressively declines with age, headache occurring in 35.4% of men and 53.2% of women age 55–64 years, to 22.5% in men and 38.3% in women aged 85–94 [9].

Tension-type headache

Epidemiology of TTH in the elderly

The 1-year prevalence of TTH in individuals age aged 55 years or over is 35.8% (27.8% in men, 42.4% in women) [9]. In the general population, the 1-year prevalence of episodic TTH (ETTH) peaks in women (46.9%) and men (42.3%) in their 30s, but declines to 27.1% in women and 25.6% in men by age 60–65. The prevalence of chronic tension-type headache (CTTH) peaks later, at 4.2% in women age 50–59 and 1.9% in men age 40–49, decreasing to 2.7% in women and 1.5% in men older than 60 years of age [7].

TTH incidence declines with age; in the 25–34 years of age group, the incidence for women is 40 per 1000 person–years and for men is 15 per 1000 person–years. Incidence declines in both sexes to less than 5 per 1000 person–years at 55–64 years

of age [10]. Despite this decline, most elderly persons with new-onset headache are most likely to have TTH [1].

Management of TTH in the elderly

Management of TTH in the elderly is similar to that in all other age groups, and includes not only trigger avoidance, but also the use of both acute and preventive medications, for which non-steroidal anti-inflammtory drugs (NSAIDs) and tricyclic antidepressants (TCAs) have the best evidence. In addition, nonpharmacologic treatments such as biofeedback and relaxation training have good evidence supporting their efficacy [11].

Acute treatments

In patients with TTH, treatment of acute attacks consists of nonspecific simple analgesics such as acetaminophen or aspirin and NSAIDs. This distinguishes TTH from migraine therapeutically, specific treatments such as ergotamine-containing compounds and triptans being effective for migraine. Opioids and barbiturates are generally discouraged in TTH, and if a patient is using these agents, they likely already need prophylactic therapy. Caffeine combination products have demonstrated efficacy in TTH treatment [12], but in patients with frequent TTH they should be used cautiously as excessive caffeine intake is a known risk factor for the development of chronic daily headache (CDH) [13].

There is ample evidence for the efficacy of a variety of NSAIDs for TTH, including ibuprofen, naproxen, and ketoprofen [14]; however, there is no clear evidence for using one NSAID over another [15]. The adverse effects of NSAIDs, including provocation or aggravation of pre-existing peptic ulcer disease [16], are highly relevant to the elderly population, and NSAIDs should not be used in conjunction with anticoagulants because of the increased risk of gastrointestinal bleeding [16, 17]. They should also be avoided in patients with renal dysfunction, as they can cause acute renal failure, interstitial nephritis, hypercalcemia, proteinuria, and fluid retention [18]. NSAIDs may increase the risk of cardiovascular disease, particularly with cyclooxygenase-2 (COX-2) inhibitors and agents that interact with acetylsalicylic acid taken concomitantly [19].

Prophylactic treatments

In treating TTH in the elderly, only the minority of patients may require prophylaxis. It should strongly be considered in patients with frequent attacks impeding daily quality of life (frequent ETTH and CTTH), or when contraindications, side effects, failure, or the overuse of acute treatments is present.

The main prophylactic agents used in TTH are the TCAs. For TTH, the first-generation TCA amitriptyline has the best evidence, particularly at daily doses of 75–150 mg, although it may be more effective for CTTH than ETTH [20]. Other TCAs that have less evidence but are used in clinical practice include nortriptyline, protriptyline, and doxepin. A related antidepressant, mirtazapine, may also have evidence in CTTH prophylaxis, with better tolerability [21].

Adverse effects often limit the use of TCAs. Anticholinergic effects such as sedation, dry mouth, constipation, and urinary retention are common [22]. In elderly men with benign prostatic hypertrophy, TCAs may induce urinary retention. Their sedating properties can occasionally be helpful in patients with insomnia. In the elderly, TCAs, via sedation and orthostatic hypotension, are associated with an increased risk of falls [23]. They may also cause weight gain, as well as tachycardia and ECG changes such as QT interval prolongation [22]. TCAs may lower the seizure threshold in epilepsy patients. In the elderly, they should be started at a low dose, such as 10 mg nightly, and can be slowly titrated to avoid side effects. If a patient is also taking a selective serotonin reuptake inhibitor, the metabolism of a TCA may be inhibited [24], and it should be particularly titrated slowly and with a lower target dose. Nortriptyline, a secondary amine, may be better tolerated than amitriptyline, although there is less evidence supporting its use [22].

Other agents have been studied in TTH prophylaxis but show limited or no benefit, including tizanadine [25], topiramate [26], memantine [27], and OnabotulinumtoxinA [28]. Peripheral nerve blockade has also limited evidence in successful TTH treatment [29].

Other aspects of TTH management

In older patients with frequent ETTH or CTTH, addressing modifiable risk factors for headache progression (and perhaps perpetuation) is equally important, particularly when medication use is limited by medical comorbidities or polypharmacy. Biofeedback and relaxation techniques are a particularly important treatment modality in the elderly patient for the same reasons, and may not only work in isolation, but also have added effects to prophylactic agents [14].

Migraine

Epidemiology of migraine in the elderly

In the USA, the 1-year prevalence of migraine in individuals aged 60 years or over was 6.4% in women and 2.1% in men [8], with similar estimates in Europe [9]. As with TTH, the incidence of migraine declines with increasing age. Five-year incidence estimates decline progressively from 8.2 cases per 1000 person–years in women age 20–24, to 0.9 per 1000 person–years in women age 65–69, and to 0.3 per 1000 person–years in women age 80 or over. In men, the 5-year incidence peaks earlier, at 6.2 cases per 1000 person–years at age 15–19, decreasing to 0.1 at age 65–69, and 0.0 at age 80 and over [30]. This trend confirms that new-onset headache resembling migraine is rare in the elderly, particularly in men, and warrants an exhaustive search for secondary causes.

Migraine symptomatology may also change with advancing age. Although aura can remit or persist in older individuals, many older patients (with or without a migraine history) can experience aura symptoms without headache or newly with headache, termed "late-life migraine accompaniments," leading to confusion with transient ischemic attacks and partial seizures [31]. Aura prevalence may also escalate with increasing age [32].

★ TIPS AND TRICKS

Migraine attacks in elderly patients often feature a different pattern of associated symptoms. Older patients are less likely to have unilateral pain, photophobia, and phonophobia [32] and are more likely to have vegetative symptoms, including pallor, dry mouth, and anorexia [33].

Management of migraine in the elderly

Migraine treatment in the older adult can be complex and multifaceted. Pharmacologic acute and preventive treatments are the mainstay. As in TTH, trigger avoidance and behavioral therapies also play major roles, and interventional techniques are becoming more prominent as well.

Acute treatments

Acute migraine attacks can be treated with migraine-specific and migraine-nonspecific medications. The most commonly used specific acute treatment class is the triptans. Clinical trials of triptans for migraine have excluded patients over the age of 65 years [34]. Because of their potential for vasoconstriction, triptans are contraindicated in any patient with known coronary artery disease (CAD) or a history of ischemic stroke. In the absence of cardiovascular risk factors, there is abundant evidence that triptans are safe [35]. Triptans are not recommended for patients likely to have silent myocardial ischemia, but defining this group is difficult. Patients can be stratified as low, intermediate, or high risk for CAD and ischemic stroke by using the Adult Treatment Panel report of the National Cholesterol Education Program [36]. Age, 45 years or over in men and 55 years or over in women, is

considered one of the risk factors. Patients with just one risk factor are considered low risk, but patients with two or more risk factors are considered intermediate risk [37]. One recent study demonstrated that a cardiovascular work-up is not needed for most patients prior to initiating triptan therapy, and if the probability of CAD were high enough, a work-up was likely indicated anyway [38].

Ergotamine compounds have largely been supplanted by triptans, but remain available and are very effective. Ergot alkaloids, consisting of ergotamine tartrate and dihydroergotamine, have a more broad mechanism of action than triptans. These compounds also may constrict cerebral, coronary, and peripheral blood vessels, and should not be used in patients with a history of or any uncontrolled risk factors for CAD, ischemic stroke, or peripheral vascular disease.

Antiemetics are often helpful in migraine treatment, working largely by dopaminergic blockade. They increase gastric motility, yield a greater gastrointestinal absorption of other agents, reduce nausea, and have antiheadache properties themselves. Oral metoclopramide may be a useful adjunctive medication. Prochlorperazine, particularly rectal, may be effective for moderate to severe migraine attacks, even as monotherapy [39]. These medications can cause sedation, orthostatic hypotension, and movement disorders including akathisia, parkinsonism, and acute dystonic reactions [40, 41].

☟ CAUTION!

Although acute extrapyramidal syndromes may occur less commonly in the elderly [42], antiemetic-induced parkinsonism may occur more commonly [43], and elderly patients should be cautioned to use agents like metoclopramide judiciously.

Prophylactic treatments

In migraine, prophylactic treatment is indicated for the same reasons as TTH, and chronic migraine (CM) certainly warrants prophylaxis. In addition, prophylaxis may be useful in treating bothersome aura symptoms [39], which may apply to elderly patients experiencing migrainous late-life accompaniments [31]. Although elderly patients may be more prone to the adverse effects of preventive medications, many cannot take migraine-specific acute medications because of cardiovascular comorbidites, and the risk of gastrointestinal or renal side effects with NSAIDs may preclude their use. In these elderly patients, using preventive medications is particularly justified. Table 23.3 demonstrates the benefits and concerns of various migraine prophylactic agents in the elderly.

TCAs are a first-line treatment for migraine prevention. For migraine, amitriptyline is best studied, and is used at doses similar to those for treating TTH [39, 44]. Other TCAs that have been less studied for migraine but may be effective are nortriptyline, protriptyline, and doxepin.

Antiepileptics are widely used in migraine prophylaxis. Divalproex sodium is very efficacious [39, 45], but its use in the elderly is often limited by an unfavorable side effect profile, including gastrointestinal symptoms (nausea, anorexia, and diarrhea), tremor, weight gain, sedation, alopecia, thrombocytopenia, ataxia, and transaminitis [46]. Rare and severe side effects include fulminant hepatitis, hyperammonemia, and pancreatitis [46]. A suggested regimen is to start a nightly dose of 250 mg of the enteric-coated formulation, increasing to an initial target dose of 500 or 750 mg over a period of several weeks [45].

Topiramate is efficacious in treating episodic migraine and CM [46, 47]. Unfortunately, it too has a distinctive adverse effect profile that may limit its use in some elderly individuals, including paresthesias, anorexia, taste perversion, nausea, dizziness, and sedation. Cognitive side effects may occur, which are dose-related and reversible, and include language difficulties, inattention, and short-term memory problems [46]. It is a weight-neutral drug and even causes weight loss in a minority of patients, which makes it an appealing agent in overweight individuals. It may reduce tremor in elderly patients with coexisting essential tremor [40]. Serious adverse effects include acute angle-closure glaucoma, nephrolithiasis, metabolic acidosis, and anhydrosis [46]. Largely because of cognitive side effects, it is best to titrate the medication slowly in elderly individuals, starting at 12.5 mg daily and increasing by 12.5 mg every 2 weeks until the target dose, often 100 mg daily, is reached.

Although gabapentin is less well studied, it has two randomized placebo-controlled studies supporting its efficacy [48, 49]. Common adverse effects include sedation and dizziness, and it can be a cumbersome drug to take, requiring three times daily dosing [46]. Nonetheless, its lack of drug interactions makes it an appealing choice in elderly patients taking multiple other medications. Zonisamide [46], lamotrigine [50, 51], and levetiracetam [52] have limited evidence in migraine prophylaxis. Levetiracetam, an extremely well-tolerated anticonvulsant with no hepatic metabolism or drug interactions like gabapentin, is an extremely appealing prophylactic agent for use in the elderly if controlled studies confirm its efficacy. Both levetiracetam and gabapentin require dose adjustments in the setting of decreased creatinine clearance.

Beta-adrenergic receptor antagonists (beta-blockers), along with TCAs and anticonvulsants, are first-line agents in migraine prophylaxis. Propranolol and timolol have excellent evidence, but metoprolol, nadolol, and atenolol may also be effective [39]. The side effects of beta-blockers include lethargy, depression, exercise intolerance, impotence, weight gain, hypotension, and bradycardia [53]. In the elderly, beta-blockers may particularly be sedating, and should be started at low doses with slow titration schedules. They may be useful when an elderly patient needs to also be started on an agent for blood pressure control or essential tremor, avoiding polypharmacy [40].

Beta-blockers are often not prescribed in patients with certain comorbid illnesses. They may alter glycemic control in diabetics, and blunt the sympathetic response to hypoglycemia. Although the evidence for beta-blockers inducing or exacerbating depression is poor, they should be used cautiously in elderly depressed patients. In patients with chronic obstructive pulmonary disease or asthma, nonselective beta-blockers can aggravate airway disease [22]. Beta-blockers can now likely be used safely in patients with congestive heart failure [54]. In small studies of patients with prolonged aura symptoms, beta-blockers may induce more frequent aura and even cause irreversible neurologic injury such as stroke, and at this point should be avoided [55].

Other classes of prophylactic medications may be quite helpful in elderly migraine patients.

Table 23.3. Migraine prophylactic agents in the elderly

Prophylactic treatments	Potential nonheadache benefits	Concerns
Antiepileptics		
Topiramate	Epilepsy, obesity, essential tremor	Cognitive impairment, somnolence, metabolic acidosis, nephrolithiasis, angle-closure glaucoma
Divalproex sodium	Epilepsy, bipolar disorder	Weight gain, somnolence, tremor, thrombocytopenia
Gabapentin	Epilepsy, neuropathic pain	Dizziness, somnolence, peripheral edema
Beta-adrenergic antagonists		
Propranolol, timolol, metoprolol	Hypertension, essential tremor, anxiety	Asthma, chronic obstructive pulmonary disease, depression, impotence
TCAs		
Amitriptyline	Neuropathic pain, insomnia, depression	Constipation, urinary retention, sedation, delirium, weight gain, tachycardia, arrhythmias
Nortriptyline	Neuropathic pain, insomnia, depression	Same as amitriptyline, but better tolerated
Calcium-channel antagonists		
Verapamil	Hypertension, tachyarrhythmias	Bradycardia, heart block, constipation
Flunarizine	Raynaud's syndrome	Parkinsonism, sedation, depression, weight gain
Serotonin antagonists		
Methysergide	—	Hypertension, peripheral vascular disease, pulmonary disease, valvular heart disease, hepatic or renal insufficiency
Cyproheptadine	Allergic rhinitis, conjunctivitis, spasticity	Sedation, delirium
ACE inhibitors and angiotensin receptor antagonists		
Lisinopril	Hypertension, congestive heart failure	Cough, angioedema
Candesartan, telmisartan	Hypertension	Less cough, angioedema than ACE inhibitors
NMDA antagonists		
Memantine	Dementia	Diarrhea or constipation, multiple sclerosis aggravation
Nutraceuticals		
Petasites hybridus extract	—	Burping, gastroesophageal reflux
Riboflavin	—	Polyuria
Magnesium	Constipation	Diarrhea, renal failure
Neurotransmitter release antagonists		
Onabotulinumtoxin A	Blepharospasm	Labor intensive, neuromuscular disease, rare dysphagia or dysarthria

Calcium-channel blockers, particularly vera-pamil, are effective agents [39]. Flunarizine is another calcium-channel blockers used for migraine, although it is not available in the USA. Common adverse effects include somnolence, depression, and weight gain [56]. In addition, via central dopaminergic receptor blockade, it can cause prolactinemia and parkinsonism, which is a concern in elderly patients. Although the sero-tonin receptor antagonist methysergide is very effective in migraine prophylaxis [39, 57], it is not recommended in the elderly, as it has a multitude of contraindications and side effects, and requires a 1-month drug holiday every 6 months because of the risk of retroperitoneal, pleural, and peri-cardial fibrosis [58].

Although not designated as first-line agents for migraine prophylaxis, the angiotensin-converting enzyme (ACE) inhibitor lisinopril [59] and the angiotensin receptor antagonists candesartan [60] and telmisartan [61] have shown efficacy in migraine prophylaxis, and are appealing agents in elderly patients with comorbid hypertension. These medications are typically very well toler-ated in elderly individuals, although ACE inhibi-tors carry the risk of cough and angioedema.

Memantine, a noncompetitive N-methyl-D-aspartate (NMDA) receptor antagonist, was origi-nally developed as an agent to treat moderate to severe Alzheimer's disease [62]. However, it has been recently evaluated as a headache prophy-lactic agent, as NMDA receptors are involved in initiating and maintaining central sensitization [27], and it was effective in two small open-label studies, with one study also finding a benefit in a cognitive task [63, 64]. In clinical trials on demen-tia, memantine is well tolerated in elderly patients, although agitation, falls, dizziness, flu-like symptoms, and diarrhea may occur in a small minority [62]. Memantine may reversibly worsen symptoms of multiple sclerosis [65].

Nutraceutical agents are an attractive prophy-lactic treatment choice in the elderly, as they gen-erally are well tolerated with few side effects. The extract from the *Petasites hybridus* root (butter-bur) has shown excellent efficacy in two well-designed placebo-controlled trials, with burping as the most frequently reported adverse effect [66]. The plant has toxic alkaloids which must be well extracted. Vitamin B_2 (riboflavin) and coen-zyme Q10 may also be effective and are safe [66,

67]. One disadvantage of these agents can be their cost.

As a nonoral prophylactic agent, periodic craniocervical OnabotulinumtoxinA injections are an appealing agent for use in elderly patients, as drug–drug interactions are minimal with its use. Data from two separate double-blind studies suggests that this agent is effective in CM [68, 69, 70]. A 2008 American Academy of Neurology practice parameter has deemed Onabotulinum-toxinA probably ineffective in episodic migraine [71]. Reimbursement is also a limiting factor.

Other aspects of migraine management

One technique gaining increasing use in treating migraine is peripheral nerve blockade, although the evidence for its efficacy is not yet sound beyond open-label studies. Treatment consists of localized injections of a local anesthetic agent with or without a corticosteroid into the greater occipital, lesser occipital, auriculotemporal, supratrochlear, or supraorbital regions. Overall, they are safe, and often afford immediate pain relief. This is an appealing technique in the elderly as there are few known contraindications, aside from a known skull defect. It can be per-formed repetitively as an acute treatment or as a transitional treatment while prophylactic agents are added or increased [29].

Migraine is a disorder that can progress from an episodic to a chronic form, and many risk factors for this transformation have been identi-fied (Table 23.4). Managing these risk factors in migraine patients may prevent progression to CM, and may increase the possibility of CM regressing to episodic migraine. Among these risk factors, comorbid depression and anxiety can be treated effectively with not only psycho-tropic medications, but also with approaches such as biofeedback, relaxation training, and stress management techniques that are effec-tive for migraine prevention even in the ab-sence of prophylactic medications [11]. Equally important is addressing medication overuse, and transitioning away from butalbital- and opioid-containing analgesics [72]. In the elderly, where treatment options are limited because multiple acute and preventive medications are often con-traindicated or poorly tolerated, addressing these and other modifiable risk factors is especially important [73].

Table 23.4. Potentially modifiable risk factors for headache transformation

Modifiable risk factor	Potential interventions
Excessive caffeine intake	Reducing dietary consumption, switch to acute therapies lacking caffeine
Baseline headache frequency	Trigger avoidance, prophylactic medications
Medication overuse	Detoxification, preventive medications, switch acute medications away from opioids and barbiturates
Overweight/obesity	Weight loss, avoid weight-gaining prophylactic medications
Snoring/obstructive sleep apnea	Weight loss, nocturnal positive-pressure ventilation
Comorbid pain disorders	Treating other painful disorders
Depression and anxiety	Treating comorbid illness using pharmacologic and nonpharmacologic techniques
Allodynia	Early treatment with triptans, prophylactic medications, avoid opiates

Trigeminal autonomic cephalalgias including cluster headache

Epidemiology of cluster headache in the elderly

The trigeminal autonomic cephalalgias encompass a group of less common primary headache disorders that feature short attacks of unilateral pain, usually in the distribution of the first division of the trigeminal nerve, accompanied by ipsilateral autonomic features [74]. Cluster headache (CH) is the most common trigeminal autonomic cephalalgias [75], and unlike many primary headache disorders, CH is more common in men, with a male:female ratio of 4:1 [75].

In the only study where new cases of CH in both men and women were captured, the incidence peaked from 40 to 49 years in men and from 60 to 69 years in women [76]. Most of the older literature suggests that the age of onset is younger, from 26 to 30 years of age [57]. Clinic-based studies may underestimate the age of onset due to selective consultation for the more severe early-onset cases. New-onset CH has occasionally been reported in individuals in their seventh, eighth, and ninth decades [77, 78, 79]. A secondary form of CH should particularly be suspected if a patient has a prolonged (>4 hours) attack duration, an absence of circannual or circadian periodicity, interictal pain, an inadequate response to treatment, or an abnormal examination [80]. Neoplastic etiologies, which would often be more prevalent in the elderly, most com-

monly involve the ipsilateral cavernous sinus [81]. Cerebral neuroimaging targeting the sellar and cavernous sinus regions, preferably with MRI, should be explored in all elderly patients with new-onset CH [82].

Management of the elderly CH patient

Once the diagnosis has been established, the treatment of CH encompasses acute, transitional, and preventive treatments (Table 23.5).

Acute treatments

Triptans, particularly those administered via nonoral routes, are considered first-line agents in the acute treatment of CH. Subcutaneous sumatriptan is most effective [83], but intranasal zolmitriptan also aborts attacks rapidly [84].

Oxygen has been used since the 1950s for the acute treatment of CH. One randomized, placebo-controlled study has recently been performed, demonstrating its efficacy and safety [85]. Oxygen should be administered at a flow rate of at least 12 L per minute for at least 15 minutes, using a nonrebreather face mask, with the patient sitting upright [85]. Oxygen is an obvious choice for an abortive agent in the elderly CH patient because of its safety and ease of repetitive use. It should be avoided in elderly patients with chronic obstructive pulmonary disease as it can reduce the hypoxic drive to breathe, leading to carbon dioxide retention [86].

Table 23.5. Pharmacologic management of CH

Acute	Transitional	Prophylaxis

Triptans
  Sumatriptan (subcutaneous,
  nasal)
  Zolmitriptan (nasal)
	Oral corticosteroids	Calcium-channel antagonists
		  Verapamil
		  Flunarizine

Ergotamine compounds
  Dihydroergotamine (i.m, i.v.,
  nasal)
	Greater occipital nerve
	block with steroid and local
	anesthetic
		Antiepileptics
		  Valproic acid
		  Topiramate
		  Gabapentin

Oxygen, high flow via
nonrebreather face mask
	Triptans with long half-lives
	  Naratriptan
	Ergotamine compounds
	Dihydroergotamine (i.m.,
	  i.v., nasal)
		Serotonin antagonists
		  Methysergide
		Lithium
		Melatonin

i.m., intramuscular; i.v., intravenous.

Transitional treatments

The purpose of transitional treatments is to rapidly suppress CH attacks while prophylactic agents are increased. Corticosteroids are the traditional transitional treatment of choice in patients with CH. A variety of steroid regimens, including prednisone, prednisolone, and dexamethasone, are used in a 2- to 3-week tapering course [57]. They should be used cautiously or avoided in patients with comorbid psychiatric disorders, osteoporosis, diabetes, and hypertension [57].

> **✋ CAUTION!**
>
> Aseptic osteonecrosis of the femoral head has occurred after receiving short courses of high-dose oral steroids for headache [87], and elderly patients should be particularly made aware of this risk.

In CH, there is good evidence demonstrating the efficacy of unilateral greater occipital nerve blockade with a local anesthetic and corticosteroid [88]. In elderly CH patients in whom systemic corticosteroid use is contraindicated, occipital nerve blockade seems safe and reasonable.

Prophylactic treatments

The main prophylactic agent used in CH treatment is verapamil. For CH, an initial target dose of verapamil is 240 mg daily, but higher doses may be required. Common adverse effects include constipation, dizziness, bradycardia, hypotension, peripheral edema, and impotence [89]. Particularly in elderly patients who may also be taking other antihypertensive agents, verapamil should be titrated no faster than 80 mg weekly. Verapamil interacts with many medications based on its hepatic cytochrome P450-3A inhibition, including simvastatin, atorvastatin, and carbamazepine, three agents that are often used in elderly patients.

> **✋ CAUTION!**
>
> ECG abnormalities are not uncommon, occurring in at least 19% of CH patients receiving the drug; most abnormalities are first-degree heart block and junctional rhythm [90]. Elderly patients should have a baseline ECG prior to both verapamil initiation and each subsequent dosage increase.

Second-line agents for CH prophylaxis include lithium, divalproex sodium [57], topiramate [91], gabapentin, methysergide [57], and melatonin [92].

Hypnic headache

Hypnic headache, nicknamed "alarm clock headache," is characterized as an idiopathic recurrent headache disorder with minimal associated features, exclusively developing during sleep [74, 93, 94, 95], in any stage [96]. Of all the primary headache disorders, hypnic headache is the only entity that has its onset almost exclusively in older individuals, with a mean age of 61 years [96]. This disorder is quite rare, even in tertiary care [96]. Hypnic headache can be treated symptomatically or prophylactically; caffeine or even a nightly caffeinated beverage can prevent or abort an attack. Nightly doses of lithium, indomethacin, melatonin, or flunarizine may also be beneficial [94, 95, 96].

Although lithium carbonate may be the most effective prophylactic agent, it has many side effects that are cumbersome, including tremor, nausea, thirst, visual and speech disturbance. Hypothyroidism and diabetes insipidus may also occur, necessitating baseline thyroid and renal function tests prior to its use [57]. Lithium levels can be increased by many medications used in the elderly, including NSAIDs, diuretics, and carbamazepine [57].

Chronic daily headache

CDH is an umbrella term referring to headache disorders occurring on 15 days or more per month, where headache lasts 4 hours or more on each day of pain. This group encompasses four disorders: CM, CTTH, hemicrania continua (HC), and new daily persistent headache (NDPH) [97]. Of these, CM and CTTH are the most common across all age groups, including the elderly. The prevalence of CDH across multiple population-based studies is consistent at 3%–4% [1, 98, 99, 100, 101]. The prevalence in the elderly may actually be slightly higher, at 4.4% overall, 6.0% in women, and 2.5% in men. In this population, CM occurred in 2.5% and CTTH in 1.5% [1] of individuals. Management of CM and CTTH relies on preventive and behavioral treatments that are similarly used to treat their episodic counterparts, as well as addressing risk factors for headache progression.

HC features strictly unilateral continuous pain, accompanied by ipsilateral cranial autonomic features during painful exacerbations. This disorder demonstrates an absolute response to indomethacin [74]. The population prevalence of HC is unknown, as the diagnosis relies on a response to a specific medication. The average age of onset is 28 years, but it has been reported in patients 60–70 years of age [102]. HC can be secondary to an underlying structural or vascular cause, and an older age of HC onset is a risk factor for such an underlying etiology. These patients should at least have appropriate neuroimaging and an ESR [103]. HC is treated with indomethacin, which may be difficult to prescribe in elderly patients with renal insufficiency and gastrointestinal disturbances. In such patients, alternative agents such as COX-2 inhibitors, lamotrigine, gabapentin, lithium, or melatonin can be tried [83].

NDPH is a primary headache disorder in which patients have continuous head pain from the onset, without any antecedent headache disorder escalating in frequency [74]. NDPH is uncommon, occurring in 0.03% [104] to 0.1% [101] of the population, but has been described in patients aged 70 and over [105, 106]. In men, the peak age may be 41–50 years of age [105]. NDPH can be mimicked by a multitude of secondary causes, and, particularly in the elderly, an exhaustive search for an underlying etiology should be undertaken, including thyroid function tests [107]. NDPH is managed similarly to CM and CTTH, although its long-term prognosis is uncertain [108].

Conclusion

Making the diagnosis of a primary headache disorder in the elderly patient requires careful a consideration and exclusion of secondary causes, as new-onset headache in this age group is by default an automatic red flag. A wealth of acute and prophylactic medication treatment options for elderly patients exist for primary headache disorders. Knowledge of the full armamentarium of prophylactic agents in particular is important in this age group, where the ability to use many of the first-line medications is often limited. Management of risk factors for headache progression is of paramount importance in the elderly, as medical comorbidities and polypharmacy often preclude pharmacologic management alone.

References

1. Prencipe M, Casini A, Ferretti C, et al. Prevalence of headache in an elderly population: attack frequency, disability, and use of med-

ication. *J Neurol Neurosurg Psychiatry* 2001;**70**(3):377–81.

2. Solomon G, Kunkel RJ, Frame J. Demographics of headache in elderly patients. *Headache* 1990;**30**(5):273–6.

3. Schievink W. Spontaneous spinal cerebrospinal fluid leaks and intracranial hypotension. *JAMA* 2006;**295**(19):2286–96.

4. Salvarani C, Cantini F, Boiardi L, Hunder G. Polymyalgia rheumatica and giant-cell arteritis. *N Engl J Med* 2002;**347**(4): 261–71.

5. Salvarani C, Hunder G. Giant cell arteritis with low erythrocyte sedimentation rate: frequency of occurence in a population-based study. *Arthritis Rheum* 2001;**45**(2): 140–5.

6. Solomon S, Cappa K. The headache of temporal arteritis. *J Am Geriatr Soc* 1987; **35**(2):163–5.

7. Schwartz B, Stewart W, Simon D, Lipton R. Epidemiology of tension-type headache. *JAMA* 1998;**279**(5):381–3.

8. Lipton RB, Bigal ME, Diamond M, Freitag F, Reed ML, Stewart WF. Migraine prevalence, disease burden, and the need for preventive therapy. *Neurology* 2007;**68**(5):343–9.

9. Schwaiger J, Kiechl S, Seppi K, et al. Prevalence of primary headaches and cranial neuralgias in men and women aged 55–94 years (Bruneck Study). *Cephalalgia* 2009; **29**(2):179–87.

10. Lyngberg A, Rasmussen B, Jørgensen T, Jensen R. Incidence of primary headache: a Danish epidemiologic follow-up study. *Am J Epidemiol* 2005;**161**(11):1066–73.

11. Buse DC, Andrasik F. Behavioral medicine for migraine. *Neurol Clin* 2009;**27**(2): 445–65.

12. Shapiro R. Caffeine and headaches. *Curr Pain Headache Rep* 2008;**12**(4):311–5.

13. Scher AI, Stewart WF, Lipton RB. Caffeine as a risk factor for chronic daily headache: a population-based study. *Neurology* 2004; **63**(11):2022–7.

14. Bigal M, Rapoport A, Hargreaves R. Advances in the pharmacologic treatment of tension-type headache. *Curr Pain Headache Rep* 2008;**12**(6):442–6.

15. Verhagen A, Damen L, Berger M, Passchier J, Merlijn V, Koes B. Is any one analgesic superior for episodic tension-type headache? *J Fam Pract* 2006;**55**(12):1064–72.

16. Griffin MR, Piper JM, Daugherty JR, Snowden M, Ray WA. Nonsteroidal anti-inflammatory drug use and increased risk for peptic ulcer disease in elderly persons. *Ann Intern Med* 1991;**114**(4):257–63.

17. Dodick D. Indomethacin-responsive headache syndromes. *Curr Pain Headache Rep* 2004;**8**(1):19–26.

18. Suleyman H, Demircan B, Karagoz Y. Anti-inflammatory and side effects of cyclooxygenase inhibitors. *Pharmacol Rep* 2007; **59**(3):247–58.

19. Farkouh M, Greenberg B. An evidence-based review of the cardiovascular risks of nonsteroidal anti-inflammatory drugs. *Am J Cardiol* 2009;**103**(9):1227–37.

20. Cerbo R, Barbanti P, Fabbrini G, Pascali MP, Catarci T. Amitriptyline is effective in chronic but not in episodic tension-type headache: pathogenetic implications. *Headache* 1998;**38**(6):453–7.

21. Bendtsen L, Jensen R. Mirtazapine is effective in the prophylactic treatment of chronic tension-type headache. *Neurology* 2004; **62**(10):1706–11.

22. Buchanan T, Ramadan N. Prophylactic pharmacotherapy for migraine headaches. *Semin Neurol* 2006;**26**(2):188–98.

23. Darowski A, Chambers S, Chambers D. Antidepressants and falls in the elderly. *Drugs Aging* 2009;**26**(5):381–94.

24. Baumann P. Pharmacokinetic-pharmacodynamic relationship of the selective serotonin reuptake inhibitors. *Clin Pharmacokinet* 1996;**31**(6):444–69.

25. Bettucci D, Testa L, Calzoni S, Mantegazza P, Viana M, Monaco F. Combination of tizanidine and amitriptyline in the prophylaxis of chronic tension-type headache: evaluation of efficacy and impact on quality of life. *J Headache Pain* 2006;**7**(1):34–6.

26. Lampl C, Marecek S, May A, Bendtsen L. A prospective, open-label, long-term study of the efficacy and tolerability of topiramate in the prophylaxis of chronic tension-type headache. *Cephalalgia* 2006;**26**(10):1203–8.

27. Lindelof K, Bendtsen L. Memantine for prophylaxis of chronic tension-type headache—a double-blind, randomized,

crossover clinical trial. *Cephalalgia* 2009; **29**(3):314–21.

28. Harden RN, Cottrill J, Gagnon CM, et al. Botulinum toxin a in the treatment of chronic tension-type headache with cervical myofascial trigger points: a randomized, double-blind, placebo-controlled pilot study. *Headache* 2009;**49**(5):732–43.

29. Ashkenazi A, Blumenfeld A, Napchan U, et al. Peripheral nerve blocks and trigger point injections in headache management— a systematic review and suggestions for future research. *Headache* 2010;**50**(6): 943–52.

30. Stewart WF, Wood C, Reed ML, Roy J, Lipton RB. Cumulative lifetime migraine incidence in women and men. *Cephalalgia* 2008; **28**(11):1170–8.

31. Fisher CM. Late-life migraine accompaniments—further experience. *Stroke* 1986; **17**(5):1033–42.

32. Bigal ME, Liberman JN, Lipton RB. Age-dependent prevalence and clinical features of migraine. *Neurology* 2006;**67**(2):246–51.

33. Martins KM, Bordini CA, Bigal ME, Speciali JG. Migraine in the elderly: a comparison with migraine in young adults. *Headache* 2006;**46**(2):312–6.

34. Haan J, Hollander J, Ferrari MD. Migraine in the elderly: a review. *Cephalalgia* 2007; **27**(2):97–106.

35. Dodick D, Lipton R, Martin V, et al. Consensus statement: cardiovascular safety profile of triptans (5-HT agonists) in the acute treatment of migraine. *Headache* 2004; **44**(5):414–25.

36. Executive Summary of the Third Report of the National Cholesterol Education Program (NCEP) Expert Panel on Detection, Evaluation, and Treatment of High Blood Cholesterol in Adults (Adult Treatment Panel III). *JAMA* 2001;**285**(19):2486–97.

37. Papademetriou V. Cardiovascular risk assessment and triptans. *Headache* 2004; **44**(Suppl. 1):S31–9.

38. Orlando LA, Matchar DB. When to stress over triptans: a Markov analysis of cardiovascular risk in migraine treatment. *Headache* 2004;**44**(7):652–60.

39. Silberstein SD. Practice parameter: evidence-based guidelines for migraine headache (an evidence-based review): report of the Quality Standards Subcommittee of the American Academy of Neurology. *Neurology* 2000;**55**(6):754–62.

40. Sarchielli P, Mancini M, Calabresi P. Practical considerations for the treatment of elderly patients with migraine. *Drugs Aging* 2006;**23**(6):461–89.

41. MacGregor E. Anti-emetics. *Curr Med Res Opin* 2001;**17**(Suppl. 1):s22–5.

42. Aguilar E, Keshavan M, Martínez-Quiles M, Hernández J, Gómez-Beneyto M, Schooler N. Predictors of acute dystonia in first-episode psychotic patients. *Am J Psychiatry* 1994;**151**(12):1819–21.

43. Thanvi B, Treadwell S. Drug induced parkinsonism: a common cause of parkinsonism in older people. *Postgrad Med J* 2009; **85**(1004):322–6.

44. Ad hoc committee of the Italian Society for the Study of Headaches (SISC). Diagnostic and therapeutic guidelines for migraine and cluster headache. *J Headache Pain* 2001; **2**(3):105–92.

45. Silberstein SD. Divalproex sodium in headache: literature review and clinical guidelines. *Headache* 1996;**36**(9):547–55.

46. Kaniecki R. Neuromodulators for migraine prevention. *Headache* 2008;**48**(4):586–600.

47. Diener HC, Dodick DW, Goadsby PJ, et al. Utility of topiramate for the treatment of patients with chronic migraine in the presence or absence of acute medication overuse. *Cephalalgia* 2009;**29**(10):1021–7.

48. Di Trapani G, Mei D, Marra C, Mazza S, Capuano A. Gabapentin in the prophylaxis of migraine: a double-blind randomized placebo-controlled study. *Clin Ter* 2000; **151**(3):145–8.

49. Mathew NT, Rapoport A, Saper J, et al. Efficacy of gabapentin in migraine prophylaxis. *Headache* 2001;**41**(2):119–28.

50. Steiner TJ, Findley LJ, Yuen AW. Lamotrigine versus placebo in the prophylaxis of migraine with and without aura. *Cephalalgia* 1997;**17**(2):109–12.

51. Wheeler S. Lamotrigine efficacy in migraine prevention. *Cephalalgia* 2001;**21**:374.

52. Brighina F, Palermo A, Aloisio A, Francolini M, Giglia G, Fierro B. Levetiracetam in the prophylaxis of migraine with aura: a

6-month open-label study. *Clin Neuropharmacol* 2006;**29**(6):338–42.

53. Silberstein SD. Preventive treatment of migraine. *Trends Pharmacol Sci* 2006;**27**(8): 410–5.

54. McMurray JJ. Clinical practice. Systolic heart failure. *N Engl J Med* 2010 ;**362**(3): 228–38.

55. Evans RW, Rizzoli P, Loder E, Bana D. Beta-blockers for migraine. *Headache* 2008; **48**(3):455–60.

56. Leone M, Grazzi L, La Mantia L, Bussone G. Flunarizine in migraine: a minireview. *Headache* 1991;**31**(6):388–91.

57. Matharu MS, Goadsby PJ. Trigeminal autonomic cephalalgias: diagnosis and management. In Silberstein SD, Lipton RB, Dodick DW (eds.), *Wolff's Headache and Other Head Pain* (8th edn.). New York: Oxford University Press; 2008: pp. 379–430.

58. Koehler PJ, Tfelt-Hansen PC. History of methysergide in migraine. *Cephalalgia* 2008;**28**(11):1126–35.

59. Schrader H, Stovner LJ, Helde G, Sand T, Bovim G. Prophylactic treatment of migraine with angiotensin converting enzyme inhibitor (lisinopril): randomised, placebo controlled, crossover study. *BMJ* 2001;**322**(7277):19–22.

60. Tronvik E, Stovner LJ, Helde G, Sand T, Bovim G. Prophylactic treatment of migraine with an angiotensin II receptor blocker: a randomized controlled trial. *JAMA* 2003; **289**(1):65–9.

61. Diener HC, Gendolla A, Feuersenger A, et al. Telmisartan in migraine prophylaxis: a randomized, placebo-controlled trial. *Cephalalgia* 2009;**29**(9):921–7.

62. Farlow M, Graham S, Alva G. Memantine for the treatment of Alzheimer's disease: tolerability and safety data from clinical trials. *Drug Saf* 2008;**31**(7):577–85.

63. Charles A, Flippen C, Romero Reyes M, Brennan K. Memantine for prevention of migraine: a retrospective study of 60 cases. *J Headache Pain* 2007;**8**(4): 248–50.

64. Bigal M, Rapoport A, Sheftell F, Tepper D, Tepper S. Memantine in the preventive treatment of refractory migraine. *Headache* 2008;**48**(9):1337–42.

65. Villoslada P, Arrondo G, Sepulcre J, Alegre M, Artieda J. Memantine induces reversible neurologic impairment in patients with MS. *Neurology* 2009;**72**(19):1630–3.

66. Sun-Edelstein C, Mauskop A. Foods and supplements in the management of migraine headaches. *Clin J Pain* 2009;**25**(5): 446–52.

67. Sándor P, Di Clemente L, Coppola G, et al. Efficacy of coenzyme Q10 in migraine prophylaxis: a randomized controlled trial. *Neurology* 2005;**64**(4):713–5.

68. Aurora S, Dodick D, Turkel C, et al. OnabotulinumtoxinA for treatment of chronic migraine: Results from the double-blind, randomized, placebo-controlled phase of the PREEMPT 1 trial. *Cephalalgia* 2010; **30**(7):793–803.

69. Diener H, Dodick D, Aurora S, et al. OnabotulinumtoxinA for treatment of chronic migraine: results from the double-blind, randomized, placebo-controlled phase of the PREEMPT 2 trial. *Cephalalgia* 2010; **30**(7):804–14.

70. Dodick D, Turkel C, DeGryse R, et al. OnabotulinumtoxinA for treatment of chronic migraine: pooled results from the double-blind, randomized, placebo-controlled phases of the PREEMPT clinical program. *Headache* 2010;**50**(6):921–36.

71. Naumann M, So Y, Argoff CE, et al. Assessment: botulinum neurotoxin in the treatment of autonomic disorders and pain (an evidence-based review): report of the Therapeutics and Technology Assessment Subcommittee of the American Academy of Neurology. *Neurology* 2008;**70**(19):1707–14.

72. Bigal ME, Serrano D, Buse D, Scher A, Stewart WF, Lipton RB. Acute migraine medications and evolution from episodic to chronic migraine: a longitudinal population-based study. *Headache* 2008;**48**(8): 1157–68.

73. Bigal ME, Lipton RB. Clinical course in migraine: conceptualizing migraine transformation. *Neurology* 2008;**71**(11):848–55.

74. The International Classification of Headache Disorders: 2nd edition. *Cephalalgia* 2004;**24**(Suppl. 1):9–160.

75. Fischera M, Marziniak M, Gralow I, Evers S. The incidence and prevalence of cluster

headache: a meta-analysis of population-based studies. *Cephalalgia* 2008;**28**(6): 614–8.

76. Swanson JW, Yanagihara T, Stang PE, et al. Incidence of cluster headaches: a population-based study in Olmsted County, Minnesota. *Neurology* 1994;**44**(3 Pt 1): 433–7.

77. Evers S, Frese A, Majewski A, Albrecht O, Husstedt IW. Age of onset in cluster headache: the clinical spectrum (three case reports). *Cephalalgia* 2002;**22**(2):160–2.

78. Fischera M, Anneken K, Evers S. Old age of onset in cluster-headache patients. *Headache* 2005;**45**(5):615.

79. Seidler S, Marthol H, Pawlowski M, Heckmann JG. Cluster headache in a ninety-one-year-old woman. *Headache* 2006;**46**(1): 179–80.

80. Dodick D, Capobianco D. Treatment and management of cluster headache. *Curr Pain Headache Rep* 2001;**5**(1):83–91.

81. Carter D. Cluster headache mimics. *Curr Pain Headache Rep* 2004;**8**(2):133–9.

82. Favier I, van Vliet JA, Roon KI, et al. Trigeminal autonomic cephalgias due to structural lesions: a review of 31 cases. *Arch Neurol* 2007;**64**(1):25–31.

83. Matharu MS, Boes CJ, Goadsby PJ. Management of trigeminal autonomic cephalgias and hemicrania continua. *Drugs* 2003; **63**(16):1637–77.

84. Hedlund C, Rapoport A, Dodick D, Goadsby P. Zolmitriptan nasal spray in the acute treatment of cluster headache: a meta-analysis of two studies. *Headache* 2009; **49**(9):1315–23.

85. Cohen A, Burns B, Goadsby P. High-flow oxygen for treatment of cluster headache: a randomized trial. *JAMA* 2009;**302**(22): 2451–7.

86. Bateman N, Leach R. ABC of oxygen. Acute oxygen therapy. *BMJ* 1998;**317**(7161): 798–801.

87. Hussain A, Young WB. Steroids and aseptic osteonecrosis (AON) in migraine patients. *Headache* 2007;**47**(4):600–4.

88. Tobin J, Flitman S. Occipital nerve blocks: when and what to inject? *Headache* 2009;**49**(10):1521–33.

89. Tfelt-Hansen P, Tfelt-Hansen J. Verapamil for cluster headache. Clinical pharmacology and possible mode of action. *Headache* 2009;**49**(1):117–25.

90. Cohen AS, Matharu MS, Goadsby PJ. Electrocardiographic abnormalities in patients with cluster headache on verapamil therapy. *Neurology* 2007;**69**(7):668–75.

91. Wheeler S, Carrazana E. Topiramate-treated cluster headache. *Neurology* 1999;**53**(1): 234–6.

92. Leone M, D'Amico D, Moschiano F, Fraschini F, Bussone G. Melatonin versus placebo in the prophylaxis of cluster headache: a double-blind pilot study with parallel groups. *Cephalalgia* 1996;**16**(7):494–6.

93. Raskin NH. The hypnic headache syndrome. *Headache* 1988;**28**(8):534–6.

94. Newman L, Lipton R, Solomon S. The hypnic headache syndrome: a benign headache disorder of the elderly. *Neurology* 1990; **40**(12):1904–5.

95. Dodick D, Mosek A, Campbell J. The hypnic ("alarm clock") headache syndrome. *Cephalalgia* 1998;**18**(3):152–6.

96. Evers S, Goadsby PJ. Hypnic headache: clinical features, pathophysiology, and treatment. *Neurology* 2003;**60**(6):905–9.

97. Silberstein S, Lipton R, Sliwinski M. Classification of daily and near-daily headaches: field trial of revised IHS criteria. *Neurology* 1996;**47**(4):871–5.

98. Wang S, Fuh J, Lu S, et al. Chronic daily headache in Chinese elderly: prevalence, risk factors, and biannual follow-up. *Neurology* 2000;**54**(2):314–9.

99. Scher A, Stewart W, Liberman J, Lipton R. Prevalence of frequent headache in a population sample. *Headache* 38(7):497–506.

100. Lu S, Fuh J, Chen W, Juang K, Wang S. Chronic daily headache in Taipei, Taiwan: prevalence, follow-up and outcome predictors. *Cephalalgia* 2001;**21**(10):980–6.

101. Castillo J, Muñoz P, Guitera V, Pascual J. Kaplan Award 1998. Epidemiology of chronic daily headache in the general population. *Headache* 1999;**39**(3):190–6.

102. Peres MF, Silberstein SD, Nahmias S, et al. Hemicrania continua is not that rare. *Neurology* 2001;**57**(6):948–51.

103. Prakash S, Shah ND, Soni RK. Secondary hemicrania continua: case reports and a literature review. *J Neurol Sci* 2009; **280**(1–2):29–34.

104. Grande RB, Aaseth K, Lundqvist C, Russell MB. Prevalence of new daily persistent headache in the general population. The Akershus study of chronic headache. *Cephalalgia* 2009;**29**(11):1149–55.

105. Li D, Rozen TD. The clinical characteristics of new daily persistent headache. *Cephalalgia* 2002;**22**(1):66–9.

106. Meineri P, Torre E, Rota E, Grasso E. New daily persistent headache: clinical and sero-logical characteristics in a retrospective study. *Neurol Sci* 2004;**25**(Suppl. 3):S281–2.

107. Tepper D, Tepper S, Sheftell F, Bigal M. Headache attributed to hypothyroidism. *Curr Pain Headache Rep* 2007;**11**(4):304–9.

108. Robbins M, Grosberg B, Napchan U, Crystal S, Lipton R. Clinical and prognostic sub-forms of new daily-persistent headache. *Neurology* 2010;**74**(17):1358–64.

109. Swanson JW, Caopbianco DJ, Evers S. Headaches in the elderly. In Silberstein SD, Lipton RB, Dodick DW (eds.), *Wolff's Headache and Other Head Pain* (8th edn.). New York: Oxford University Press; 2008: pp. 711–20.

Index

Headache, First Edition. Edited by Matthew S. Robbins, Brian M. Grosberg, and Richard B. Lipton.
© 2013 John Wiley & Sons, Ltd. Published 2013 by John Wiley & Sons, Ltd.